Principles of Musculoskeletal Treatment and Management

For my mother and father (NJP)
For my wife Claudia and children Sam, Alfie and Matilda (KB)

For Elsevier

Content Strategist: Rita Demetriou-Swanwick
Content Development Specialist: Sally Davies, Nicola Lally
Senior Project Manager: Kamatchi Madhavan
Designer/Design Direction: Maggie Reid
Illustration Manager: Amy Faith Heyden
Illustrator: MPS

Principles of Musculoskeletal Treatment and Management

A HANDBOOK FOR THERAPISTS

Third Edition

EDITED BY

NICOLA J PETTY DPT MSc GradDipPhys FMACP FHEA

Associate Professor, School of Health Sciences, University of Brighton, Eastbourne, UK

KIERAN BARNARD MSc BSc(Hons) MCSP MMACP

Advanced Practitioner Physiotherapist, Hip and Knee Clinical Lead, Sussex MSK Partnership, Brighton, UK; Private Practitioner, Flex Physiotherapy, Horsham, UK

FOREWORD BY

JEREMY LEWIS PhD FCSP

Consultant Physiotherapist, Professor of Musculoskeletal Research, Sonographer and Independent Prescriber, www.LondonShoulderClinic.com; Professor (adjunct) of Musculoskeletal Research, Clinical Therapies, University of Limerick, Ireland; Reader in Physiotherapy, School of Health and Social Work, University of Hertfordshire, Hatfield, Hertfordshire, UK

ELSEVIER   Edinburgh   London   New York   Oxford   Philadelphia   St Louis   Sydney   Toronto   2018

ELSEVIER

First edition 2004
Second edition 2011
Third edition 2018

ISBN 978-0-7020-6719-8

British Library Cataloguing in Publication Data
A catalogue record for this book is available from the British Library

Library of Congress Cataloging in Publication Data
A catalog record for this book is available from the Library of Congress

Notices

Knowledge and best practice in this field are constantly changing. As new research and experience broaden our understanding, changes in research methods, professional practices or medical treatment may become necessary.

Practitioners and researchers must always rely on their own experience and knowledge in evaluating and using any information, methods, compounds or experiments described herein. In using such information or methods they should be mindful of their own safety and the safety of others, including parties for whom they have a professional responsibility.

With respect to any drug or pharmaceutical products identified, readers are advised to check the most current information provided (i) on procedures featured or (ii) by the manufacturer of each product to be administered, to verify the recommended dose or formula, the method and duration of administration and contraindications. It is the responsibility of practitioners, relying on their own experience and knowledge of their patients, to make diagnoses, to determine dosages and the best treatment for each individual patient and to take all appropriate safety precautions.

To the fullest extent of the law, neither the Publisher nor the authors, contributors or editors assume any liability for any injury and/or damage to persons or property as a matter of products liability, negligence or otherwise, or from any use or operation of any methods, products, instructions or ideas contained in the material herein.

 your source for books, journals and multimedia in the health sciences
www.elsevierhealth.com

  Working together to grow libraries in developing countries

www.elsevier.com • www.bookaid.org

The publisher's policy is to use paper manufactured from sustainable forests

Printed in China

Last digit is the print number: 9 8 7 6 5 4 3 2 1

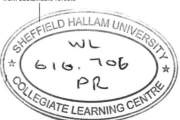

CONTENTS

FOREWORD

■ ■

Through its 10 chapters, the 12 highly respected and expert clinicians who have authored *Principles of Musculoskeletal Treatment and Management* skilfully guide the reader through the complexity of managing an individual presenting with a musculoskeletal condition.

The value of such a text is easily understood when reflecting upon the findings of research that have evaluated the impact of those experiencing musculoskeletal conditions. Taylor (2015) concluded that, for some, musculoskeletal pain is common, disabling and associated with subjective quality-of-life scores that are comparable with complicated diabetes mellitus, chronic liver disease prior to liver transplantation and terminal cancer. These findings should encourage and motivate every clinician to learn more, know more, do better and to be more compassionate and understanding. *Principles of Musculoskeletal Treatment and Management* supports clinicians in their journey to achieve these important goals.

Musculoskeletal management has moved on from the days of the 'magic manipulation' that aligns a segmental fault in the skeletal system, from a belief that there is one ideal posture that everyone should aim to achieve, that the clinician knows best and that currently we can with certainty know where the individual's symptoms are coming from. Our knowledge base is constantly evolving and, just as we know that the world is not flat and that bloodletting is not a cure for pneumonia, our research has also taught us that across the spectrum of all health conditions, for the one associated with the highest number of years lived with disability, low-back pain, bed rest is not a cure (Vos et al., 2012). *Principles of Musculoskeletal Treatment and Management* contributes to our knowledge and synthesizes research and clinical experience within a biopsychosocial framework that would conceivably take a clinician years to

acquire. For that we are indebted to Nicola Petty and Kieran Barnard and the team of skilled authors they have assembled for the invaluable information we now have access to and can learn from to improve our clinical practice. For this book to achieve its goals and aims, as an essential and important clinical resource, it must not remain in the pristine condition in which it arrived. It demands that its pages become well thumbed, creased, highlighted with reference tabs, annotated, reflected upon, discussed with colleagues, and the information contained within its pages compared to new and emerging research, when it is published and becomes available, and always with consideration to the most important person in the healthcare system, the patient.

Currently, we do not talk about 'cures' for many healthcare conditions such as diabetes, asthma, many mental health conditions, such as schizophrenia, infectious diseases, such as HIV/AIDs, and even certain skin conditions, such as psoriasis. We talk about managing these conditions. Management includes education, advice and providing the individual with the range of management options, together with their risks and benefits. We discuss what we, as healthcare providers, may offer and provide, and what the individual should consider doing. We do our best to improve health literacy through a variety of methods. We may assess the quality of our interventions by ensuring that individuals understand their condition more thoroughly, by helping them self-manage, by increasing time between 'flare-ups' and by reducing the impact, duration and intensity of the next flare-up until someone 'finds a cure'. In addition, we provide the best treatment we can, informed by all the tenets of evidence-based practice.

For some reason many involved in the management of musculoskeletal conditions still only talk of a 'cure'. Our knowledge base clearly informs us that this is not possible. Maybe if we changed 'our' philosophical approach and contributed to better balanced educational approaches, many people with musculoskeletal problems, like the individual diagnosed with diabetes, would better understand the journey that lies ahead.

The new edition of *Principles of Musculoskeletal Treatment and Management* contributes to this. It tells us that we must be active listeners, be empathetic, that we must be very careful and thoughtful with the language we use so that we are not contributing to the individual's distress and concern. It discusses the importance of clinical reasoning and shared decision making. These are essential skills for every clinician, whether newly qualified or experienced. As such, all clinicians will find value within its pages. In addition, *Principles of Musculoskeletal Treatment and Management* is packed with anatomy, biomechanics, physiology, pain science and clinical management principles, and this new, updated edition will be an invaluable resource for all involved in the management of those with conditions involving the musculoskeletal system.

JEREMY LEWIS
2017

REFERENCES

Taylor, W., 2015. Musculoskeletal pain in the adult New Zealand population: prevalence and impact. N. Z. Med. J. 118, U1629.

Vos, T., Flaxman, A.D., Naghavi, M., et al., 2012. Years lived with disability (YLDs) for 1160 sequelae of 289 diseases and injuries 1990–2010: a systematic analysis for the Global Burden of Disease Study 2010. Lancet 380, 2163–2196.

PREFACE

This new edition has been significantly updated and has benefited from being co-edited with Kieran Barnard. There are new contributors to this edition, with only the editor, Kieran Barnard and Colette Ridehalgh continuing from the previous edition, and this provides the opportunity to gain fresh perspectives. Each chapter reflects contemporary practice with the addition of new treatment and management processes and removal of outdated ones. There are two new chapters covering principles of communication and principles of rehabilitation that help to reflect the importance of these areas in current musculoskeletal therapy. All the contributors are well known within the musculoskeletal world and bring with them specialist knowledge and expertise in both clinical and educational practice. We are grateful, not only for the valuable input each contributor has made to the text, but also for their energy and enthusiasm in completing the job under tight timescales.

Thanks must go to Elsevier and in particular Rita Demetriou-Swanwick, Sally Davies and Nicola Lally for their guidance and support throughout the publishing process.

The overall aim of the book is to provide a clear and accessible text for pre-registration students that provides theory and research evidence underpinning musculoskeletal treatment and management; it is not a manual of how to treat and manage, rather it provides the principles of how to do this. We hope this provides the reader with the underpinning theory to be able to work creatively to meet the needs of individual patients.

Nicola J Petty
Kieran Barnard
Eastbourne and Brighton 2016

CONTRIBUTORS

KIERAN BARNARD BSc(Hons) MSc MCSP MMACP

Advanced Practitioner Physiotherapist, Hip and Knee Clinical Lead, Sussex MSK Partnership, Brighton, UK; Private Practitioner, Flex Physiotherapy, Horsham, UK

PAUL COMFORT BSc(Hons) MSc PhD

Senior Lecturer and Programme Leader, Directorate of Sport, Exercise and Physiotherapy, University of Salford, Salford, Greater Manchester, UK

CLAIR HEBRON BSc(Hons) PgCERT MSc PhD MMACP FHEA

Senior Physiotherapy Lecturer and Physiotherapist, School of Health Sciences, University of Brighton, Eastbourne, UK

CATHERINE HENNESSY BSc(Hons) MSc PgCAP

Teaching Fellow in Anatomy, Department of Anatomy, Brighton Sussex Medical School, Brighton, UK

LEE HERRINGTON BSc(Hons) MSc PhD

Senior Lecturer in Sports Rehabilitation, School of Health Sciences, University of Salford, Salford, Greater Manchester, UK; Technical Lead Physiotherapist, Physiotherapy, English Institute of Sport, Manchester, UK

NEIL LANGRIDGE BSc(Hons) MSc DClinP MCSP MMACP

Consultant Physiotherapist, Musculoskeletal Services, Lymington New Forest Hospital, Southern Health NHS Foundation Trust, Lymington, Hants, UK

IOANNIS PANERIS BSc(Hons) MSc MCSP MMACP

Advanced Practitioner, Musculoskeletal Physiotherapy and Tier II Clinic, Central Manchester University Hospitals NHS Foundation Trust, Manchester, UK

NICOLA J PETTY DPT MSc GradDipPhys FMACP FHEA

Associate Professor, School of Health Sciences, University of Brighton, Eastbourne, UK

COLETTE RIDEHALGH BSc(Hons) MSc PhD MMACP

Senior Lecturer, School of Health Sciences, University of Brighton, Eastbourne, East Sussex, UK

LISA ROBERTS PhD PFHEA FCSP

Associate Professor, Faculty of Health Sciences, University of Southampton, Southampton, UK; Consultant Physiotherapist, Therapy Services, University Hospital Southampton NHS Foundation Trust, Southampton, UK

SIMON SPENCER BSc MSc

Head of Physiotherapy, The English Institute of Sport, Lilleshall National Sports Centre, near Newport, Shropshire, UK

HUBERT VAN GRIENSVEN BSc DipAc MSc(Pain) PhD

Senior Lecturer in Pain, Department of Allied Health Professions and Midwifery, School of Health and Social Work University of Hertfordshire, Hatfield, UK

1

INTRODUCTION

NICOLA J. PETTY ■ KIERAN BARNARD

■ ■ ■ ■ ■ ■ ■ ■ ■ ■ ■ ■ ■ ■ ■ ■ ■ ■ ■

The aim of this book is to make explicit the underlying principles behind the treatment and management of patients with musculoskeletal disorders. It has been written as a companion text to the examination and assessment of the musculoskeletal system (Petty & Ryder 2017).

This chapter aims to help the reader understand how the information has been laid out, by giving a brief résumé of what is contained within each chapter. Broadly, the book is divided into two sections: principles of tissue management (Chapters 2–7) and principles of patient management (Chapters 8–10).

Chapter 2 provides key information on the anatomy, biomechanics, physiology and movement of joint structures, and, on the basis of this summary of joint function, classifies and discusses common clinical presentations of joint dysfunction. Using this classification of dysfunction, Chapter 3 provides the principles underpinning joint treatment.

Chapter 4 provides key information on the anatomy, biomechanics and physiology of muscle and tendon, and, from this summary of function, classifies and discusses common clinical presentations of muscle and tendon dysfunction. Using this classification of dysfunction, Chapter 5 provides the principles underpinning muscle treatment.

Chapter 6 provides key information on the anatomy, biomechanics, physiology and movement of nerves, and, from this summary of nerve function, classifies and discusses common clinical presentations of nerve dysfunction. Using this classification of dysfunction, Chapter 7 provides the principles underpinning nerve treatment.

In this text, a 'joint treatment' is defined as a 'treatment to effect a change in a joint'; that is, the intention of the clinician is to produce a change in a joint, and therefore it is described as a joint treatment. Similarly, where a technique is used to effect a change in a muscle, it will be referred to as a 'muscle treatment', and where a technique is used to effect a change in a nerve, it will be referred to as a 'nerve treatment'. Thus, techniques are classified according to which tissue the clinician is predominantly attempting to affect. What is emphasized throughout the text is the impossibility of affecting only one tissue in isolation; treatment will always affect all three tissues.

Treatment is very often aimed to relieve pain and, for this reason, Chapter 8 provides information related to understanding and managing people with persistent pain. However, treatment of an individual patient is not simply the physical treatment of joint, muscle and nerve to relieve pain and other symptoms. The patient is a person with mind and spirit, as well as body, and the person lives within a particular context, all of which need to be taken into account when managing people with musculoskeletal conditions. This potent combination creates a complex therapeutic relationship, which defies a simple cause-and-effect analysis of our therapeutic interaction. Chapter 8 discusses these issues and provides an overview of the principles of managing patients with persistent pain. This leads to Chapter 9, which outlines the all-important topic of communication and how that relates to clinical reasoning. This chapter is new for this edition and reflects the greater appreciation of communication in managing people with musculoskeletal conditions. Finally,

Chapter 10 considers the principles of exercise rehabilitation, that is so critical for full recovery and preventing recurrence of musculoskeletal problems.

In terms of content, it may be helpful to make some general comments here. Anatomy, biomechanics, physiology and pathology textbooks provide general information that is often articulated in a straightforward manner; textbooks often aim to enhance the broad understanding of the reader. In contrast, articles published in scientific journals often awaken the reader to a more complex and uncertain view of the subject. Anatomy journals, for example, describe variations in joint architecture, muscle attachments and nerve pathways, demonstrating the uniqueness of individuals. So, while anatomy textbooks describe what is generally true, they do not describe what is particularly true for any one individual. This has important implications for clinical practice. Each individual patient presenting for treatment may not have the anatomical structure that has been described in textbooks. The same might be said of biomechanics, physiology and pathology texts. The content of this textbook is no different: it provides general information on joint, nerve and muscle function and dysfunction, and may not be directly applicable to an individual patient.

Much of what is known about the musculoskeletal system of the human body is based on animal research studies. While in general it may be assumed that the findings would be similar in the human body, it cannot be assumed to be identical.

Our knowledge of the musculoskeletal system is far from complete. Research often focuses on one area, which is then assumed to reflect other similar areas. For example, the quadriceps muscle group has been used to investigate the principles of muscle strengthening and the cat knee joint has been used to investigate the behaviour of joint afferent activity during movement. The research provides knowledge of one area, and indirect knowledge of other similar areas. So, for example, the behaviour of joint afferent activity in the cat is presumed to be similar to that of the human, and is presumed to reflect afferent activity in other joints. These are logical and reasonable assumptions to make, but we must be aware that we are making these assumptions.

Research articles are used widely within the text to support or refute arguments. Details of the research carried out and a critical evaluation of the research are not provided in the text, as this would limit the flow of the arguments. Readers are encouraged to refer to these articles so that their own understanding is enhanced. For those completing degree-level study, reference to the original article will be vital.

One final point to highlight is that all patients enter the treatment room with their own thoughts, feelings, hopes and fears. Whilst an understanding of the theoretical underpinning of musculoskeletal management is crucial, we must not lose sight of patients themselves.

REFERENCE

Petty, N.J., Ryder, D., 2017. Musculoskeletal examination and assessment: a handbook for therapists, fifth ed. Elsevier, Edinburgh.

Section 1

PRINCIPLES OF TISSUE MANAGEMENT

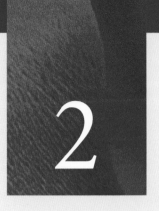

2

FUNCTION AND DYSFUNCTION OF JOINTS

CATHERINE M. HENNESSY ■ IOANNIS PANERIS

CHAPTER CONTENTS

In this text, the term 'joint' refers to both the intraarticular and periarticular structures. The function of the neuromusculoskeletal system is to produce movement. This is dependent on each component of the system, that is, normal function of joint, nerve and muscle. This interrelationship is depicted in Fig. 2.1, which shows a theoretical model originally devised to describe stability of the spine (Panjabi 1992a) but which is applicable to the entire neuromusculoskeletal system. Similarly, the stability of the knee joint has been described as 'a synergistic function in which bones, joint capsules, ligaments, muscles, tendons, and sensory receptors and their spinal and cortical neural projects and connections function in harmony' (Solomonow & Krogsgaard 2001). This description could equally be applied to all peripheral joints, so, while this chapter is concerned with the function of joints, it is important to highlight that the joint does not function in isolation but in a highly interdependent way with muscle and nerve.

For a joint to function optimally there must be normal functioning of the relevant muscles and nerves. One example of this close relationship between joint, nerve and muscle functioning together to stabilize joints can be observed in the lumbar spine where the deep fibres of the multifidus muscle blend with the zygapophyseal joint capsule (Jemmett et al. 2004) and dysfunction of the lumbar multifidus is associated with low-back pain (MacDonald et al. 2006). Stability of a joint is a function of joint stiffness (Panjabi 1992b), and this is provided not only by the joint capsule but also by skin, muscle and tendon. In the human lumbar spine, a number of the ligaments are considered too weak to contribute significantly to joint stiffness and are regarded as transducers serving a proprioceptive function (Panjabi 1992a; Adams et al. 2013), while muscle augments segmental stability during functional movement (McGill et al. 2003). There is substantial evidence throughout the body that stability of joints is enhanced by muscle (Hortobagyi & DeVita 2000; Solomonow & Krogsgaard

2001; Delahunt et al. 2006; Veeger & Van Der Helm 2007).

The nervous system underpins this joint stability function of muscle. For example, stimulation of afferents of the dorsal scapholunate interosseous ligament in the wrist causes activation of muscles adjacent to it (flexor carpi radialis, flexor carpi ulnaris and extensor carpi radialis brevis). This is thought to be a protective reflex to avoid excessive ligamentous tension (Hagert et al. 2009). In the lumbar spine, the supraspinous ligament contains mechanoreceptors which, when stimulated, cause a reflex contraction of the multifidus muscle; this is thought to improve spinal stability (Solomonow et al. 1998, 2003). Collectively, this research clearly links the interdependent relationship of joint, nerve and muscle in providing joint stability.

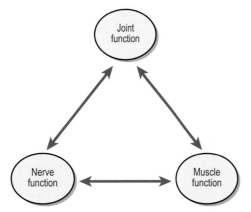

FIG. 2.1 ■ Interdependence of the function of joint, nerve and muscle for normal movement. Normal function of the neuromusculoskeletal system requires normal function of joint, nerve and muscle. *(After Panjabi 1992a, with permission.)*

JOINT FUNCTION

The previous section has highlighted the complex, interdependent nature of joint, muscle and nerve. This should be borne in mind when reading the next section on aspects of joint function. Aspects of joint function that will be discussed are:

- classification of joints
- anatomy, biomechanics and physiology of joints
- nerve supply of joints
- classification of synovial joints
- joint movement
- biomechanics of joint movement.

A joint is the junction between two or more bones, and the function of a joint is to permit limited movement and to transfer force from one bone to another (Nigg & Herzog 2007).

Classification of Joints

Joints can be classified as either synarthrosis (not synovial) or diarthrosis (synovial) (Levangie & Norkin 2011). Synarthrosis joints are further divided into fibrous and cartilaginous joints (Fig. 2.2).

Fibrous joints can be further subdivided into suture joints, as in the joints of the skull, gomphosis joints, as in the joints between a tooth and the mandible or maxilla, and a syndesmosis joint between the shaft of the radius and ulna (Fig. 2.3A). As the name suggests, in each type of joint fibrous tissue unites the joint surfaces and, as a result, only a small amount of movement is possible.

Cartilaginous joints can be further subdivided into symphysis, as in the symphysis pubis and the interbody joint (two vertebral bodies and the intervening disc) in the vertebral column (Fig. 2.3B), and synchondroses,

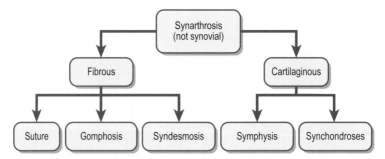

FIG. 2.2 ■ Classification of synarthrosis joints. *(From Levangie & Norkin 2011.)*

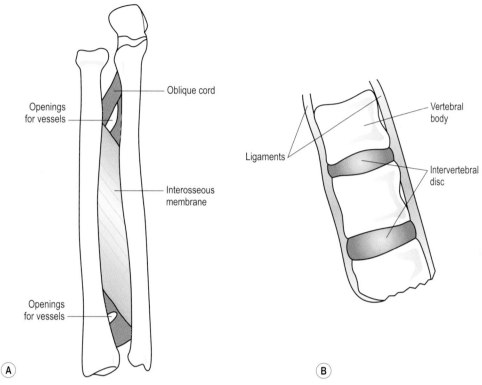

FIG. 2.3 ■ (A) The syndesmosis joint between the shaft of the radius and ulna; the fibrous interosseous membrane unites the two bones. (B) The symphysis joint between the vertebral bodies in the spine. *(From Palastanga & Soames 2012, with permission.)*

as in the first chondrosternal joint. In this type of joint, fibrocartilage or hyaline cartilage directly unites the bone and, again, only a small amount of movement is possible.

Diarthrosis or synovial joints are characterized by having no tissue uniting each end of the bone; rather, a joint space exists, thus allowing movement to occur. Synovial joints are characterized by a fibrous joint capsule lined with a synovial membrane, the bone end being covered by hyaline cartilage with a film of synovial fluid. Fat pads lie within the synovial membrane, filling the irregularities and potential spaces within the joint, and ligaments and tendons lie either within or adjacent to the joint. There may be a meniscus, for example in the knee joint, fibroadipose meniscoids in the zygapophyseal joints, a labrum in the glenohumeral or hip joints, an intervertebral disc in the temporomandibular joint and in some cases bursae within the joint. Fig. 2.4 identifies the features of two synovial joints, one with an intraarticular disc and one without.

Anatomy, Biomechanics and Physiology of Joint Tissues

Ligaments

Ligaments attach directly from one bone to another and may be:

- named parallel bundles of the outer fibrous capsule
- intraarticular, as in the cruciate ligaments of the knee, the ligamentum teres of the hip and the intraarticular ligament of the costovertebral joint
- periarticular, as in the lateral collateral ligament of the knee.

Ligaments consist of approximately two-thirds water and one-third solids, with the solids made up of 75% collagen and the balance being made up of elastin, proteoglycans and other proteins and glycoproteins (Frank 2004).

The collagen fibres in ligament are arranged in parallel bundles which have an undulated or 'crimping'

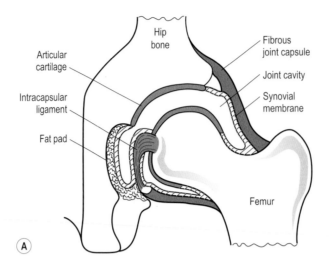

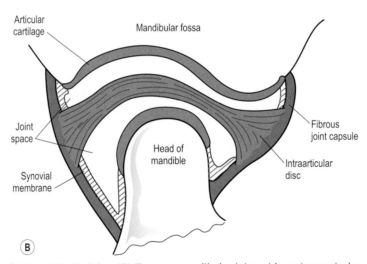

FIG. 2.4 ■ Two synovial joints. (A) Hip joint. (B) Temporomandibular joint with an intraarticular disc. *(From Palastanga & Soames 2012, with permission.)*

appearance under the microscope (Frank & Shrive 1999; Stanish 2000) when they are relaxed. The ligament buckles under compression, and so it is only the stretching of ligament with tensile loading that is functionally important (Panjabi & White 2001). The crimping gives some slack to the ligament during minimal tensile loading (longitudinal stretching), and as it straightens out it provides some resistance (Frank & Shrive 1999).

Fig. 2.5 demonstrates the change in fibre alignment during lengthening of a typical ligament.

The strength of connective tissue to tensile loading can be depicted on a force (or load)–displacement curve, shown in Fig. 2.6. The load or force is plotted against the stretch or deformation. In both load–displacement and stress–strain curves, the slope of the curve is the modulus of elasticity and is a measure of the 'stiffness'

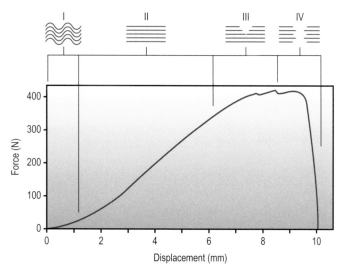

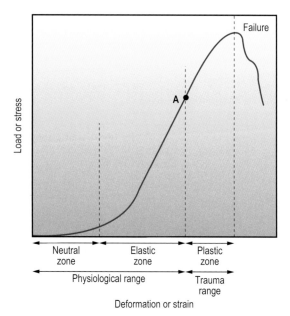

FIG. 2.5 ■ A typical force–displacement curve for a ligament. I, toe region where the collagen is crimped (schematic representation); II, linear region where the collagen is straightened out; III, microfailure; IV, failure region. *(After Frank & Shrive 1999, with permission.)*

FIG. 2.6 ■ Load (or force)–displacement curve or stress–strain curve of connective tissue. The physiological range is divided into an initial neutral zone followed by an elastic zone. Further force causes trauma and enters the plastic zone. Point A is the junction between the elastic and temporary displacement, and the plastic and permanent displacement. This point is known as the yield stress and is the minimum stress necessary to cause a residual strain in the material. *(After Panjabi & White 2001, with permission.)*

of the ligament (Panjabi & White 2001). It can be seen in Fig. 2.6 that very little force is initially required to deform the ligament, a region referred to as the 'neutral zone' (Panjabi & White 2001). Stiffness then increases, so that greater force is required to deform the ligament; this region is referred to as the elastic zone (Panjabi & White 2001). Forces within the elastic zone will result in no permanent change in length; as soon as the force is released the tissue returns to its preload shape and size (Panjabi & White 2001). The neutral zone and elastic zone fall within the normal physiological range of forces and deformation on ligament during everyday activities (Nordin & Frankel 2012).

Towards the end of a joint's physiological range the force and deformation may be sufficient to cause microtrauma of individual ligament collagen fibres since microfailure of connective tissue begins at approximately 3% elongation and macrofailure at approximately 8% (Noyes et al. 1983; Lundon 2007). The point at which there is permanent deformation is termed the 'yield stress', and the region beyond this point is known as the plastic zone (Panjabi & White 2001; Lundon 2007). A further increase in force will lead to trauma and eventually failure of the ligament, i.e. a strain injury.

The progressive failure of the human anterior cruciate ligament of the knee can be seen in the force–displacement curve in Fig. 2.7. The early part of the

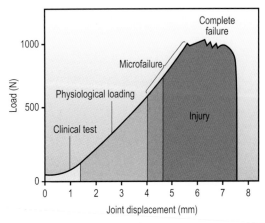

FIG. 2.7 ■ Load (or force)–displacement curve or stress–strain curve of connective tissue. The force–displacement curve during the anterior drawer test is depicted in the early toe region, with physiological loading in the linear region, followed by eventual microfailure and complete failure. *(From Nordin & Frankel 1989, with permission.)*

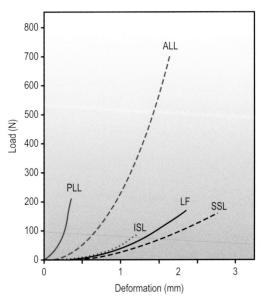

FIG. 2.8 ■ Load–displacement curves for various spinal ligaments. The slope of the curve of the posterior longitudinal ligament (*PLL*) is greatest, demonstrating greatest stiffness. Stiffness values gradually lessen with the anterior longitudinal ligament (*ALL*), interspinous ligament (*ISL*), ligamentum flavum (*LF*) and finally supraspinous ligament (*SSL*). *(From Panjabi & White 2001, with permission.)*

curve relates to clinical testing of the anterior drawer test for the knee. During normal functional activities, forces occur within the physiological loading zone. Greater forces than this result in microfailure, injury and eventually failure of the ligament. Fig. 2.8 depicts various force–displacement curves for other ligaments in the body. It can be readily seen that there are quite large variations between ligaments, reflecting differences in function.

If the strength of a ligament is to be compared with another tissue, then a stress–strain curve can be drawn, where stress is the force per unit area (measured in Pa or N/m^2) and strain is the percentage change in length (from the resting length). The stress–strain tensile properties of ligament compared with bone, cartilage, muscle and nerve are shown in Table 2.1. The stress–strain curve of collagen, of which ligament is mostly composed, is shown in Fig. 2.6.

Ligaments are viscoelastic, that is, they have time-dependent mechanical properties. These properties affect the behaviour of ligaments to movement and forces and are therefore important principles for clinicians. They can be summarized as:

- elastic nature
- viscous nature
- creep phenomena

TABLE 2.1
Tensile Properties of Ligament Compared With Bone, Cartilage, Muscle and Nerve (Panjabi & White 2001)

Tissue	Stress at Failure (MPa)	Strain at Failure (%)
Ligament	10–40	30–45
Cortical bone	100–200	1–3
Cancellous bone	10	5–7
Cartilage	10–15	80–120
Tendon	55	9–10
Muscle (passive)	0.17	60
Nerve roots	15	19

- stress relaxation
- load-dependent
- hysteresis.

The elastic nature means that ligaments will stretch and return to their original shape like an elastic band.

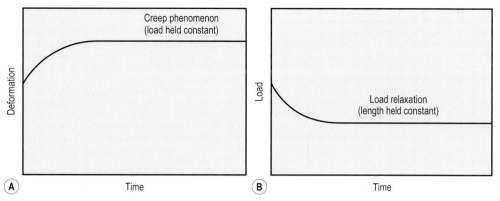

FIG. 2.9 ■ Creep and load relaxation. (A) Creep is the increase in deformation that occurs when a constant load is applied over time. (B) Load relaxation is the decrease in stress within a ligament when a constant force is applied over a period of time. *(From Nordin & Frankel 1989, with permission.)*

The viscous nature means that ligaments will gradually elongate over a period of time, when a constant force is applied. The ability of ligaments to elongate gradually with a constant force (or load) is known as creep and is depicted in Fig. 2.9A (Panjabi & White 2001). The magnitude of the force is below the linear region of the load–displacement curve. The phenomenon of stress relaxation means that ligaments undergo load (or stress) relaxation. When the deformation is kept constant (Fig. 2.9B), the force (or stress) within ligament decreases over time (Panjabi & White 2001).

Ligaments share load-dependent properties, that is, the stress–strain (or load–displacement) curve depends on the rate of loading. When the ligament is loaded quickly it will be stiffer and will deform less than when it is loaded more slowly (Fig. 2.10). This is relevant when applying therapeutic force, as a slower rate will result in less resistance and more movement. The additional effect of having load-dependent properties is that the failure point of the ligament will be higher with a higher loading rate; in other words, the ligament will be stronger and less likely to rupture when the force is applied at a faster rate.

Ligaments demonstrate the phenomenon of hysteresis – energy loss during loading and unloading of the tissue, which results in elongation (Fig. 2.11) (Panjabi & White 2001). If the force applied is less than the yield stress, then the elongation will be temporary, and if it is the same as, or greater than, the yield stress the elongation will be permanent.

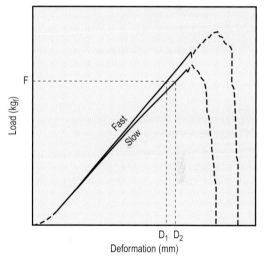

FIG. 2.10 ■ Ligament is load-dependent. It can be seen that a given force (F) applied quickly will produce a certain deformation (D_1), and if applied more slowly will produce a greater deformation (D_2). *(After Noyes et al. 1974, with permission.)*

The biomechanical properties of ligaments change with age; in younger subjects (16–26 years) ligaments fail after 44% elongation while in older subjects (over 60 years), failure occurs at 30% elongation (Noyes & Grood 1976). Ageing causes changes in collagen and elastin which result in reduced compliance of ligamentous structures, thus making them more susceptible to injury. This effect can be reduced or retarded to an extent by exercise (Menard 2000).

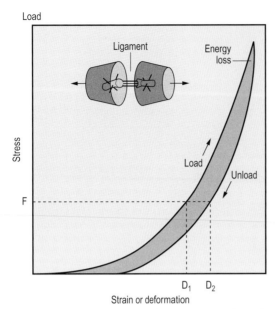

FIG. 2.11 ▪ Loading and unloading curves to indicate hysteresis. The shaded area depicts the loss of energy with deformation and is a measure of hysteresis. The unloading curve does not return to the same point on the strain or deformation axis; there is an increase in length as a result of the application of load. For a given force (F) there is a lengthening from the loading curve (D_1) to the unloading curve (D_2). *(After Panjabi & White 2001, with permission.)*

Fibrous Joint Capsules and Synovial Membranes

The outer layer of a fibrous capsule is composed of dense irregular and regular fibrous tissue and completely surrounds the bone ends, attaching into the periosteum of the bone. Where the fibrous tissue is arranged in regular fashion, in parallel bundles, it is referred to as a named ligament. Fibrous capsules have a poor blood supply but are highly innervated. They are often reinforced by adjacent ligamentous and musculotendinous structures. The inner layer of the fibrous capsule forms the synovial membrane, which is composed of areolar connective tissue and elastic fibres, and is highly vascularized.

Articular Cartilage

Articular cartilage is white dense connective tissue covering the bone ends of synovial joints and is between 1 and 5 mm in thickness. The function of articular cartilage is to distribute load, minimize friction of opposing joint surfaces and provide shock absorption from impact forces (Mow et al. 1989; Nigg 2000). It is composed largely of water, chondrocytes, collagen and proteoglycans, and it contains no blood or lymph vessels or nerve supply in normal joints. It obtains nutrients from synovial fluid, and during movement nutrients are pumped through the cartilage (O'Hara et al. 1990; Wong & Carter 2003). Cyclic loading of joints, as in walking, has been found to increase the pumping of large solutes such as growth factors, hormones and enzymes into articular cartilage – although it has no effect on the transport of small solutes such as glucose and oxygen (O'Hara et al. 1990; Wong & Carter 2003).

Microscopically, articular cartilage has a layered appearance. The most superficial layer is densely packed with collagen fibrils which are oriented parallel to the articular surface. This arrangement is thought to help resist shear forces at the joint (Shrive & Frank 1999). The middle layer is characterized by the collagen fibrils being further apart, and the deepest layer has fibrils lying at right angles to the articular surface (Fig. 2.12). The collagen fibrils in this layer cross the interface between the articular cartilage and the underlying calcified cartilage beneath, a region known as the tidemark. This arrangement anchors the cartilage to the underlying bone.

This varying orientation of collagen fibre layers allows for tensile forces to be distributed across the articular surface (Nigg 2000; Wong & Carter 2003) since collagen fibrils are able to resist high tensile forces (Fig. 2.13). Meanwhile the water and proteoglycans surrounding the collagen fibrils create a fluid-filled matrix that has the mechanical characteristics of a solid object (Mow et al. 1989).

Articular cartilage is viscoelastic, therefore displaying creep, stress relaxation and hysteresis, and has a sensitivity to the rate of loading.

Compressive Loading of Articular Cartilage. The compressive properties of articular cartilage depend on which layer is tested; the deepest layer is the stiffest because of its higher glycosaminoglycan and type II collagen content (Wong & Carter 2003). The creep response of articular cartilage when a constant compressive force is applied is due to exudation of fluid (Fig. 2.14). The rate of fluid loss reduces over time until the compressive stress within the cartilage equals the applied

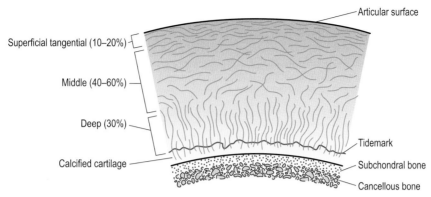

FIG. 2.12 ▪ Longitudinal section of articular cartilage demonstrating the varied orientation of collagen fibrils in the superficial, middle and deep layers. *(After Mow et al. 1989, with permission.)*

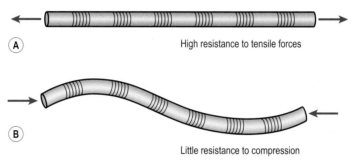

FIG. 2.13 ▪ Mechanical properties of collagen fibrils. (A) Resistance to tension. (B) Resistance to compression. *(From Mow et al. 1989, with permission.)*

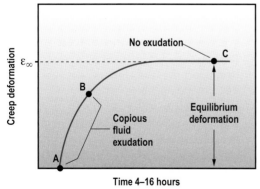

FIG. 2.14 ▪ Creep response of articular cartilage with a constant compressive load. *(After Mow et al. 1989, with permission.)*

compressive load so that equilibrium is reached. At this point the compressive load is resisted by the matrix of collagen and proteoglycan.

The stress relaxation of articular cartilage is shown in Fig. 2.15. A compressive force is applied to the cartilage until a specific amount of deformation is reached; the force is then held constant. During the initial compression phase the stress within the cartilage increases (to point B), but, once the force is held constant, there is a gradual reduction in stress (from point B to point E). Point E indicates the point where equilibrium is reached.

The effect of hysteresis on articular cartilage is ultimately a reduction in cartilage thickness; however, this is dependent on the rate of loading: the faster the rate of loading, the stiffer the articular cartilage becomes and the less deformation occurs; with slower rates of

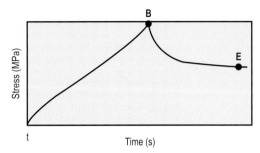

FIG. 2.15 ■ Stress relaxation of articular cartilage with a constant rate of compression. Point B is the maximum stress within the tissue, followed by the gradual reduction in stress until equilibrium is reached at point E. *(After Mow et al. 1989, with permission.)*

loading the articular cartilage is more compliant and there is greater deformation (Shrive & Frank 1999).

Synovial Fluid

Synovial fluid contains surface-active phospholipid (SAPL), which is adsorbed as the outermost layer of articular cartilage (Hills & Crawford 2003). The term 'adsorb' refers to how the articular cartilage holds SAPL to its surface to form a thin film. This film creates, in engineering terms, boundary lubrication, which prevents the adjacent articular surfaces contacting each other and reduces friction during movement, even under high-load-bearing activities (Hills & Crawford 2003). SAPL has also been shown to have antiwear properties (Hills 1995). SAPL has been found to be deficient in osteoarthritic joints (Hills & Monds 1998), which is thought to explain the associated joint stiffness in osteoarthritis (Hills & Thomas 1998; Hills & Crawford 2003), since injection treatment of osteoarthritic joints with exogenous SAPL has been encouraging (Vecchio et al. 1999).

Movement of the joint increases the production of synovial fluid (Levick 1983) and helps to distribute synovial fluid over the articular cartilage (Levick 1984). The flow of synovial fluid into the joint cavity depends, to some extent, on the intraarticular fluid pressure and on the removal of fluid via the synovial lymphatic system (Levick 1984). Intraarticular fluid pressure depends on a large number of factors, including the volume of fluid, rate of change of volume, joint angle, age of the person and muscle action (Levick 1983). Joint movement is also required to remove fluid via the synovial lymphatic

system. Lack of movement will reduce the removal of synovial fluid and so will result in an increase in intraarticular volume and pressure. Moderate amounts of movement will increase both the volume of synovial fluid and also the removal of fluid via the lymphatic system. Excessive movement causes a greater increase in the volume of synovial fluid than the removal of fluid, resulting in increased intraarticular volume and pressure (Levick 1984).

Synovial Joint Lubrication.

A variety of mechanisms are thought to ensure that synovial joints are able to maintain almost friction-free movement under a variety of functional activities. These mechanisms include the following.

Boundary Lubrication.

SAPL is adsorbed as the outermost layer of articular cartilage. This layer prevents the adjacent articular surfaces contacting each other and reduces friction during movement, even under high loading (Hills 1995; Hills & Crawford 2003).

Fluid Lubrication.

A thin film of lubricant separates the adjacent articular surfaces and is thought to operate under low loads and high speeds (Nordin & Frankel 2012) using the following three mechanisms:

1. Hydrodynamic lubrication occurs when the articular surfaces do not lie parallel and then one articular surface slides on the other. A wedge of viscous fluid provides a lifting pressure to support the load (Fig. 2.16).
2. Squeeze film lubrication occurs when the two articular surfaces move towards each other – the fluid pressure between them increases and helps to support the load (Fig. 2.17).
3. Elastohydrodynamic lubrication occurs due to the fact that articular cartilage is not rigid. This allows fluid pressures developed from the previous two mechanisms to cause deformation of the articular surface, which increases its surface area. This increases the time taken for the fluid to be squeezed out and therefore enhances the ability to withstand load.

Fat Pads

Fat pads are generally considered to act like cushions, occupying the potential spaces which often occur

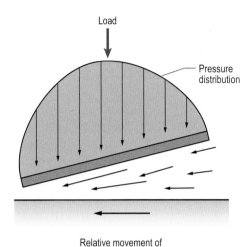

FIG. 2.16 ■ Hydrodynamic lubrication. *(From Nordin & Frankel 1989, with permission.)*

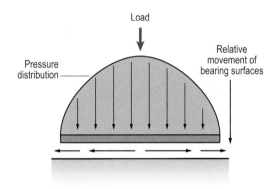

FIG. 2.17 ■ Squeeze film lubrication. *(From Nordin & Frankel 1989, with permission).*

between the synovial membrane and capsule as synovial joints move. At the elbow, for example, there are a number of fat pads, including one in the olecranon, coronoid and radial fossae which accommodate the related bony prominences during elbow flexion and extension (Drake et al. 2015).

Menisci and Meniscoids

Fibrocartilage menisci are found in the temporomandibular, knee and sternoclavicular joints. The menisci in the knee joint increase the congruence between the articular surfaces of the femur and tibia, distribute weight-bearing forces, act as shock absorbers and reduce friction (Levangie & Norkin 2011; Palastanga & Soames 2012). Messner and Gao (1998) summarized that a further important function of menisci is to provide proprioceptive feedback, particularly at the extremes of joint range, due to the presence of mechanoreceptors and free nerve endings, with greatest density at the anterior and posterior horns (Albright et al. 1987). Fibroadipose meniscoids in the zygapophyseal joints are thought to protect the joint by preventing articular surface apposition during movement and by reducing friction (Bogduk 2005).

Bursae

Bursae are sacs made of connective tissue lined by a synovial membrane and filled with fluid similar to synovial fluid. A bursa acts as a cushion to reduce friction. Bursae can be found between skin and bone, muscle and bone, tendon and bone, and ligament and bone. Some named bursae include the subacromial bursa, lying between the acromion and the glenohumeral joint capsule, and the prepatellar bursa, lying between the tendon skin and the patella (Drake et al. 2015).

Labra

Two joints in the human body contain a labrum: the glenohumeral joint and the hip joint. They form a fibrocartilaginous wedge-shaped rim around the glenoid and acetabular fossae, respectively. They deepen the articulating socket and may aid lubrication of the joints (Drake et al. 2015).

Intervertebral Disc

Intervertebral discs comprise an outer ring of thick fibrous cartilage, the annulus fibrosus, which contains the gelatinous inner core, the nucleus pulposus, with the superior and inferior cartilaginous end-plates completing the structure.

Discs are vulnerable to injury, particularly in spinal flexion and rotation (Gordon et al. 2001), which can lead to annular tears and end-plate fracture and subsequent herniation of annular material. Degenerative changes cause a loss of hydration, reduction in disc height, neural ingrowth and a loss of ability to resist compressive load – this can shift greater load bearing to the facet joints, predisposing them to arthritic change (Fujiwara et al. 1999).

Nerve Supply of Joints

Most of the components of joints, such as capsule, ligament, articular disc, meniscus, fat pad and articular blood vessels, are innervated; in fact the only structure that is not innervated is the avascular articular cartilage (Messner 1999).

The nerve endings in joints can be classified into four types:

1. Ruffini end-organs
2. Pacinian corpuscles
3. Golgi endings
4. free nerve endings.

Ruffini End-Organs

These are encapsulated (covered in a capsule) mechanoreceptors that lie around collagen fibres and are stimulated by displacement of collagen (Fig. 2.18A). They signal static joint position, direction, amplitude and velocity of joint movement and change in intraarticular pressure (Messner 1999). Activation of Ruffini end-organs has been found to affect the tone of the overlying muscle directly (Freeman & Wyke 1967a). Ruffini end-organs innervate the posterior capsule of the cat knee joint, almost exclusively, and are extremely sensitive to a change in capsule stretch (Fuller et al.

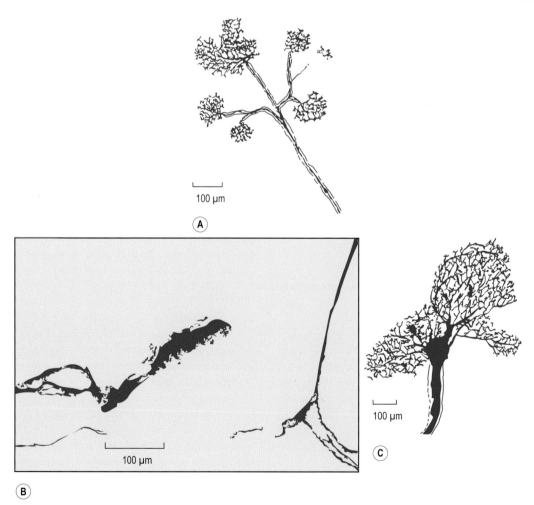

100 μm

(A)

100 μm

(B)

100 μm

(C)

FIG. 2.18 ■ Three types of nerve ending. (A) Ruffini end-organs (type I). (B) Pacinian corpuscles (type II). (C) Golgi endings (type III). *(From Skoglund 1956, with permission.)*

1991). For this reason they are thought to signal the limit of knee extension (Grigg & Hoffman 1982).

Pacinian Corpuscles

These are also encapsulated mechanoreceptors (Fig. 2.18B) but are stimulated by dynamic movement, signalling the start and end of a movement, deceleration and acceleration and a change in stress applied to the tissue in which they occur (Messner 1999). In the cat they are stimulated throughout knee joint movement, particularly during end-range and combined movements (Clark 1975; Krauspe et al. 1992). Activation of Pacinian corpuscles also directly affects the tone of the overlying muscle (Freeman & Wyke 1967a).

Golgi Endings

These are encapsulated mechanoreceptors (Fig. 2.18C) that signal extreme ranges of movement (Zimny 1988).

Free Nerve Endings

Free nerve endings do not have a capsule. They signal pain and are therefore classed as nociceptors. Their afferent fibres can be classified according to their conduction velocity as Aα, Aβ, Aδ myelinated fibres or C unmyelinated fibres (Palastanga & Soames 2012), the latter having a lower conduction velocity. The various descriptive names for each type of nerve ending, along with its function, anatomical position and afferent nerve, are given in Table 2.2.

In the cat, free nerve endings are continuous with group III and IV axons, or afferents (Heppelmann et al. 1990). In the cat knee joint, group III and IV afferents have a limited response to joint movement, with rather more response to end-range positions (Clark & Burgess 1975; Schaible & Schmidt 1983; Krauspe et al. 1992). While group III and IV afferents respond to movement, their sensitivity is low, suggesting a limited role in proprioception and perhaps more of a nociceptor role (Schaible & Schmidt 1983; Grigg 1994).

Effect of Joint Afferent Activity on Muscle

Joint afferent activity directly affects overlying muscle activity. Passive dorsiflexion of an anaesthetized cat ankle joint causes activation of mechanoreceptors in the posterior joint capsule, which produces a reflex facilitation of gastrocnemius motor neurons and inhibition of tibialis anterior (Freeman & Wyke 1967a).

Similarly, passive plantarflexion causes activation of mechanoreceptors in the anterior joint capsule, which facilitates tibialis anterior and inhibits gastrocnemius (Freeman & Wyke 1967a). Thus, when the joint capsule is put on a stretch, the mechanoreceptors cause activation of muscle that would, on contraction, reduce this stretch, and inhibition of the muscle that would increase the stretch. The mechanoreceptors stimulated were slowly adapting type I fibres which are activated during the ankle movement and continue to be active once the movement has stopped, and rapidly adapting type II fibres which are activated only during the ankle movement. The type III fibres in the ankle ligaments and the type IV fibres distributed throughout the capsule, ligaments, fat pad and blood vessels are not activated during passive ankle movements (Freeman & Wyke 1967a).

The converse has also been demonstrated, that is, that muscle activity can directly affect mechanoreceptor activity (Ferrell 1985). In the cat knee joint, it has been found that, at extreme flexion and extension positions, and with passive movement, mechanoreceptor activity can be influenced (increased or decreased) by muscle contraction around the knee (Ferrell 1985).

Effect of Joint Afferent Activity on Pain

Stimulation of the joint mechanoreceptors causes a reduction in transmission of nociceptor activity from the free nerve endings (Wyke 1970).

From Table 2.2 it can be seen that type I, II and III nerve endings are supplied by Aβ fibres, while type IV nerve endings are supplied by group Aδ and C fibres.

The nerve supply to the skin is also relevant, as this will be involved in any joint movement. Details of skin sensation can be found under nerve function in Chapter 6.

Classification of Synovial Joints

While all synovial joints share the features described above, they vary a great deal in terms of the shape of the articular surfaces and subsequent movement that occurs.

Joint surfaces can be classified as flat, ovoid and sellar (MacConaill 1966, 1973):

- Flat is where the articular surfaces are flat, or plane, although no surface is completely flat.

TABLE 2.2				
Nerve Endings and Afferents Supplying Joints				
Type of Nerve Ending	Descriptive Name for Nerve Ending	Function	Position	Afferent Nerve
Type I	Ruffini endings Golgi–Mazzoni endings Meissner corpuscles Spray-type endings Basket endings Ball-of-thread endings Bush-like endings	Low-threshold slowly adapting static and dynamic mechanoreceptors – signal static joint position, changes in intraarticular pressure and direction, amplitude and velocity of joint movement	Joint capsule (superficial layer) Ligaments Meniscus Articular disc	Aβ fibre, myelinated, diameter 5–10 μm or group II afferent
Type II	Pacinian corpuscle Krause's Endkörperchen Vater'schen Körper Vater–Pacinian corpuscle Modified Pacini(an) corpuscle Simple Pacinian corpuscle Paciniform corpuscle Golgi–Mazzoni body Meissner corpuscle Gelenknervenkörperchen Corpuscle of Krause Club-like ending Bulbous corpuscle Corpuscula nervosa articularia	Low-threshold rapidly adapting dynamic mechanoreceptors – signal beginning and end of movement, deceleration and acceleration, change in vibration or stress	Joint capsule (deeper layer) Ligaments Meniscus Articular disc Fat pads Synovium	Aβ fibre, myelinated diameter 8–12 μm or group II afferent
Type III	Golgi endings Golgi–Mazzoni corpuscles	High-threshold, very slowly adapting mechanoreceptors – signal extreme ranges of movement or when there is considerable stress	Ligaments Meniscus Articular disc	Aβ fibre, myelinated diameter 13–17 μm Group II axons
Type IVa	Free nerve terminals	High-threshold, non-adapting pain receptors	Joint capsule (superficial and deep layers) Ligaments Meniscus Articular disc Fat pads	C fibre, unmyelinated, diameter 1–2 μm and thinly myelinated A fibre, diameter 2–4 μm Type III and IV axons
Type IVa	Free nerve endings	High-threshold, non-adapting pain receptors	Articular blood vessels	Aδ fibre, myelinated diameter 2–5 μm Group II/III axons
Type IVb	Free nerve endings	Vasomotor function	Articular blood vessels	C fibre, unmyelinated diameter <2 μm Group IV axons

(Freeman & Wyke 1967b; Wyke 1970; Kennedy et al. 1982; Albright et al. 1987; Zimny & St Onge 1987; Strasmann & Halata 1988; Zimny 1988; Messner 1999; Palastanga & Soames 2012)

- Ovoid is where the articular surfaces are wholly concave or wholly convex.
- Sellar is where the articular surfaces are concave in one plane and convex in another.

Synovial joints are classified as gliding, hinge, pivot, condyloid or ellipsoidal, saddle and ball and socket (Fig. 2.19):

- Gliding joints include intercarpal and intertarsal joints, zygapophyseal joints in the cervical and thoracic spine, patellofemoral and the costotransverse and costovertebral joints in the lower ribs. The articular surfaces are more or less flat (MacConaill 1953), and, as the name suggests, simple gliding or translational movement can occur.

- Hinge joints include tibiofemoral, humeroulnar, talocrural and interphalangeal joints in the hand and foot. One articular surface is convex and the other concave, allowing rotational flexion and extension movement.
- Pivot joints include the atlantoaxial and the superior radioulnar joints (MacConaill 1973). One articular surface is round and sits within a ring formed partly by bone and partly by ligament. Rotational movement is around the longitudinal axis of the bone, producing, for example, in the forearm, pronation and supination.
- Condyloid or ellipsoidal joints include the radiocarpal joint and the metacarpophalangeal joints. One articular surface is oval and the other elliptical; movement can occur in two planes.

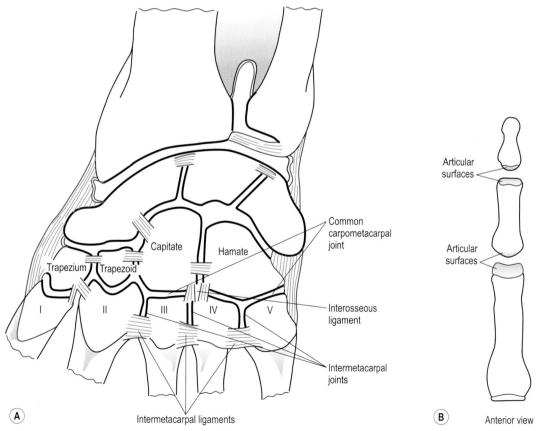

FIG. 2.19 ■ Types of synovial joint. (A) Gliding joints of the intercarpal joints at the wrist. (B) Hinge: interphalangeal joints.
Continued

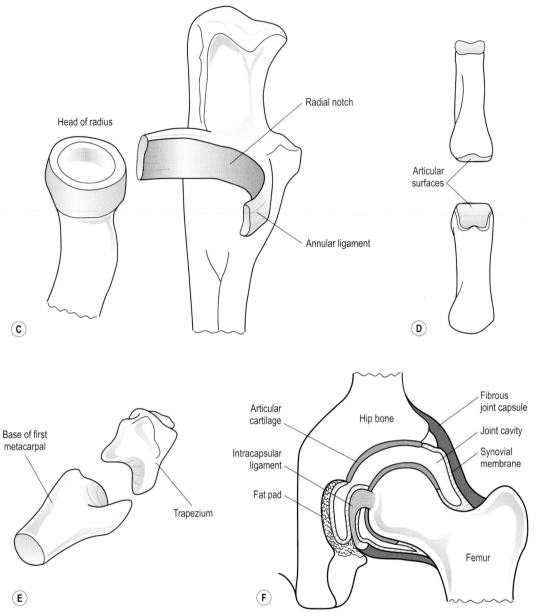

FIG. 2.19, cont'd ■ (C) Pivot: superior radioulnar joint. (D) Condyloid: metacarpophalangeal joint of the thumb. (E) Saddle: carpometacarpal of the thumb. (F) Ball and socket: hip joint. *(After Palastanga & Soames 2012, with permission.)*

For example, at the radiocarpal joint, there is both flexion and extension and radial and ulnar deviation.

- Saddle joints include the first carpometacarpal joint, pisotriquetral joint and lumbar zygapophyseal joints (MacConaill 1953). The shape of the articular surfaces is like the saddle on a horse: each articular surface is reciprocally concave in one plane and convex in another, sometimes referred to as sellar (MacConaill 1953). Like the condyloid joints, movement occurs in two planes, allowing flexion and extension and abduction and adduction.
- Ball and socket joints include the glenohumeral and hip joints. One articular surface is shaped like a ball and the other articular surface is shaped as a hand, which holds the ball. Movement occurs in three planes of movement, allowing flexion and extension, abduction and adduction, and medial and lateral rotation.

Joint Movement

The study of the movement of joint surfaces is termed arthrokinematics. The type of movement at a joint surface can be classified as slide, roll or spin:

- Slide or glide is a pure translation of one surface on another.
- Roll is when the bone rolls or rotates over the articular surface as a wheel rolls along the ground.
- Spin is pure rotation; it occurs at the humeroulnar joint during pronation and supination and at the hip and glenohumeral joint during flexion and extension (MacConaill 1966).

The movement that occurs at a plane (or gliding) joint is slide or glide, but at all the other types of joint (hinge, pivot, condyloid, saddle, ball and socket) movement is a combination of slide with roll or spin.

Movement at a joint is further complicated by conjunct rotation, where a secondary rotation occurs during a rotational movement. For example, during flexion of the elbow and the knee joint, there is lateral rotation of the humerus and femur, respectively (MacConaill 1966).

At any joint, there are potentially six degrees of freedom (Fig. 2.20), which can be described in terms of movement in a plane, or according to the axis of

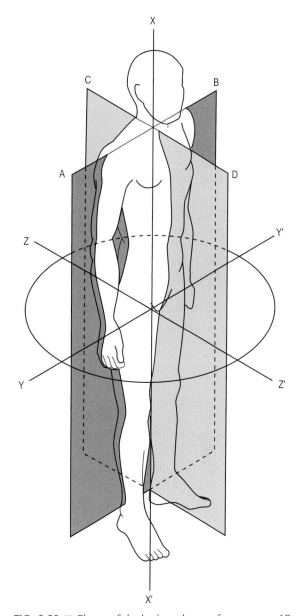

FIG. 2.20 ■ Planes of the body and axes of movement. AB is the coronal plane, CD is the sagittal plane and the horizontal circle surrounding the person depicts the horizontal plane; XX′ is the vertical axis, YY′ is the frontal axis and ZZ′ is the sagittal axis. *(From Middleditch & Oliver 2005, with permission.)*

movement (Middleditch & Oliver 2005). Movements according to the plane of movement are:

- rotation and translation in the sagittal plane
- rotation and translation in the coronal plane
- rotation and translation in the horizontal plane.

During lumbar spine flexion, for example, there is at each spinal level a combination of anterior sagittal rotation and anterior sagittal translation; during extension there is posterior sagittal rotation and posterior sagittal translation. More information and measurements of these movements can be obtained from Pearcy et al. (1984) and Pearcy and Tibrewal (1984).

Joint Glide During Physiological Movements

Movement at a joint is a combination of roll or spin with a glide or translation; for example, during elbow flexion, the radial head rotates around the capitulum of the humerus and translates (that is, slides) anteriorly. During knee flexion, non-weight bearing, the tibia rotates posteriorly around the femur and slides posteriorly. Because movement consists of both a roll or spin and a glide, the axis of movement constantly changes and is referred to as the instantaneous axis of rotation. Table 2.3 identifies, for each joint movement, the direction of the bone translation.

The direction in which the bone glides (or translates) depends upon the shape of the moving articular surface (Fig. 2.21) (MacConaill 1973; Kaltenborn 2014). When the joint surface of the moving bone is concave, the glide usually occurs in the same direction as the bone is moving so that, with flexion on the knee joint (in non-weight bearing), posterior glide of the tibial condyles occurs on the femoral condyles. When the joint surface is convex, the glide is usually in the opposite direction to the bone movement so that, with ankle dorsiflexion, there is a posterior glide of the talus on the inferior tibia and fibula. There is some evidence to suggest that this rule may not be valid in relation to movement of the glenohumeral joint (Brandt et al. 2007).

Another consideration is the relative size of the articular surfaces; for example, at the glenohumeral joint the head of the humerus has a much larger surface area than the glenoid cavity. The effect of this is that the head of the humerus, as it rolls, would run out of

TABLE 2.3
Direction of Bone Translation During Active Physiological Movements

Movement	Translation
Glenohumeral	
Flexion	Anterior and superior
Extension	Posterior and inferior
Abduction	Inferior
Elbow: Humeroulnar	
Flexion	Anterior
Extension	Posterior
Elbow: radiohumeral	
Flexion	Anterior
Extension	Posterior
Forearm: Superior Radioulnar	
Pronation	Posterior
Supination	Anterior
Forearm: Inferior Radioulnar	
Pronation	Anterior
Supination	Posterior
Wrist: Proximal Row of Carpus on Radius and Ulnar	
Flexion	Posterior
Extension	Anterior
Radial deviation	Medial
Ulnar deviation	Lateral
Thumb: Base of First Metacarpal on Trapezium	
Flexion	Anterior
Extension	Posterior
Abduction	Medial
Adduction	Lateral
Hip	
Flexion	Posterior
Extension	Anterior
Abduction	Medial
Adduction	Lateral
Knee, Non-Weight Bearing	
Flexion	Posterior
Extension	Anterior
Ankle, Non-Weight Bearing Talus on Tibia and Fibula	
Dorsiflexion	Posterior
Plantarflexion	Anterior

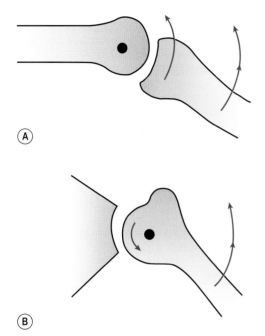

FIG. 2.21 ■ Movement of articular surfaces during physiological movements. The single arrow depicts the direction of movement of the articular surface and the double arrow depicts the physiological movement. (A) With knee extension (non-weight bearing), the concave articular surface of the tibia slides superiorly on the convex femoral condyles. (B) With shoulder elevation through abduction, the convex articular surface of the humerus slides inferiorly on the concave glenoid cavity. *(After Kaltenborn 2014, with permission.)*

articular surface on the glenoid. This is overcome by a glide and also by accompanying movement of the scapula, during humeral movements (Levangie & Norkin 2011).

The examples given above refer to peripheral joints. The spinal joints follow the same principles but are worth describing separately here. Each spinal segmental level, between C2 and S1, consists of an interbody joint (two vertebral bodies and the intervening intervertebral disc) and two zygapophyseal joints (Middleditch & Oliver 2005), functionally a triad joint. The shape and direction of the articular surface of the zygapophyseal joints influence the gliding movement available at that segmental level (Table 2.4). The shape and direction of the articular surfaces vary throughout the spine (Table 2.5 and Fig. 2.22).

The upper cervical spine, C0–C1 (between the occiput and atlas) and C1–C2 (between C1 and the axis) are, anatomically, rather different from the rest of the spine. The superior articular facets of C1 are concave and face upwards and medially; in addition, the lines of the two facets, when viewed superiorly, converge anteriorly (Fig. 2.23A). The occipital condyles are reciprocally shaped. The shape of the facets at C0–C1 facilitates flexion and extension movement. As the head rotates forwards on C1, the occipital condyles slide (or translate) in a posterior direction, following the above principle of a convex surface moving on a concave surface (Fig. 2.23B). With extension of the head on C1, the occipital condyles slide in an anterior direction.

The superior articular facets of C2 are large, oval and convex, and they lie in an anteroposterior direction. They face superiorly and laterally (Fig. 2.24A). The inferior articular facets of C1 are reciprocally shaped. The shape of the facets at C1–C2 facilitates rotation. With rotation to the right, the right inferior facet of C1 glides posteriorly and slightly downwards (Fig. 2.24B). The posterior movement produces the rotation movement, and the downward (inferior) movement produces a right lateral flexion movement. Thus, at this segmental level, rotation to the right is accompanied by ipsilateral (right) lateral flexion. During flexion, the inferior facets of C1 glide backward on the superior facets of C2. During extension, the inferior facets of C1 glide forward.

In the cervical spine (C3–C7 levels) the superior articular facets are oval and flat and face upwards and backwards (Fig. 2.22). During cervical spine flexion, the inferior articular facets of each cervical vertebra slide upward and forward on the superior articular facets of the vertebra below. For example, the inferior facets of C5 slide upward and forward on the superior facets of C6. On extension the reverse occurs throughout the cervical spine, so, for example, at C5–C6, the inferior facets of C5 slide downward and backward on the superior facets of C6.

On right lateral flexion, the left inferior articular facets of each cervical vertebra slide upward but also forward on the vertebra below, and on the right-hand side the inferior articular facets slide downward but also backward. Thus, in the cervical spine, right lateral flexion is accompanied by right (ipsilateral) rotation

TABLE 2.4

Glide of Inferior Articular Facets During Physiological Movements of the Spine. Movement in Parentheses Denotes Minimal Amount of Movement

	Flexion	Extension	Left Lateral Flexion	Right Lateral Flexion	Left Rotation	Right Rotation
C2–C7						
Left inferior articular facet	Upward Forward	Downward Backward	Downward Backward	Upward Forward	Downward Backward medial	Upward Forward lateral
Right inferior articular facet	Upward Forward	Downward Backward	Upward Forward	Downward Backward	Upward Forward lateral	Downward Backward medial
T1–T12						
Left inferior articular facet	Upward (forward)	Downward (backward)	Downward (backward)	Upward (forward)	Medial	Lateral
Right inferior articular facet	Upward (forward)	Downward (backward)	Upward (forward)	Downward (backward)	Lateral	Medial
L1–S1						
Left inferior articular facet	Upward (forward)	Downward (backward)	Downward (backward)	Upward (forward)		
Right inferior articular facet	Upward (forward)	Downward (backward)	Upward (forward)	Downward (backward)		

TABLE 2.5

Shape and Direction of the Superior Articular Surfaces of the Zygapophyseal Joints in the Spine

Spinal Level	Shape of Superior Facets	Direction of Superior Facets	Movement Facilitated by Direction of Facets
C1	Concave	Upwards and medial	Flexion and extension
C2	Large, oval, convex	Upwards and lateral	Rotation
C2–C7	Oval, flat	Upwards and backwards	All directions
T1–T12	Triangular, flat	Backwards, slightly upwards and lateral	Rotation Lateral flexion
L1–L5	Concave	Backwards and medial	Flexion, extension, lateral flexion

(Fig. 2.25). It is the forward movement of the left inferior articular facet that produces the right rotation movement, and its upward movement produces a right lateral flexion movement.

On cervical rotation to the right, the left inferior articular facets at each cervical level glide upward, forward and laterally on the superior facet of the vertebra below (Fig. 2.25) and on the right-hand side the inferior articular facets glide downward, backward and medially on the vertebra below, therefore producing right (ipsilateral) lateral flexion.

In summary, then, cervical lateral flexion is accompanied by ipsilateral rotation, and rotation is accompanied by ipsilateral lateral flexion.

In the thoracic spine the flat, triangular superior articular facets face backward and slightly upward and lateral (Fig. 2.22). During thoracic flexion, the inferior articular facets at each level glide essentially upward, with some forward translation (Fig. 2.26). On thoracic extension, the inferior articular facets glide downward with some backward translation. On left lateral flexion, the right inferior articular facets glide upward and

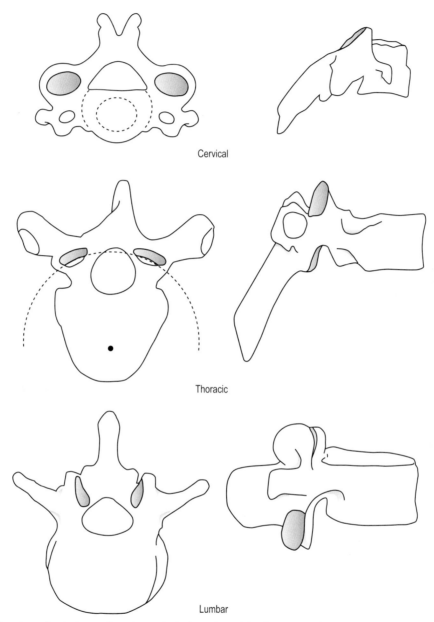

Cervical

Thoracic

Lumbar

FIG. 2.22 ■ Direction of articular surfaces in cervical, thoracic and lumbar spine. The superior articular facets of the cervical vertebrae face upwards and backwards, those of the thoracic vertebrae backwards and laterally, and those of the lumbar vertebrae backwards and medially. *(From Palastanga & Soames 2012, with permission.)*

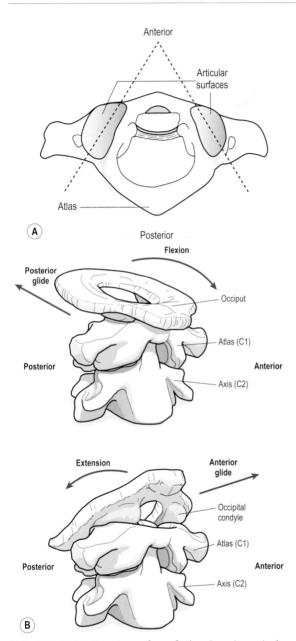

FIG. 2.23 ■ (A) Superior surface of atlas. Superior articular facets of C1 are concave and face upwards and medial. The lines of the two facets, when viewed superiorly, converge anteriorly. *(From Palastanga & Soames 2012, with permission.)* (B) Flexion and extension at the C0–C1 joint. During flexion the occipital condyles glide posteriorly, whereas during extension they glide anteriorly. *(After Edwards 1999, with permission.)*

slightly forward; the upward movement produces the lateral flexion, the forward movement produces a rotation movement to the left (ipsilateral). The combination of rotation and lateral flexion movements in the thoracic spine is not as straightforward as in the cervical spine. The coupled movements vary in different regions of the thoracic spine. At T2, lateral flexion is accompanied by ipsilateral rotation, whereas at T6 and T11 lateral flexion can be accompanied by ipsilateral rotation or contralateral rotation.

In the lumbar spine, the superior articular facets are concave, facing backwards and medially (Fig. 2.22). During lumbar flexion, the inferior articular facets glide upward and forward. On extension, the inferior articular facets glide downward and backward (Fig. 2.27). The movement of the articular facets during lateral flexion is less clear. With lateral flexion, there may be ipsilateral or contralateral rotation (Pearcy & Tibrewal 1984). On lumbar rotation to the left (moving the trunk), the inferior articular facet on the right glides anteriorly and laterally to impact on to the superior articular facet of the vertebra below. The left inferior articular facet glides in a posterior and medial direction, so there is gapping of the joint space. Rotation of the lumbar spine from L1 to L4 is accompanied by contralateral lateral flexion, whereas rotation at L5–S1 is accompanied by ipsilateral lateral flexion (Pearcy & Tibrewal 1984).

Normal function of any synovial joint, then, requires the moving bone to rotate and translate. Each of these movements, rotation and translation, if normal, would be full-range, symptom-free, and with normal through-range and end-range resistance; normal muscle and nerve function is assumed. In the examination of a patient, normal rotation and translation are examined during active and passive physiological movements, and normal translation is examined during accessory movements; this is described in detail elsewhere (Hengeveld & Banks 2014a, b; Petty & Ryder 2017).

A knowledge of the normal rotation and translation of bone during movement of a joint is important when attempting to restore normal joint function. The following examples may highlight this. With the patient lying prone, to facilitate an increase in cervical flexion at the C4–C5 level, a central posteroanterior force with a cephalad inclination could be used on the C4 spinous process. This accessory movement will also enhance extension at the C3–C4 segmental level. In the same

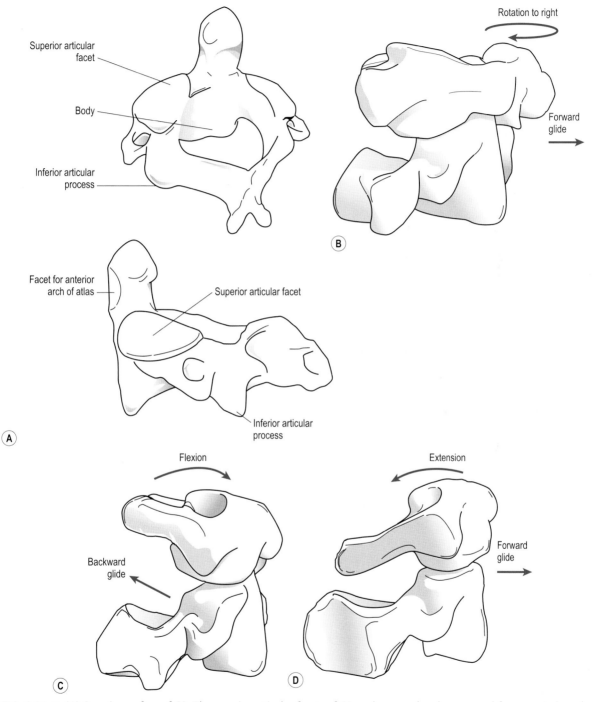

FIG. 2.24 ■ (A) Superior surface of C2. The superior articular facets of C2 are large, oval and convex and face superiorly and laterally. *(After Middleditch & Oliver 2005, with permission.)* (B) Rotation to the right at the C1–C2 joint. The right inferior facet of C1 glides posteriorly and slightly downwards, while the left inferior facet of C1 glides anteriorly and slightly upwards. *(After Edwards 1999, with permission).* (C) Flexion at the C1–C2 joint: the inferior facets of C1 glide backward on the superior facets of C2. (D) Extension at the C1–C2 joint: the inferior facets of C1 glide forward on the superior facets of C2.

way, to facilitate cervical lateral flexion or rotation to the right at the C4–C5 level, a unilateral posteroanterior pressure with a cephalad inclination could be applied on the left C4 articular pillar. This accessory movement would also enhance ipsilateral lateral flexion and rotation

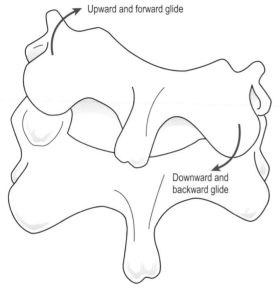

FIG. 2.25 ■ Cervical rotation to the right is accompanied by lateral flexion to the right. The left inferior articular facet glides upward and forward, while the right inferior articular facet glides downward and backward. *(After Middleditch & Oliver 2005, with permission)*

at the C3–C4 level. Similar accessory movements can be applied to the thoracic and lumbar spine joints and to the peripheral joints (for further information, see Hengeveld & Banks 2014 a, b).

Another concept is that of close pack and loose pack position of a joint. Close pack is where there is maximal congruency of joint surfaces, maximal tension in the joint capsule and ligaments, and least joint play; it is usually found at the extreme of range. Loose pack is any position other than close pack, where the joint capsule and ligaments are relatively slack and there is some joint play. Joint play is the amount of slack, or give, in the joint.

Knowledge of the close-packed and loose-packed positions of a joint helps with determining which joint movements cause compression and which cause distraction of the adjacent articular surfaces. The position of the joint at the time of injury can ultimately predict the injury that occurs. For example, in a close-packed position, the application of force is likely to lead to a bony injury, as, in this position, the congruency of the adjoining bones enables the force to be taken up through the bone rather than the supporting ligaments/capsular structures, e.g. a Colles fracture sustained by a fall on the outstretched hand and the wrist joint in extension. With the wrist in flexion, a loose-packed position, it is more likely that a capsular or ligamentous injury will occur as the force of impact is taken up by the supporting soft-tissue structures. In the lower limb, for example,

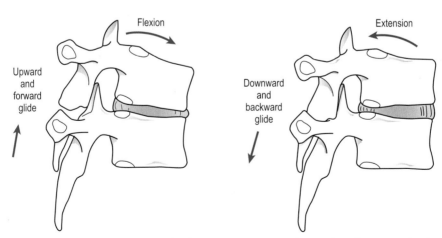

FIG. 2.26 ■ Flexion and extension movements in the thoracic spine. During flexion the inferior articular facets glide upward and slightly forward, and on extension the inferior articular facets glide downward and slightly backward. *(After Palastanga & Soames 2012, with permission.)*

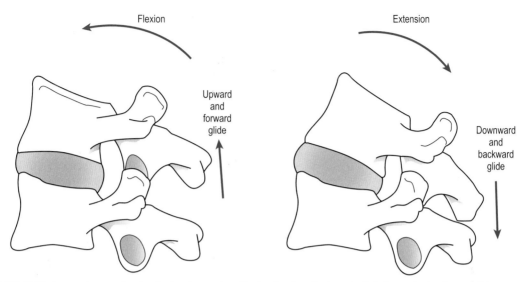

FIG. 2.27 ■ Flexion and extension in the lumbar spine. During lumbar flexion the inferior articular facets glide upward and forward, while on extension they glide downward and backward. *(After Palastanga & Soames 2012, with permission.)*

an anterior cruciate ligament tear may be sustained with the knee in a flexed and rotated position (Hertling & Kessler 2006a).

Biomechanics of Normal Joint Movement

The normal function of most joints is to allow full-range movement of the adjacent bones. As the bones move towards the end-range of joint movement, resistance to movement increases (Wright & Johns 1961; Nigg & Herzog 2007) as the surrounding joint capsule, ligaments and muscles become taut (Wright & Johns 1961), eventually causing movement to stop. This is a protective mechanism so that the joint does not sublux or dislocate. More information on the forces required during accessory movements can be found in Petty et al. (2002).

End-Feel. Different joints are limited by different structures at the end of a particular range of movement. For example, elbow extension is limited by bony opposition of the olecranon process of the ulna in the olecranon fossa, knee flexion is limited by soft-tissue opposition between the calf and the thigh, and wrist flexion is limited by the wrist dorsal ligaments as well as the bony configuration of the carpus. This resistance at the end of range of a joint movement and when felt by a clinician is referred to as end-feel. End-feel varies for different movements in different joints, whether pathology is present or not. It is used in clinical assessment of joint movement. The testing of end-feel can be performed for both physiological and accessory movements.

Classification of end-feel as normal or pathological is based on the ability to interpret the movement occurring at the joint, in conjunction with anatomical knowledge and the point in the range at which the resistance is felt. End-feel can be normal or indicative of pathology, and therefore requires interpretation by an experienced clinician.

- Capsular end-feel: a firm, leathery feeling (Cyriax 1982; Hertling & Kessler 2006b; Atkins et al. 2010; Kaltenborn 2014), considered normal when felt at the end of some ranges of movement, e.g. lateral rotation of the shoulder/hip. It is considered abnormal when felt early in the range, and may be indicative of early degenerative changes in a joint.
- Bony end-feel: occurs normally at end-range when there is bony apposition of approximating surfaces, e.g. full-range elbow extension. This end-feel is considered abnormal when occurring before expected end-range and may indicate degenerative change or malunion of an intraarticular fracture.

- Soft-tissue end-feel: a soft feeling at the end of range occurs when muscular tissue is approximated, as in elbow flexion and knee flexion. It may be considered abnormal if joint range of motion is restricted due to muscle hypertrophy (Cyriax 1982; Hertling & Kessler 2006b; Kaltenborn 2014).
- Ligamentous end-feel: this is a firm end-feel with no appreciable give, and may be felt when applying an abduction/adduction force to an extended knee. Any notable give may be due to ligamentous damage.

Abnormal end-feel may be categorized as follows:

- Hard end-feel: seen in capsular and degenerative pathology. End-feel is harder than expected and/or occurs earlier in the range (Hertling & Kessler 2006b; Atkins et al. 2010).
- Springy end-feel: often occurs in the presence of a loose body; full range of joint movement is not achieved and an abnormal 'bouncy' feeling is experienced by the clinician at the end of the available range (Atkins et al. 2010).
- Muscle spasm end-feel: often occurs with pain; end-feel is that of an abrupt stop to movement, often with visible muscle contraction present as a 'guarding' mechanism to prevent further movement.
- Empty end-feel: rare, but of high clinical significance. The sensation is described as 'empty' as the examiner experiences no resistance to continuation of movement, but the patient halts the movement due to severe pain. Interpretation of this response must be treated with caution but may be indicative of neoplasm, fracture, septic arthritis or acute bursitis.

Functional Movement

While movement at an individual joint can occur, functional activities often involve movement throughout the limb. For example, in standing, when a person bends at the knees this will be accompanied by hip flexion and ankle dorsiflexion. This predictable movement pattern can be referred to as a closed kinematic chain, a term used in engineering for linkages that make up a system. In contrast, the unpredictable movement patterns that can occur in the upper limb (and the lower limb when not weight bearing) can be termed an open kinematic chain. The concept of open and closed kinematic chains is useful in that it highlights that movement involves a number of joints, and rarely does a joint move in isolation. Furthermore, these patterns are used in clinical practice in varying stages of rehabilitation to mimic normal functional movement.

Proprioception

Joint stability occurs through the integration of dynamic and mechanical restraints (Myers et al. 2006; Munn et al. 2010). Dynamic restraints pertain to the joint capsule, ligaments, bony anatomy and intraarticular pressures while mechanical restraints include muscle activation and the force produced from this muscle activity. These dynamic and mechanical restraints are mediated by the sensorimotor system, which includes sensory, motor, central integration and processing components. When functioning optimally, this provides a feedforward/feedback system, where mechanical restraints provide neural feedback via efferent motor pathways to the central nervous system. This in turn provides feedback to the dynamic restraints (Myers et al. 2006; Munn et al. 2010).

Proprioception is part of this sensorimotor system and forms the afferent feedback from joint and soft-tissue mechanoreceptors, present in muscle, ligaments, joint capsule and fascia, through mechanical and dynamic restraints. Proprioception, by definition, is a perception of position and movement (Boisgontier & Swinnen 2014) gained from skin, joint and muscle receptors (Hewett et al. 2002). It has three main components: joint position sense, kinaesthesia and sensation of force. Damage to the joint, ligaments, muscle or skin can affect this feedback system and thus cause a loss of proprioception which may ultimately lead to muscle, joint and/or nerve dysfunction.

JOINT DYSFUNCTION

Just as the function of joints depends on the function of muscles and nerves, so dysfunction of joints can lead to dysfunction in muscles and nerves. They are dependent on each other in both normal and abnormal conditions, and this relationship is depicted in Fig. 2.28. The following examples explore how joint

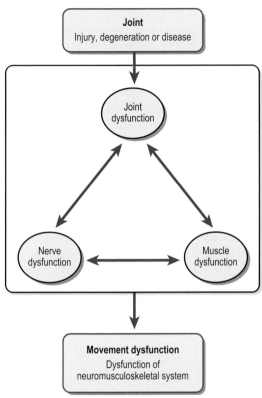

FIG. 2.28 ■ Dysfunction of joint can produce muscle and/or nerve dysfunction.

dysfunction is often accompanied by muscle and/or nerve dysfunction.

Joint Pathology and Muscle/Nerve Dysfunction

Joint pathology can lead to weakness of the overlying muscle and deficits in neuromuscular control (Myers & Lephart 2000; Callaghan et al. 2014). This has been demonstrated in the presence of a variety of pathologies: patellofemoral pain syndrome (Callaghan & Oldham 2004); patellofemoral osteoarthritis (Callaghan et al. 2014); and ligamentous injuries (Urbach & Awiszus 2002) following meniscectomy (Malliou et al. 2012). The presence of effusion has been shown to result in muscle inhibition in the knee (Palmieri-Smith et al. 2007) and in the hip joint (Freeman et al. 2013). However other research has failed to find a direct association between joint distension and muscle inhibition (Callaghan et al. 2014). The inhibition of muscle

is thought to be due to inhibitory (Suter & Herzog 2000; Torry et al. 2000) or abnormal (Rice et al. 2011) input from joint afferents. Thus, joint pathology leads to altered nervous system activity, which leads to altered muscle activity.

Joint Immobilization and Muscle/Nerve Dysfunction

Joint immobilization can also have a negative effect on muscular and neural function. Joint immobilization for 3 weeks has been shown to cause a reduced maximal voluntary contraction of the muscle around the joint, and a decrease in the maximal firing rate of motor neurons supplying muscle (Seki et al. 2001; Kazuhiko & Hiroshi 2007). Thus, immobilization of a joint leads to muscle weakness and altered nervous system activity.

Joint Instability and Muscle/Nerve Dysfunction

Joint instability and ligament insufficiency have been shown to alter nervous system activity, which leads to altered muscle activity. In the ankle joint, arthrogenic muscle inhibition was found to be present post ankle sprain (McVey et al. 2005) and at the knee, anterior cruciate ligament deficiency has been found to alter activity of quadriceps and hamstring muscle groups during knee movement (Suarez et al. 2016), gait (Serrancoli et al. 2016) and negotiating stairs (Hall et al. 2015). A cycle of events leading to dysfunction in ligament, muscle and nerve is shown in Fig. 2.29 (Suter & Herzog 2000). Thus, ligamentous injury leads to altered nervous system activity, which leads to altered muscle activity, altered neuromuscular control and altered proprioception.

Proprioceptive deficits have been identified in human arthritic conditions, and are attributed to reduced activity of the joint, local muscle atrophy (Cuomo et al. 2005) and the presence of pain, where increased nociceptor activity causes a reduction in proprioception (Safran et al. 2001; Fortier & Basset 2012) and joint swelling. Although it was previously thought that swelling had a negative influence on proprioception, it is now believed that the loss of proprioception in the presence of swelling is more likely to be due to the nature of the fluid contents or the length of time the effusion is present, e.g. arthritic conditions (Palmieri et al. 2003), or the presence of pain (Callaghan et al. 2014).

It has also been hypothesized that loss of proprioceptive mechanisms either due to age or due to decreased muscle mass may initiate or accelerate arthritic damage through its effect on a joint's dynamic and mechanical restraints (Ikeda et al. 2005; Kim et al. 2016). This is well acknowledged in the literature, where ligamentous injury such as damage to the anterior cruciate ligament can affect postural control in both the injured and uninjured side (Ageberg 2002), and joint damage, such as in arthritic conditions, may evoke abnormal articular afferent information, causing subsequent loss of muscle activation and altered neuromuscular control (Myers & Lephart 2000). Problems with muscle activation are

also reported following joint injury and proprioceptive loss and can contribute to recurrent instability problems, through suppressed reflexive activation and slow co-activation patterns from muscles with stabilizing roles (Myers et al. 2006).

Joint Nociception and Muscle Dysfunction

Joint nociceptor activity directly affects muscle activity. Joint pain is directly associated with muscle inhibition and weakness. Quadriceps muscle inhibition was found to be directly associated with the severity of pain from osteoarthritic patellofemoral joints (Callaghan et al. 2014) and more than 3 months' history of pain caused by lumbar disc herniation is linked to reduction in the cross-sectional area of multifidus (Kim et al. 2011).

Conversely, dysfunction in muscle is thought to lead to joint dysfunction (Suter & Herzog 2000). For example, quadriceps muscle weakness is thought to alter knee joint loading which may, in the long term, lead to osteoarthritis in the joint (Herzog & Longino 2007; Hall et al. 2012). Thus, joint dysfunction may occur as a result of a muscle dysfunction and this sequence of events is outlined in Fig. 2.30.

Classification of Joint Dysfunction

The function of a joint is to transfer force from one bone to another and to permit limited movement (Nigg & Herzog 2007). Some joints, such as the sacroiliac joint (SIJ), transmit very high forces and have hardly any movement, whereas other joints, such as the glenohumeral joint, transmit less force and have a large range of movement. The signs and symptoms of joint

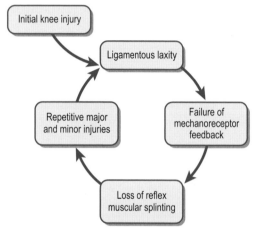

FIG. 2.29 ■ A proposed cycle of progressive knee instability following an initial ligament injury. *(From Kennedy et al. 1982, with permission.)*

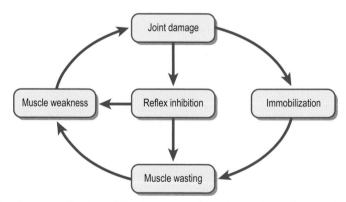

FIG. 2.30 ■ Effect of joint damage and/or immobilization on muscle and nerve tissue. *(From Stokes, M., Young, A. 1984 Clinical Science 67:7–14. © The Biochemical Society and the Medical Research Society, with permission.)*

dysfunction are directly related to these functions, that is, there may be one or more of the following: reduced range of joint movement (hypomobility), increased range of joint movement (hypermobility), altered quality of movement or production of symptoms. These signs and symptoms can occur in isolation or in any combination. A particular mix of these signs and symptoms occurs with a ligamentous sprain, and for clarity this is discussed in a separate section at the end of this chapter. Box 2.1 highlights these characteristics of joint function and dysfunction.

Hypomobility

Hypomobility can affect accessory or physiological movements. It seems reasonable to suggest that if there is a reduced range of translation this will affect, to some degree, the range of rotation of the bone. In the same way, if there is a reduced range of rotation movement, this will affect the range of translation movement.

Limited range of accessory or physiological movement is often associated with an altered quality of movement. This is most commonly increased resistance to movement or production of symptoms; these are depicted in Fig. 2.31.

Traumatized or pathological tissues, which may produce alteration to the movement quality, include intraarticular structures, such as joint capsule, a torn meniscus or a loose body, and periarticular structures such as ligament, muscle or nerve overlying the joint. Each joint has its own unique range and resistance to movement owing to its particular intraarticular and periarticular arrangement. In the upper and lower limbs,

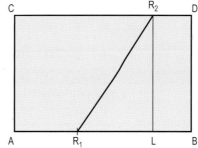

Resistance is first felt (R_1) between ¼ and ½ range and increases to limit range (R_2) just beyond ¾ range (L)

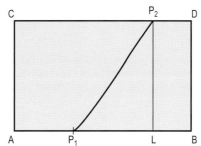

Pain is first felt (P_1) between ¼ and ½ range and increases to limit range (P_2) just beyond ¾ range (L)

FIG. 2.31 ■ Movement diagram of hypomobility due to resistance or production of symptoms, where L is the limit of range, R_1 is the first point of resistance felt by the examiner, R_2 is the maximum intensity of resistance which limits further movement, P_1 is the point in the range where pain is first felt and P_2 is the maximum intensity of pain which limits further movement.

the clinician compares the left and right side to determine normality for the patient, comparing the range of movement and the through-range and end-range resistance to movement (Petty & Ryder 2017). The clinician judges any difference, while bearing in mind that range of movement varies from side to side in normal asymptomatic subjects. Where there is no other side with which to compare, as with central posteroanterior pressures of the vertebrae, the clinician can compare movement at adjacent levels, but again bearing in mind that there are normal differences in the range of movement at different segmental levels (Middleditch & Oliver 2005).

Limited range of accessory or physiological movements may be caused by the production of symptoms. Symptoms can be any sensation felt by the patient and can include pain, ache, pulling, pins and needles, numbness, a sense of something crawling along the skin, as well as apprehension by the patient to move further into range.

Hypomobility can be more fully appreciated by exploring the effects of immobilization on joint structures, as this produces the most profound joint hypomobility.

Immobilization

Knowledge of the effects of immobilization on joint tissue has come about largely from research on animals.

The timescales involved in tissue changes with knee joint immobilization on the joint space, articular cartilage and subchondral bone are summarized in Table 2.6. Changes include the formation of adhesions between the connective tissue and the articular cartilage, ulceration of the articular cartilage and erosion of subchondral bone. All the knees investigated following immobilization had reduced range of movement and joint stiffness due to the connective tissue and adhesion formation in the joint space (Ando et al. 2010, Lee et al. 2010; Iqbal et al. 2012). The detailed changes of articular cartilage following immobilization (Box 2.2) include reduced proteoglycan synthesis, softening of the articular cartilage, softening and reduced thickness, adhesions to the fibrofatty connective tissue in the joint space and pressure necrosis where adjacent surfaces are in contact with chondrocyte death (Vanwanseele et al. 2002).

However, the effects of immobilization to the articular cartilage can be minimized by exercise before immobilization, whilst exercise can increase cartilage thickness (Maldonado et al. 2013).

TABLE 2.6			
Effect of Immobilization on Joint			
Tissue	**Time**	**Effect**	**Study**
Joint space	15 days; well established at 1 month	Fibrofatty connective tissue within the joint space	Evans et al. (1960)
Adhesions	2 weeks	Adhesions between synovial membrane and meniscus	Ando et al. (2010)
	4 weeks	Adhesions bridged the synovial membrane meniscus and articular cartilage	
	Between 8 and 16 weeks	Adhesions become hypocellular and fibrous	
Articular cartilage	1 month	Cartilage thinning with necrotic areas and erosion	Iqbal et al. (2012)
	2 months	Atrophy of unapposing cartilage and ulceration of the articular cartilage	Evans et al. (1960)
Subchondral bone	2 months	Proliferation of vascular connective tissue under areas of articular cartilage lesion and erosion of subchondral bone	Evans et al. (1960)
Synovial membrane	2–4 weeks	Shortening	Ando et al. (2010)
	16 weeks	Non-distinguishable synovial membrane	
Joint capsule	3 days	Cell proliferation hypoxia and inflammation	Yabe et al. (2013)
	8 and 16 weeks	Shortening	Ando et al. (2010)

The detailed effect of immobilization on joint capsule, synovial membrane, ligament and articular cartilage has also been investigated. In the first few days after immobilization the joint capsule connective tissue shows conditions of hypoxia and inflammation (Yabe et al. 2013). In the first 2 weeks the synovial membrane becomes shorter and forms adhesions (Ando et al. 2010). The collagen fibres of the capsule become disorganized and the range of motion decreases (Lee et al. 2010). The adhesions become fibrous and hypocellular in 8–16 weeks (Ando et al. 2010) whilst at 16 weeks the connective tissue becomes hypocellular as well (Lee et al. 2010; Yabe et al. 2013). The ligament undergoes alterations in its water and glycosaminoglycan content, degradation in collagen synthesis, increase in collagen cross-links after 9 weeks, bone resorption at the bone–ligament junction, reduced stiffness and increased extensibility of the ligament and a reduction in load to failure (Box 2.3). The substantial change in the load–displacement curve of the rabbit femur–medial collateral ligament–tibia complex, after 9 weeks of immobilization, compared with a control group is depicted in Fig. 2.32 (Woo et al. 1988). The structural and mechanical effects of immobilization and remobilization of the bone–ligament–bone complex are depicted in Fig. 2.33 (Woo et al. 1987).

Hypermobility

Joint hypermobility is a condition in which synovial joints move excessively beyond normal limits, even after age, gender and race are taken into account (Grahame 2003). Joint hypermobility may be inherited (Ferrell et al. 2004) or acquired through years of training or stretching (Grahame 2003). In many cases it causes no

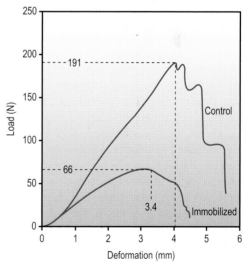

FIG. 2.32 ■ The load-displacement curve of the rabbit femur–medial collateral ligament–tibia complex after 9 weeks of immobilization compared with a control group. *(From Woo, S., Buckwalter, J. 1988 Injury and repair of the musculoskeletal soft tissues. Rosemont, IL: American Academy of Orthopaedic Surgeons, with permission.)*

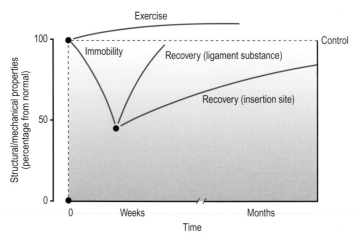

FIG. 2.33 ■ The structural and mechanical properties of bone–ligament–bone complex following immobilization and recovery. *(From Woo et al. 1988, with permission of the American Academy of Orthopaedic Surgeons.)*

symptoms and in some cases is considered advantageous in areas such as the performing arts (Hakim & Grahame 2003). It is important to note that the presence of joint hypermobility with symptoms is given the term benign joint hypermobility syndrome (BJHS), but symptom-free presentation of joint hypermobility is simply referred to as joint hypermobility (Hakim & Grahame 2003; Simmonds & Keer 2007). BJHS refers to the existence of physical signs and symptoms in persons with generalized joint laxity in the absence of systemic rheumatological disease (Aktas et al. 2008). For those individuals who do have symptoms, these may include soft-tissue injury, arthralgias, myalgias, widespread pain, joint stiffness, clunking, popping, subluxations, dislocations, instability, as well as paraesthesiae, tiredness, faintness, feeling unwell, flu-like symptoms, skin fragility and laxity (Grahame 2003; Simmonds & Keer 2007).

There may be hypermobility of one or more accessory movements and/or physiological movements in one or more joints. This increased range of motion may cause an increase in the range of translation of the joint surfaces and vice versa. This type of hypermobility may be inherited or may be due to injury/recurrent injury causing symptoms of increased joint range on active or passive testing.

Joint Instability

Joint instability may be due to a deficit in the ligamentous, muscular and/or neural functioning around a joint.

Instability refers to a significant reduction in the spine's ability to maintain the intervertebral neutral zones within their normal physiological boundaries, thus avoiding pain, deformity and neurological damage (Panjabi 1992a). This definition was put forward to describe instability of the vertebral column; however, it can be extended to include any joint. Instability may be further described as mechanical or functional in nature. Mechanical instability refers to laxity of a joint due to injury of the ligamentous tissues which support the joint (Hertel & Kaminski 2005). Functional instability refers to deficits in proprioceptive and neuromuscular control secondary to joint injury (Hertel & Kaminski 2005). This is hypothesized to be due to the damage of the mechanoreceptors within the ligamentous structures following injury, which causes a reduction in perception of movement and particularly changes in direction (Hughes & Rochester 2008). The relationship between the two is unclear, although mechanical instability can cause functional instability over time (Richie 2001).

Instability can occur in any region of the spine, but may be more common in the cervical and lumbar regions due to the anatomical arrangement of the joints, particularly in the cervical spine, which may predispose to instability owing to the large range of movement available. Instability of the spine occurs when the size of the neutral zone increases, causing uncontrolled or unstable movement patterns with an altered quality of movement, which the stabilizing subsystems are unable to control (Panjabi 1992a; Olsen & Joder 2001). The causes of the increase in the neutral zone size include degenerative change and/or mechanical injury (Panjabi 1992a). As no clinical or diagnostic tests have been found to produce valid and reliable results for this condition, diagnosis can be challenging and requires careful interpretation by an experienced clinician (Cook et al. 2005). In a study by Cook et al. (2005) there was general agreement amongst physiotherapists that the diagnosis of clinical cervical spine instability would be considered when symptoms such as reduced tolerance to prolonged static postures, fatigue, decreased ability to hold the head up, improvement of symptoms with external support, frequent acute attacks and sharp pain triggered by quick movements were reported. Physical examination findings, including poor muscular control, poor muscle recruitment and dissociation of cervical movement, increased joint play on manual testing and poor-quality movement patterns including hinging/pivoting were reported as the most common physical signs that would lead a clinician to consider this diagnosis.

Regarding the lumbar spine, the signs and symptoms that could lead to the diagnosis of instability may include a painful arc in flexion, painful arc on return, Gower's sign, poor-quality movement patterns ('catch' or sudden acceleration or deceleration) and reversal of lumbopelvic rhythm when the patient is asked to flex the trunk (Gopinath 2015). In addition, the passive lumbar extension test (Kasai et al. 2006) can be useful in confirming the diagnosis as it was found to have excellent diagnostic accuracy and good reliability (Ferrari et al. 2015). As in hypomobility, the clinician makes a judgement that a joint has more movement than 'normal', which may be based on comparing sides or, in the spine, comparing adjacent levels. The presence of increased range of accessory and/or physiological movement may be associated with altered quality of movement and can be associated with symptoms.

Altered Quality of Joint Movement

Alteration to the quality of movement encapsulates anything that is considered to be abnormal either by comparison with the other side or from the clinician's or the patient's experience of what is 'normal'. Abnormalities may include: instability; increased or decreased resistance to movement; poor control of movement; the presence of joint noise such as a clunk or crepitus; excessive effort or reluctance of the patient to move. Alterations in the quality of movement can directly or indirectly affect local or remote neuromuscular systems, leading to dysfunction, injury and musculoskeletal pathology. For example, weakness of hip abductors and external rotators can lead to increased hip internal rotation and adduction at the hip during dynamic activities and could lead to pathologies such as iliotibial band syndrome and patellofemoral joint dysfunction (Powers 2010).

Production of Symptoms

Symptoms from joint dysfunction are most commonly a pain or an ache. Other symptoms include soreness, pulling and apprehension by the patient to move further into range. Symptoms can come on at any point, or increase through the joint range of movement and/or at the end of the range of joint movement. Sometimes a symptom is felt only during a part of the range, that is, through a particular arc of the movement, and if the symptom is pain it is then commonly referred to as an 'arc or catch of pain'. This would be documented, for example, as 'active shoulder abduction 120–140° produces lateral shoulder pain'. More commonly, symptoms are produced some time during the range and increase to the limit of range. The symptom may be sufficiently intense to be the cause of the limitation in range, depicted as P_2 on a movement diagram (Fig. 2.34), or may reach a particular intensity at the limit of range (P'). Symptoms may be produced in a joint with 'normal', hypomobile or hypermobile range of movement, with or without altered quality of movement. For further information on movement diagrams, see Petty and Ryder (2017).

Nociception and Pain

Most of the tissues that make up a joint (capsule, ligament, articular disc, meniscus and fat pad) are innervated (McDougall 2006); in fact, the only structure that is not innervated is the avascular articular cartilage (McDougall & Linton 2012). All of these tissues are therefore capable of being a source of pain. The fibres that signal pain are type IV, an unmyelinated meshwork, usually associated with blood vessels, or myelinated, type III fibres with unmyelinated free nerve terminals

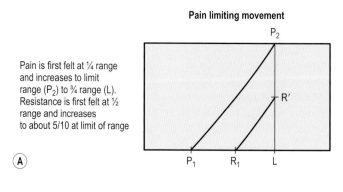

Pain is first felt at ¼ range and increases to limit range (P_2) to ¾ range (L). Resistance is first felt at ½ range and increases to about 5/10 at limit of range

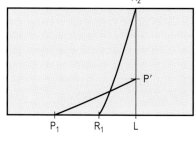

Resistance is first felt at ½ range and increases to limit range (R_2) to ¾ range (L). Pain is first felt at ¼ range and increases to about 3/10 at limit of range (where 0 is no pain and 10 is maximum pain ever felt by the patient)

FIG. 2.34 ■ Movement diagram depicting (A) P_2 with some resistance and normal range, and (B) P' and resistance limiting movement.

lying between the collagen and elastic fibres of the connective tissue in which they lie (McDougall 2006). These fibres are supplied by myelinated Aδ and unmyelinated C fibres.

Nociceptors in joint tissues can be activated by a noxious mechanical force or chemical stimulus (Jessell & Kelly 1991). To produce the sensation of pain, this noxious stimulus must be transduced to a relevant neural neurophysiological signal (Giordano 2005). The primary afferent fibres for pain are the Aδ and C fibres. The Aδ fibres are fast-conducting myelinated fibres that are modality-specific. That is, some Aδ fibres respond to intense mechanical or thermal stimulus. The Aδ fibres have a small receptive field producing sharp, localized and well-defined pain (Giordano 2005). In contrast, C fibres are thin, unmyelinated slow-conducting fibres and they have a broad receptive field and thus produce a poorly localized, burning, throbbing, gnawing pain. C fibres are polymodal, responding to mechanical, thermal and chemical stimuli (Giordano 2005).

Mechanical pain (Box 2.4) occurs when certain movements stress injured tissue or when a noxious movement or stress is applied to a joint, increasing the mechanical deformation and thus dramatically increasing the firing rate of nociceptors and which the central nervous system interprets as pain (McDougall 2006). This mechanical pain is present in the absence of inflammation and transmitted by the fast-conducting Aδ fibres. Thus, with mechanical pain, there are particular movements which aggravate and ease the pain, sometimes referred to as 'on/off pain'. The magnitude of the mechanical deformation may be directly related to the magnitude of nociceptor activity; this has been found in the skin of the cat where greater forces cause greater nociceptor activity (Garell et al. 1996).

Chemical nociceptive pain can be produced by the chemicals released as a result of inflammation, ischaemia or activity of the sympathetic nervous system (Gifford 1998).

Tissue injury causes release of fatty acids and free ions from damaged cell membranes. This release activates a chain of reactions inducing an inflammatory cascade and production of chemicals that affect the sensitivity of the nociceptors and/or modify the configurational state of their ion channels, thus reducing the nociceptors' membrane thresholds (Giordano 2005). This phenomenon is called peripheral sensitization (Cousing & Power 2003).

This sensitization of nociceptors leads to phenomena of hyperalgesia (termed 'primary hyperalgesia'), where there is heightened pain intensity as a response to a noxious stimulus, and phenomena of 'allodynia', where innocuous stimuli, over the area of peripheral sensitization, are causing pain (McDougall 2006).

Continuous stimulation of nociceptors causes an antidromic impulse causing the release of inflammatory mediators from the nerve fibre into the target tissues, causing in turn local inflammatory responses resulting in vasodilation and swelling in a process termed neurogenic inflammation (Butler 2000; Giordano 2005). Some joint afferents and some nociceptors have been found to contain proinflammatory chemicals (Levine et al. 1985a, b; Salo & Theriault 1997); this suggests that mechanoreceptors and nociceptors may contribute to the development of joint inflammation (Levine et al. 1985a; Holzer 1988).

Normally, the nociceptors' high threshold causes some of them to become 'silent nociceptors', that is, they may never fire (Butler 2000, McDougall 2006). However, joint injury and inflammation cause silent nociceptors to become active and hyperresponsive to normal and noxious movement by increasing their firing frequency. This increased sensitivity and firing frequency is interpreted by the central nervous system as pain, causing the phenomena of hyperalgesia and allodynia in acutely inflamed joints (McDougall 2006). Activated silent nociceptors and sensory nerves may also continue to fire spontaneously in the absence of any mechanical stimulation. This accounts for the pain at rest experienced by patients with arthritis (McDougall 2006).

In addition to the peripheral sensitization, prolonged nociceptive input drives changes in the dorsal horn that lead to the phenomenon of central sensitization. There is a reduction of the threshold so that stimulations arriving in the dorsal horn that are not normally noxious will activate neurons that transmit nociceptive information. Another change involves the increase in responsiveness of the neurons so that there is an increase in duration and magnitude of the stimuli. In addition, there is an expansion of the receptive field so that neurons will respond to nociceptive stimulation coming from areas outside the ones they normally serve (Butler 2000, Cousing & Power 2003). At the periphery, these changes result in an area of hyperalgesia and allodynia, with no change to thermal threshold, extending to uninjured tissues surrounding the site of injury or inflammation. This phenomenon is termed secondary hyperalgesia (Meyer 1995; Cousing & Power 2003).

Clinical features of inflammatory pain (Box 2.4) are: redness, oedema and heat, acute pain and tissue damage, a close relationship of stimulus response and pain, a diurnal pattern with pain and stiffness worst at night and, in the morning, signs of neurogenic inflammation

	TABLE 2.7	
Degenerative versus Inflammatory Arthropathy		
Parameter	Degenerative	Inflammatory
Exercise	Worse	Better
Rest	Better (but stiffness may follow prolonged periods of rest)	Worse
Morning stiffness	<30 minutes	>30 minutes
Night pain	Not disturbing sleep	Disturbing sleep
Age of onset	Usually >40 years	<40 years

(redness, swelling or symptoms in the neural zone) and a beneficial effect of antiinflammatory medication (Butler 2000). More specifically, joint inflammatory spondyloarthropathy symptoms also include pain on waking in the morning which improves with activity but gets worse with rest and disturbs night sleep (Rudwaleit et al. 2006; Sieper et al. 2009; Walker & Williamson 2009, Bailly et al. 2014). A comparison of the clinical features of degenerative (Gaskell 2013) versus inflammatory arthropathy is displayed in Table 2.7.

Ischaemic nociceptive pain is caused by a lowered pH (acidosis) in tissues (Issberner et al. 1996), which stimulates nociceptor activity (Steen et al. 1995). Lowered pH level is frequently related to both painful ischaemic conditions and painful inflammatory conditions (Steen et al. 1995; Issberner et al. 1996). Clinical features of ischaemic pain (Box 2.4) are thought to be: symptoms produced after prolonged or unusual activities, rapid ease of symptoms after a change in posture, symptoms towards the end of the day or after the accumulation of activity, a poor response to antiinflammatory medication and sometimes absence of trauma (Butler 2000). In the presence of tissue injury or inflammation, sympathetic nervous system activity can maintain the perception of pain or enhance nociception in inflamed tissue. Sympathetically maintained pain can occur with complex regional pain syndromes and may play a part in chronic arthritis and soft-tissue trauma (Raja et al. 1999).

Clinicians must also be aware of the possibility of joint infection, referred to as septic arthritis, which can occur in both natural and artificial joints. A number of possible organisms (bacterial, fungal or viral) can be responsible and possible associated factors are recent surgery or injection, human immunodeficiency virus (HIV) infection, immune deficiency, intravenous drug use or preexisting systemic inflammatory arthritis. Local signs of inflammation will be present as well as systemic signs such as fever and chills.

The commonest symptom from a joint is pain. The perception of pain occurs in the central nervous system and is multidimensional, including sensory, physiological, affective, cognitive, behavioural and sociocultural factors.

Pain Referral Areas

Cervical spine discs are capable of referring pain to distal axial and extremity regions (Slipman et al. 2005). More specifically, C2–C3 through C5–C6 discs can cause cervical and facial pain and C2–C3 through C6–C7 cervical and head pain. C4–C5, C5–C6, C6–C7 discs can cause cervical and anterior chest wall pain and C3–C4 through to C6–C7 and possibly C7–T1 cervical and upper-extremity pain (Slipman et al. 2005) (Fig. 2.35).

Pain from cervical spine zygapophyseal joints has been investigated by pain-provocative injections in the joints of normal subjects (Dwyer et al. 1990) and by pain-provocative injection and radiofrequency facet denervation on subjects suffering cervical spine pain of suspected facet joint origin (Fukui et al. 1996). Cephalad cervical spine facets refer pain closer to the same level as the painful joint. However, more caudal levels refer pain more distally and caudally, with the C5–C6 referring pain to the upper shoulder girdle and C6–C7 and C7–T1 the posterior upper and midscapular regions (Fig. 2.36).

Pain arising from the lumbar zygapophyseal joints has been investigated by diagnostic steroid and local anaesthetic facet injections (Marks 1989), radiofrequency facet denervation (Fukui et al. 1997) and pain mapping from patients with confirmed facet pathology (Jung et al. 2007). Absence of referred pain does not exclude facet joints as a cause of symptoms whilst coccygeal pain is unlikely to be caused by facet joint pathology (Marks 1989). Common areas of lumbar facet joint pain referral are shown in Figs 2.37 and 2.38. In agreement with previous studies (McCall et al. 1979; Marks 1989), Fukui et al. (1997) found significant overlap of pain referral regions from facet joints of different levels, which makes interpretation of this information in the clinical field difficult.

Information on pain from the SIJ has been explored in 10 asymptomatic subjects by radiopaque injection into the joint (Fortin et al. 1994a). Pain was felt fairly locally around the posterior superior iliac spine. In a further study, it was found that this area of referral could not be used to identify accurately patients with SIJ pain (Fortin et al. 1994b). Indeed, in a study by Dreyfuss et al. (1996), the SIJ pain pattern was found to be widespread, covering wide areas of the pelvis and lower limbs. However, in contrast with the pain arising from the lumbar spine, SIJ pain was rarely referring above the level of L5. A more recent study of mapping

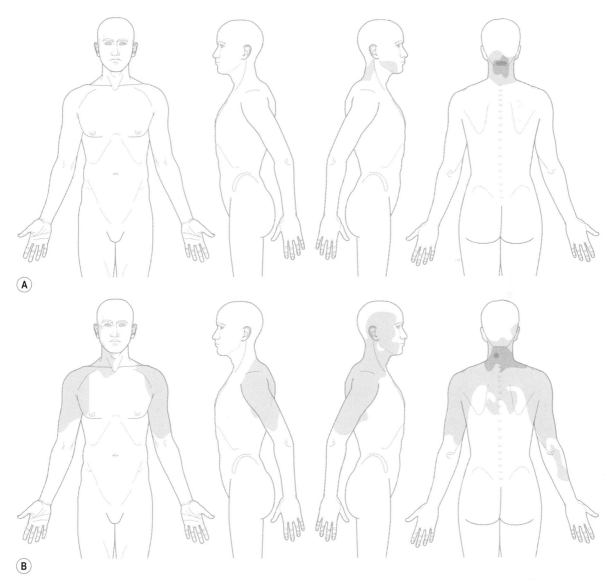

FIG. 2.35 ■ Discography-produced pain referral map. (A) C2–C3 discogram pain referral map. (B) C4–C5 discogram pain referral map. *Continued*

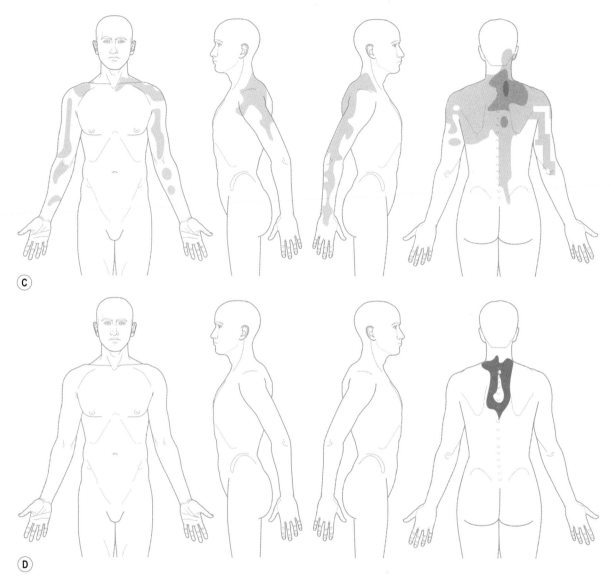

FIG. 2.35, cont'd ■ (C) C6–C7 discogram pain referral map. (D) C7–T1 discogram pain referral map. *(From Slipman et al. 2005, with permission.)*

of the pain from patients with confirmed SIJ pathology has found more concentrated but still wide pain referral areas (Jung et al. 2007) (Fig. 2.39).

Hip joint pathology tends to produce pain that is mostly localized around the groin, anterior hip joint, lateral hip and buttock (Khan et al. 2004; Lesher et al. 2008; Arnold et al. 2011). However, hip osteoarthritis can refer pain below the knee joint (Khan et al. 2004;

Lesher et al. 2008) (Fig. 2.40), whilst there are clinical cases where hip pathology can cause knee pain only (Emms et al. 2002).

Pain arising from joints in the upper or lower limb tends to be localized around the joint. A study by Bayam et al. (2011) has shown a variety of quality and distribution of pain in the upper limb produced by different shoulder girdle joint pathologies (Fig. 2.41).

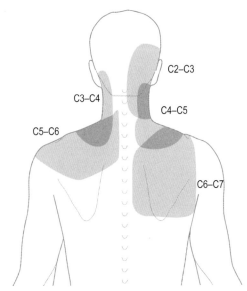

FIG. 2.36 ■ Distribution of pain following contrast medium injections in the cervical spine zygapophyseal joints of normal volunteers. *(From Dwyer et al. 1990, with permission.)*

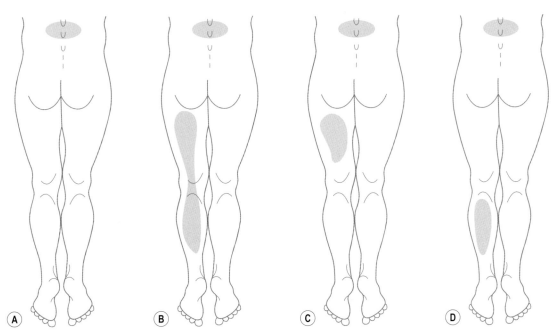

FIG. 2.37 ■ (A–D) Types of pain distribution patterns in lumbar zygapophyseal joint arthropathy. *(From Jung et al. 2007, with permission.)*

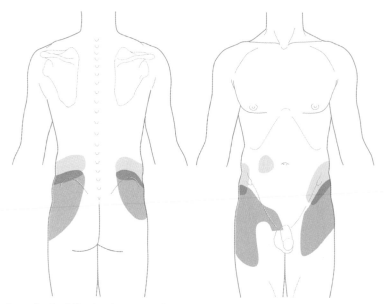

FIG. 2.38 ■ Distribution of pain following injection of saline into the L1–L2 (lighter shading) and L4–L5 (darker shading) zygapophyseal joint. *(After McCall et al. 1979, with permission.)*

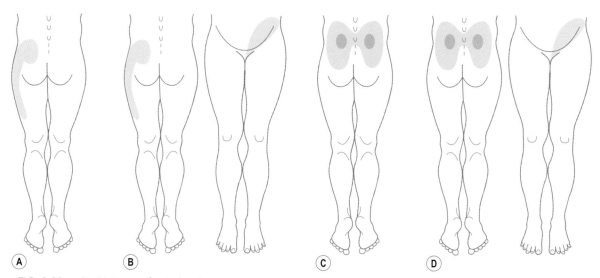

FIG. 2.39 ■ (A–D) Types of pain distribution patterns in sacroiliac joint arthropathy. *(From Jung et al. 2007, with permission.)*

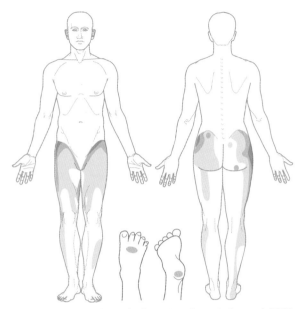

FIG. 2.40 ■ Distribution of pain from the hip joint. *(From Lesher et al. 2008, with permission.)*

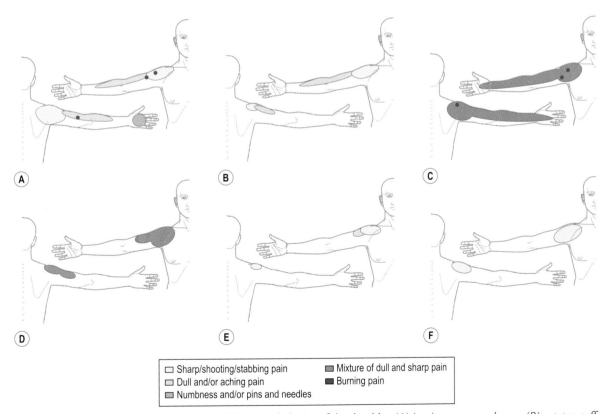

FIG. 2.41 ■ Patterns of referred pain from different pathologies of the shoulder. (A) Impingement syndrome, (B) rotator cuff tear, (C) glenohumeral joint arthritis, (D) instability, (E) acromioclavicular joint pathology and (F) calcific tendonitis. *(From Bayam et al. 2011, with permission.)*

REFERENCES

Adams, M.A., Bogduk, N., Burton, K., et al., 2013. The biomechanics of back pain, third ed. Churchill Livingstone, Edinburgh.

Ageberg, E., 2002. Consequences of a ligament injury on neuromuscular function and relevance to rehabilitation using the anterior cruciate ligament-injured knee as model. J. Electromyogr. Kinesiol. 12, 205–212.

Akeson, W.H., Woo, S.L.-Y., Amiel, D., et al., 1973. The connective tissue response to immobility: biochemical changes in periarticular connective tissue of the immobilized rabbit knee. Clin. Orthop. Relat. Res. 93, 356–362.

Akeson, W.H., Amiedl, D., Mechanic, G.L., et al., 1977. Collagen cross-linking alterations in joint contractures: changes in the reducible cross-links in periarticular connective tissue collagen after nine weeks of immobilization. Connect. Tissue Res. 5, 15–19.

Akeson, W.H., Amiel, D., Abel, M.F., et al., 1987. Effects of immobilization on joints. Clin. Orthop. Relat. Res. 219, 28–37.

Aktas, I., Ofluoglu, D., Albay, T., 2008. The relationship between benign joint hypermobility syndrome and carpal tunnel syndrome. Clin. Rheumatol. 27, 1283–1287.

Albright, D.J., Zimny, M.L., Dabezies, E., 1987. Mechanoreceptors in the human medial meniscus. Anat. Record 218, 6A–7A.

Amiel, D., Akeson, W.H., Harwood, F.L., et al., 1983. Stress deprivation effect on metabolic turnover of the medial collateral ligament collagen, a comparison between nine- and 12-week immobilization. Clin. Orthop. Relat. Res. 172, 265–270.

Ando, A., Hagiwara, Y., Onoda, Y., et al., 2010. Distribution of type A and B synoviocytes in the adhesive and shortened synovial membrane during immobilization of the knee joint in rats. Tohoku J. Exp. Med. 221, 161–168.

Arnold, D.R., Keene, J.S., Blankenbaker, D.G., et al., 2011. Hip pain referral patterns in patients with labral tears: analysis based on intra-articular anesthetic injections, hip arthroscopy, and a new pain 'circle' diagram. Phys. Sportsmed. 39, 29–35.

Atkins, E., Kerr, J., Goodlad, E., 2010. A practical approach to orthopaedic medicine: assessment, diagnosis and treatment, 3rd ed. Churchill Livingstone Elsevier, Edinburgh.

Bailly, F., Maigne, J., Genevay, S., et al., 2014. Inflammatory pain pattern and pain with lumbar extension associated with Modic 1 changes on MRI: a prospective case-control study of 120 patients. Eur. Spine J. 23, 493–497.

Bayam, L., Ahmad, M.A., Naqui, S.Z., et al., 2011. Pain mapping for common shoulder disorders. Am. J. Orthop. (Belle Mead NJ) 40, 353–358.

Bogduk, N., 2005. Clinical anatomy of the lumbar spine and sacrum, fourth ed. Elsevier Churchill Livingstone, Edinburgh.

Boisgontier, M.P., Swinnen, S.P., 2014. Proprioception in the cerebellum. Front. Hum. Neurosci. 8, 212.

Brandt, C., Sole, G., Krause, M.W., et al., 2007. An evidence-based review on the validity of the Kaltenborn rule as applied to the glenohumeral joint. Man. Ther. 12, 3–11.

Butler, D.S., 2000. The sensitive nervous system. Noigroup Publications, Adelaide, Australia.

Callaghan, M.J., Oldham, J.A., 2004. Quadriceps atrophy: to what extent does it exist in patellofemoral pain syndrome? Br. J. Sports Med. 38, 295–299.

Callaghan, M.J., Parkes, M.J., Hutchinson, C.E., 2014. Factors associated with arthrogenous muscle inhibition in patellofemoral osteoarthritis. Osteoarthritis Cartilage 22, 742–746.

Clark, F.J., 1975. Information signaled by sensory fibers in medial articular nerve. J. Neurophysiol. 38, 1464–1472.

Clark, F.J., Burgess, P.R., 1975. Slowly adapting receptors in cat knee joint: can they signal joint angle? J. Neurophysiol. 38, 1448–1463.

Cook, C., Brismée, J.M., Fleming, R., et al., 2005. Identifiers suggestive of clinical cervical spine instability: a Delphi study of physical therapists. Phys. Ther. 85, 895–906.

Cousing, M., Power, I., 2003. Acute and postoperative pain. In: Handbook of pain management: a clinical companion to Wall and Melzack's 'Textbook of pain'. Churchill Livingstone, London.

Cuomo, F., Birdzell, M.G., Zuckerman, J.D., 2005. The effect of degenerative arthritis and prosthetic arthroplasty on shoulder proprioception. J. Shoulder Elbow Surg. 14, 345–348.

Cyriax, J., 1982. Textbook of orthopaedic medicine – diagnosis of soft tissue lesions, eighth ed. Baillière Tindall, London.

Delahunt, E., Monaghan, K., Caulfield, B., 2006. Altered neuromuscular control and ankle joint kinematics during walking in subjects with functional instability of the ankle joint. Am. J. Sports Med. 34, 1970–1976.

Drake, R., Vogl, A.W., Mitchell, A.W., 2015. Gray's anatomy for students, third ed. Elsevier Churchill Livingstone, Philadelphia.

Dreyfuss, P., Michaelsen, M., Pauza, K., et al., 1996. The value of medical history and physical examination in diagnosing sacroiliac joint pain. Spine 21, 2594–2602.

Dwyer, A., Aprill, C., Bogduk, N., 1990. Cervical zygapophyseal joint pain patterns. I: A study in normal volunteers. Spine 15, 453–457.

Edwards, B.C., 1999. Manual of combined movements, second ed. Butterworth-Heinemann, Oxford.

Emms, N.W., O'Connor, M., Montgomery, S.C., 2002. Hip pathology can masquerade as knee pain in adults. Age. Ageing 31, 67–69.

Evans, E.B., Eggers, G.W.N., Butler, J.K., et al., 1960. Experimental immobilization and remobilization of rat knee joints. J. Bone Joint Surg. Am. 42A, 737–758.

Ferrari, S., Manni, T., Bonetti, F., et al., 2015. A literature review of clinical tests for lumbar instability in low back pain: validity and applicability in clinical practice. Chiropr. Man. Therap. 23, 14.

Ferrell, W.R., 1985. The response of slowly adapting mechanoreceptors in the cat knee joint to tetanic contraction of hind limb muscles. Q. J. Exp. Physiol. 70, 337–345.

Ferrell, W.R., Tennant, N., Sturrock, R.D., et al., 2004. Amelioration of symptoms by enhancement of proprioception in patients with joint hypermobility syndrome. Arthritis Rheumatol. 50, 3323–3328.

Fortier, S., Basset, F.A., 2012. The effects of exercise on limb proprioceptive signals. J. Electromyogr. Kinesiol. 22, 795–802.

Fortin, J.D., Dwyer, A.P., West, S., et al., 1994a. Sacroiliac joint: pain referral maps upon applying a new injection/arthrography technique, part I: asymptomatic volunteers. Spine 19, 1475–1482.

Fortin, J.D., Aprill, C.N., Ponthieux, B., et al., 1994b. Sacroiliac joint: pain referral maps upon applying a new injection/arthrography technique, part II: clinical evaluation. Spine 19, 1483–1489.

Frank, C.B., 2004. Ligament structure, physiology and function. J. Musculoskelet. Neuronal Interact. 4, 199.

Frank, C.B., Shrive, N.G., 1999. Ligament. In: Nigg, B.M., Herzog, W. (Eds.), Biomechanics of the musculo-skeletal system, second ed. John Wiley, Chichester, pp. 107–126.

Freeman, M.A.R., Wyke, B., 1967a. Articular reflexes at the ankle joint: an electromyographic study of normal and abnormal influences of ankle joint mechanoreceptors upon reflex activity in the leg muscles. Br. J. Surg. 54, 990–1001.

Freeman, M.A.R., Wyke, B., 1967b. The innervation of the knee joint. An anatomical and histological study in the cat. J. Anat. 101, 505–532.

Freeman, S., Mascia, A., Mcgill, S., 2013. Arthrogenic neuromusculature inhibition: a foundational investigation of existence in the hip joint. Clin. Biomech. (Bristol, Avon) 28, 171–177.

Fujiwara, A., Tamai, K., Yamato, M., et al., 1999. The relationship between facet joint osteoarthritis and disc degeneration of the lumbar spine: an MRI study. Eur. Spine J. 8, 396–401.

Fukui, S., Ohseto, K., Shiotani, M., et al., 1996. Referred pain distribution of the cervical zygapophyseal joints and cervical dorsal rami. Pain 68, 79–83.

Fukui, S., Ohseto, K., Shiotani, M., et al., 1997. Distribution of referred pain from the lumbar zygapophyseal joints and dorsal rami. Clin. J. Pain 13, 303–307.

Fuller, M.S., Grigg, P., Hoffman, A.H., 1991. Response of joint capsule neurons to axial stress and strain during dynamic loading in cat. J. Neurophysiol. 65, 1321–1328.

Garell, P.C., McGillis, S.L.B., Greenspan, J.D., 1996. Mechanical response properties of nociceptors innervating feline hairy skin. J. Neurophysiol. 75, 1177–1189.

Gaskell, L., 2013. Muskuloskeletal assessment. In: Porter, S.B. (Ed.), Tidy's physiotherapy, fifteenth ed. Churchill Livingstone, Elsevier, London.

Gifford, L., 1998. Pain. In: Pitt-Brooke, J., Reid, H., Lockwood, J., et al. (Eds.), Rehabilitation of movement, theoretical basis of clinical practice. W.B. Saunders, London, pp. 196–232.

Giordano, J., 2005. The neuroscience of pain and analgesia. In: Boswell, M.V., Cole, B.E. (Eds.), Weiner's pain management. A practical guide for clinicians, 7th ed. Informa, New York.

Gopinath, P., 2015. Lumbar segmental instability: points to ponder. J. Orthop. 12, 165–167.

Gordon, S., Yang, K.H., Mayer, P., et al., 2001. Mechanism of disc rupture: a preliminary report. Spine 16, 450–456.

Grahame, R., 2003. Hypermobility and hypermobility syndrome. In: Keer, R., Grahame, R. (Eds.), Hypermobility syndrome – recognition and management for physiotherapists. Butterworth-Heinemann, London.

Grigg, P., 1994. Peripheral neural mechanisms in proprioception. J. Sport Rehabil. 3, 2–17.

Grigg, P., Hoffman, A.H., 1982. Properties of Ruffini afferents revealed by stress analysis of isolated sections of cat knee capsule. J. Neurophysiol. 47, 41–54.

Hagert, E., Persson, J.K., Werner, M., et al., 2009. Evidence of wrist proprioceptive reflexes elicited after stimulation of the scapholunate interosseous ligament. J. Hand Surg. Am. 34, 642–651.

Hakim, A., Grahame, R., 2003. Joint hypermobility. Best Pract and Research. Clin. Rheumatol. 17, 989–1004.

Hall, M., Stevermer, C.A., Gillette, J.C., 2012. Gait analysis post anterior cruciate ligament reconstruction: knee osteoarthritis perspective. Gait Posture 36, 56–60.

Hall, M., Stevermer, C.A., Gillette, J.C., 2015. Muscle activity amplitudes and co-contraction during stair ambulation following anterior cruciate ligament reconstruction. J. Electromyogr. Kinesiol. 25, 298–304.

Hengeveld, E., Banks, K., 2014a. Maitland's vertebral manipulation: management of neuromuscular disorders, vol. 1, 8th ed. Elsevier Churchill Livingstone, Edinburgh.

Hengeveld, E., Banks, K., 2014b. Maitland's peripheral manipulation: management of neuromusculoskeletal disorders, vol. 2, 8th ed. Elsevier Churchill Livingstone, Edinburgh, p. 5.

Heppelmann, B., Messlinger, K., Neiss, W.F., et al., 1990. Ultrastructural three-dimensional reconstruction of group III and group IV sensory nerve endings ('free nerve endings') in the knee joint capsule of the cat: evidence for multiple receptive sites. J. Comp. Neurol. 292, 103–116.

Hertel, J., Kaminski, T.W., 2005. Second International Ankle Symposium, October 15–16, 2004, Newark, Delaware. J. Orthop. Sports Phys. Ther. 35, A1–A28.

Hertling, D., Kessler, R.M., 2006a. Arthrology. In: Hertling, D., Kessler, R. (Eds.), Management of common musculoskeletal disorders: physical therapy, principles and methods. Lippincott, Williams and Wilkins, Philadelphia, pp. 27–52.

Hertling, D., Kessler, R., 2006b. Assessment of musculoskeletal disorders and concepts of management. In: Hertling, D., Kessler, R.M. (Eds.), Management of common musculoskeletal disorders: physical therapy, principles and methods. Lippincott, Williams and Wilkins, Philadelphia, pp. 61–107.

Herzog, W., Longino, D., 2007. The role of muscles in joint degeneration and osteoarthritis. J. Biomech. 40 (Suppl. 1), S54–S63.

Hewett, T.E., Paterno, M.V., Myer, G.D., 2002. Strategies for enhancing proprioception and neuromuscular control of the knee. Clin. Orthop. Relat. Res. 402, 76–94.

Hills, B.A., 1995. Remarkable anti-wear properties of joint surfactant. Ann. Biomed. Eng. 23, 112–115.

Hills, B.A., Crawford, R.W., 2003. Normal and prosthetic synovial joints are lubricated by surface-active phospholipid: a hypothesis. J. Arthroplasty 18, 499–505.

Hills, B.A., Monds, M.K., 1998. Deficiency of lubricating surfactant lining the articular surfaces of replaced hips and knees. Br. J. Rheumatol. 37, 143–147.

Hills, B.A., Thomas, K., 1998. Joint stiffness and 'articular gelling': inhibition of the fusion of articular surfaces by surfactant. Br. J. Rheumatol. 37, 532–538.

Hortobagyi, T., DeVita, P., 2000. Muscle pre- and coactivity during downward stepping are associated with leg stiffness in aging. J. Electromyogr. Kinesiol. 10, 117–126.

Hughes, T., Rochester, P., 2008. The effects of proprioceptive exercise and taping on proprioception in subjects with functional ankle instability: a review of the literature. Phys. Ther. Sport 9, 136–147.

Ikeda, S., Tsumura, H., Torisu, T., 2005. Age-related quadriceps-dominant muscle atrophy and incident radiographic knee osteo-arthritis. J. Orthop. Sci. 10, 121–126.

Iqbal, K., Khan, M.Y., Minhas, L.A., 2012. Effects of immobilisation and re-mobilisation on superficial zone of articular cartilage of patella in rats. J. Pak. Med. Assoc. 62, 531–535.

Issberner, U., Reeh, P.W., Steen, K.H., 1996. Pain due to tissue acidosis: a mechanism for inflammatory and ischemic myalgia? Neurosci. Lett. 208, 191–194.

Jemmett, R.S., Macdonald, D.A., Agur, A.M.R., 2004. Anatomical relationships between selected segmental muscles of the lumbar spine in the context of multi-planar segmental motion: a preliminary investigation. Man. Ther. 9, 203–210.

Jessell, T.M., Kelly, D.D., 1991. Pain and analgesia. In: Kandel, E.R., Schwartz, J.H., Jessell, T.M. (Eds.), Principles of neural science, third ed. Elsevier, New York, pp. 385–399.

Jung, J.H., Kim, H.I., Shin, D.A., et al., 2007. Usefulness of pain distribution pattern assessment in decision-making for the patients with lumbar zygapophyseal and sacroiliac joint arthropathy. J. Korean Med. Sci. 22, 1048–1054.

Kaltenborn, F.M., 2014. Manual mobilization of the joints: joint examination and basic treatment, vol. 1, eighth ed. The extremities. Olaf Norlis Bokhandel, Oslo.

Kasai, Y., Morishita, K., Kawakita, E., et al., 2006. A new evaluation method for lumbar spinal instability: passive lumbar extension test. Phys. Ther. 86, 1661–1667.

Kazuhiko, S.K.T., Hiroshi, Y., 2007. Reduction in maximal firing rate of motoneurons after 1-week immobilization of finger muscle in human subjects. J. Electromyogr. Kinesiol. 17, 113–120.

Kennedy, J.C., Alexander, I.J., Hayes, K.C., 1982. Nerve supply of the human knee and its functional importance. Am J Sports Med 10, 329–335.

Khan, A.M., Mcloughlin, E., Giannakas, K., et al., 2004. Hip osteo-arthritis: where is the pain? Ann. R. Coll. Surg. Engl. 86, 119–121.

Kim, W.H., Lee, S.H., Lee, D.Y., 2011. Changes in the cross-sectional area of multifidus and psoas in unilateral sciatica caused by lumbar disc herniation. J. Korean Neurosurg. Soc. 50, 201–204.

Kim, H.T., Kim, H.J., Ahn, H.Y., et al., 2016. An analysis of age-related loss of skeletal muscle mass and its significance on osteoarthritis in a Korean population. Korean J. Intern. Med. 31, 585–593.

Krauspe, R., Schmidt, M., Schaible, H.G., 1992. Sensory innervation of the anterior cruciate ligament. J. Bone Joint Surg. Am. 74A, 390–397.

Lee, S., Sakurai, T., Ohsako, M., et al., 2010. Tissue stiffness induced by prolonged immobilization of the rat knee joint and relevance of AGEs (pentosidine). Connect. Tissue Res. 51, 467–477.

Lesher, J.M., Dreyfuss, P., Hager, N., et al., 2008. Hip joint pain referral patterns: a descriptive study. Pain Med. 9, 22–25.

Levangie, P.K., Norkin, C.C., 2011. Joint structure and function, a comprehensive analysis, fifth ed. F.A. Davis, Philadelphia.

Levick, J.R., 1983. Joint pressure–volume studies: their importance, design and interpretation. J. Rheumatol. 10, 353–357.

Levick, J.R., 1984. Blood flow and mass transport in synovial joints. In: Renkin, E.M., Michel, C.C. (Eds.), Handbook of physiology section 2: the cardiovascular system volume IV: microcirculation, part 2. American Physiological Society, Bethesda, MD, pp. 917–947.

Levine, J.R., Dardick, S.J., Basbaum, A.I., et al., 1985a. Reflex neurogenic inflammation. 1. Contribution of the peripheral nervous system to spatially remote inflammatory responses that follow injury. J. Neurosci. 5, 1380–1386.

Levine, J.R., Moskowitz, M.A., Basbaum, A.I., 1985b. The contribution of neurogenic inflammation in experimental arthritis. J. Immunol. 135, 843s–847s.

Lundon, K., 2007. The effect of mechanical load on soft connective tissues. In: Hammer, W. (Ed.), Functional soft-tissue examination and treatment by manual methods, third ed. Jones and Bartlett, Boston, pp. 15–30.

MacConaill, M.A., 1953. The movements of bones and joints, 5. The significance of shape. J. Bone Joint Surg. Am. 35B, 290–297.

MacConaill, M.A., 1966. The geometry and algebra of articular kinematics. Biomed. Eng. 1, 205–211.

MacConaill, M.A., 1973. A structuro-functional classification of synovial articular units. Ir. J. Med. Sci. 142, 19–26.

MacDonald, D.A., Moseley, G.L., Hodges, P.W., 2006. The lumbar multifidus: does the evidence support clinical beliefs? Man. Ther. 11, 254–263.

Maldonado, D.C., Silva, M.C., Neto Sel, R., et al., 2013. The effects of joint immobilization on articular cartilage of the knee in previously exercised rats. J. Anat. 222, 518–525.

Malliou, P., Gioftsidou, A., Pafis, G., et al., 2012. Proprioception and functional deficits of partial meniscectomized knees. Eur. J. Phys. Rehabil. Med. 48, 231–236.

Marks, R., 1989. Distribution of pain provoked from lumbar facet joints and related structures during diagnostic spinal infiltration. Pain 39, 37–40.

McCall, I.W., Park, W.M., O'Brien, J.P., 1979. Induced pain referral from posterior lumbar elements in normal subjects. Spine 4, 441–446.

McDougall, J.J., 2006. Arthritis and pain. Neurogenic origin of joint pain. Arthritis Res. Ther. 8, 220.

McDougall, J.J., Linton, P., 2012. Neurophysiology of arthritis pain. Curr. Pain Headache Rep. 16, 485–491.

McGill, S.M., Grenier, S., Kavcic, N., et al., 2003. Coordination of muscle activity to assure stability of the lumbar spine. J. Electro-myogr. Kinesiol. 13, 353–359.

McVey, E.D., Palmieri, R.M., Docherty, C.L., et al., 2005. Arthrogenic muscle inhibition in the leg muscles of subjects exhibiting functional ankle instability. Foot Ankle Int. 26, 1055–1061.

Menard, D., 2000. The ageing athlete. In: Harries, M., Williams, C., Stanish, W. (Eds.), Oxford textbook of sports medicine, second ed. Oxford University Press, Oxford, pp. 786–813.

Messner, K., 1999. The innervation of synovial joints. In: Archer, C.W., Caterson, B., Benjamin, M. (Eds.), Biology of the synovial joint. Harwood, Australia, pp. 405–421.

Messner, K., Gao, J., 1998. The menisci of the knee joint. Anatomical and functional characteristics, and a rationale for clinical treatment. J. Anat. 193, 161–178.

Meyer, R.A., 1995. Cutaneous hyperalgesia and primary afferent sensitization. Pulm. Pharmacol. 8, 187–193.

Middleditch, A., Oliver, J., 2005. Functional anatomy of the spine, 2nd ed. Elsevier Butterworth-Heinemann, Edinburgh.

Mow, V.C., Proctor, C.S., Kelly, M.A., 1989. Biomechanics of articular cartilage. In: Nordin, M., Frankel, V.H. (Eds.), Basic biomechanics of the musculoskeletal system, second ed. Lea & Febiger, Philadelphia, pp. 31–58.

Munn, J., Sullivan, S.J., Schneiders, A.G., 2010. Evidence of sensorimotor deficits in functional ankle instability: a systematic review with meta-analysis. J. Sci. Med. Sport 13, 2–12.

Myers, J.B., Lephart, S.M., 2000. The role of the sensorimotor system in the athletic shoulder. J. Athl. Train. 35, 351–363.

Myers, J.B., Wassinger, C.A., Lephart, S.M., 2006. Sensorimotor contribution to shoulder stability: effect of injury and rehabilitation. Man. Ther. 11, 197–201.

Nigg, B.M., 2000. Biomechanics as applied to sport. In: Harries, M., Williams, C., Stanish, W. (Eds.), Oxford textbook of sports medicine, second ed. Oxford University Press, Oxford, pp. 153–171.

Nigg, B.M., Herzog, W., 2007. Biomechanics of the musculo-skeletal system, third ed. John Wiley, Chichester.

Nordin, M., Frankel, V.H., 1989. Basic biomechanics of the musculoskeletal system, second ed. Lea & Febiger, Philadelphia.

Nordin, M., Frankel, V.H., 2012. Basic biomechanics of the musculoskeletal system, fourth ed. Lippincott Williams & Wilkins, Baltimore.

Noyes, F.R., Grood, E.S., 1976. The strength of the anterior cruciate ligament in humans and rhesus monkeys, age-related and species-related changes. J. Bone Joint Surg. Am. 58A, 1074–1082.

Noyes, F.R., DeLucas, J.L., Torvik, P.J., 1974. Biomechanics of anterior cruciate ligament failure: an analysis of strain-rate sensitivity and mechanisms of failure in primates. J. Bone Joint Surg. Am. 56A, 236–253.

Noyes, F.R., Butler, D.L., Paulos, L.E., et al., 1983. Intra-articular cruciate reconstruction, 1: perspectives on graft strength, vascularization, and immediate motion after replacement. Clin. Orthop. Relat. Res. 172, 71–77.

O'Hara, B.P., Urban, J.P.G., Maroudas, A., 1990. Influence of cyclic loading on the nutrition of articular cartilage. Ann. Rheum. Dis. 49, 536–539.

Olsen, K.A., Joder, D., 2001. Diagnosis and treatment of cervical spine instability. J. Orthop. Sports Phys. Ther. 31, 194–206.

Palastanga, N., Soames, R., 2012. Anatomy and human movement – structure and function, sixth ed. Churchill Livingstone Elsevier, Edinburgh.

Palmieri, R.M., Ingersoll, C.D., Cordova, M.L., et al., 2003. The effect of simulated knee joint effusion on postural control in healthy subjects. Arch. Phys. Med. Rehabil. 84, 1076–1079.

Palmieri-Smith, R.M., Kreinbrink, J., Ashton-Miller, J.A., et al., 2007. Quadriceps inhibition induced by an experimental knee joint effusion affects knee joint mechanics during a single-legged drop landing. Am. J. Sports Med. 35, 1269–1275.

Panjabi, M.M., 1992a. The stabilizing system of the spine. Part 1. Function, dysfunction, adaptation, and enhancement. J. Spinal Disord. 5, 383–389.

Panjabi, M.M., 1992b. The stabilizing system of the spine. Part II. Neutral zone and instability hypothesis. J. Spinal Disord. 5, 390–396.

Panjabi, M.M., White, A.A., 2001. Biomechanics in the musculoskeletal system. Churchill Livingstone, New York.

Pearcy, M.J., Tibrewal, S.B., 1984. Axial rotation and lateral bending in the normal lumbar spine measured by three-dimensional radiography. Spine 9, 582–587.

Pearcy, M., Portek, I., Shepherd, J., 1984. Three-dimensional X-ray analysis of normal movement in the lumbar spine. Spine 9, 294–297.

Petty, N.J., Ryder, D., 2017. Musculoskeletal examination and assessment: a handbook for therapists, fifth ed. Churchill Livingstone, Edinburgh.

Petty, N.J., Maher, C., Latimer, J., et al., 2002. Manual examination of accessory movements – seeking R1. Man. Ther. 7, 39–43.

Powers, C.M., 2010. The influence of abnormal hip mechanics on knee injury: a biomechanical perspective. J. Orthop. Sports Phys. Ther. 40, 42–51.

Raja, S.N., Meyer, R.A., Ringkamp, M., et al., 1999. Peripheral neural mechanisms of nociception. In: Wall, P.D., Melzack, R. (Eds.), Textbook of pain, fourth ed. Churchill Livingstone, Edinburgh.

Rice, D.A., Mcnair, P.J., Lewis, G.N., 2011. Mechanisms of quadriceps muscle weakness in knee joint osteoarthritis: the effects of prolonged vibration on torque and muscle activation in osteoarthritic and healthy control subjects. Arthritis Res. Ther. 13, R151.

Richie, D.H., 2001. Functional instability of the ankle and the role of neuromuscular control: a comprehensive review. J. Foot Ankle Surg. 40, 240–251.

Rudwaleit, M., Metter, A., Listing, J., et al., 2006. Inflammatory back pain in ankylosing spondylitis: a reassessment of the clinical history for application as classification and diagnostic criteria. Arthritis Rheumatol. 54, 569–578.

Safran, M.R., Borsa, P.A., Lephart, S.M., et al., 2001. Shoulder proprioception in baseball pitchers. J. Shoulder Elbow Surg. 10, 438–444.

Salo, P.T., Theriault, E., 1997. Number, distribution and neuropeptide content of rat knee joint afferents. J. Anat. 190, 515–522.

Schaible, H.G., Schmidt, R.F., 1983. Responses of fine medial articular nerve afferents to passive movements of knee joint. J. Neurophysiol. 49, 1118–1126.

Seki, K., Taniguchi, Y., Narusawa, M., 2001. Effects of joint immobilization on firing rate modulation of human motor units. J. Physiol. 530, 507–519.

Serrancoli, G., Monllau, J.C., Font-Llagunes, J.M., 2016. Analysis of muscle synergies and activation-deactivation patterns in subjects with anterior cruciate ligament deficiency during walking. Clin. Biomech. (Bristol, Avon) 31, 65–73.

Shrive, N.G., Frank, C.B., 1999. Articular cartilage. In: Nigg, B.M., Herzog, W. (Eds.), Biomechanics of the musculo-skeletal system, second ed. John Wiley, Chichester, pp. 86–106.

Sieper, J., Van Der Heijde, D., Landewe, R., et al., 2009. New criteria for inflammatory back pain in patients with chronic back pain: a real patient exercise by experts from the Assessment of SpondyloArthritis international Society (ASAS). Ann. Rheum. Dis. 68, 784–788.

Simmonds, J.V., Keer, R.J., 2007. Hypermobility and the hypermobility syndrome. Man. Ther. 12, 298–309.

Skoglund, S., 1956. Anatomical and physiological studies of knee-joint innervation in the cat. Acta Physiol. Scand. 36 (Suppl.), 124.

Slipman, C.W., Plastaras, C., Patel, R., et al., 2005. Provocative cervical discography symptom mapping. Spine J. 5, 381–388.

Solomonow, M., Krogsgaard, M., 2001. Sensorimotor control of knee stability. A review. Scand. J. Med. Sci. Sports 11, 64–80.

Solomonow, M., Zhou, B.H., Harris, M., et al., 1998. The ligamento-muscular stabilizing system of the spine. Spine 23, 2552–2562.

Solomonow, M., Baratta, R.V., Zhou, B.H., et al., 2003. Muscular dysfunction elicited by creep of lumbar viscoelastic tissue. J. Electromyogr. Kinesiol. 13, 381–396.

Stanish, W.D., 2000. Knee ligament sprains – acute and chronic. In: Harries, M., Williams, C., Stanish, W. (Eds.), Oxford textbook of sports medicine, second ed. Oxford University Press, Oxford, pp. 420–440.

Steen, K.H., Issberner, U., Reeh, P.H., 1995. Pain due to experimental acidosis in human skin: evidence for non-adapting nociceptor excitation. Neurosci. Lett. 199, 29–32.

Stokes, M., Young, A., 1984. The contribution of reflex inhibition to arthrogenous muscle weakness. Clin. Sci. 67, 7–14.

Strasmann, T., Halata, Z., 1988. Applications for 3-D image processing in functional anatomy: reconstruction of the cubital joint region and spatial distribution of mechanoreceptors surrounding this joint in *Mondelphius domestica*, a laboratory marsupial. Eur. J. Cell. Biol. 48 (25 Suppl.), 107–110.

Suarez, T., Laudani, L., Giombini, A., et al., 2016. Comparison in joint-position sense and muscle coactivation between anterior cruciate ligament-deficient and healthy individuals. J. Sport Rehabil. 25, 64–69.

Suter, E., Herzog, W., 2000. Muscle inhibition and functional deficiencies associated with knee pathologies. In: Herzog, W. (Ed.), Skeletal muscle mechanics, from mechanisms to function. Wiley, Chichester, p. 365, (Chapter 21).

Tipton, C.M., James, S.L., Mergner, W., et al., 1970. Influence of exercise on strength of medial collateral knee ligaments of dogs. Am. J. Physiol. 218, 894–902.

Torry, M.R., Decker, M.J., Viola, R.W., et al., 2000. Intra-articular knee joint effusion induces quadriceps avoidance gait patterns. Clin. Biomech. (Bristol, Avon) 15, 147–159.

Urbach, D., Awiszus, F., 2002. Impaired ability of voluntary quadriceps activation bilaterally interferes with function testing after knee injuries. A twitch interpolation study. Int. J. Sports Med. 23, 231–236.

Vanwanseele, B., Lucchinetti, E., Stussi, E., 2002. The effects of immobilization on the characteristics of articular cartilage: current concepts and future directions. Osteoarthritis Cartilage 10, 408–419.

Vecchio, P., Thomas, R., Hills, B.A., 1999. Surfactant treatment for osteoarthritis. Rheumatology 38, 1020–1021.

Veeger, H.E.J., Van Der Helm, F.C.T., 2007. Shoulder function: the perfect compromise between mobility and stability. J. Biomech. 40, 2119–2129.

Walker, B.F., Williamson, O.D., 2009. Mechanical or inflammatory low back pain. What are the potential signs and symptoms? Man. Ther. 14, 314–320.

Wong, M., Carter, D.R., 2003. Articular cartilage functional histomorphology and mechanobiology: a research perspective. Bone 33, 1–13.

Woo, S.L.-Y., Gomez, M.A., Sites, T.J., et al., 1987. The biomechanical and morphological changes in the medial collateral ligament of the rabbit after immobilization and remobilization. J. Bone Joint Surg. Am. 69A, 1200–1211.

Woo, S., Maynard, J., Butler, D., et al., 1988. Ligament, tendon, and joint capsule insertions to bone. In: Woo, S.L.-Y., Buckwalter, J. (Eds.), Injury and repair of the musculoskeletal soft tissues. American Academy of Orthopaedic Surgeons, Park Ridge, IL, pp. 133–166.

Wright, V., Johns, R.J., 1961. Quantitative and qualitative analysis of joint stiffness in normal subjects and in patients with connective tissue diseases. Ann. Rheum. Dis. 20, 36–46.

Wyke, B.D., 1970. The neurological basis of thoracic spinal pain. Rheumatol. Phys. Med. 10, 356–367.

Yabe, Y., Hagiwara, Y., Suda, H., et al., 2013. Joint immobilization induced hypoxic and inflammatory conditions in rat knee joints. Connect. Tissue Res. 54, 210–217.

Zimny, M.L., 1988. Mechanoreceptors in articular tissue. Am. J. Anat. 182, 16–32.

Zimny, M.L., St Onge, M., 1987. Mechanoreceptors in the temporomandibular articular disk. J. Dent. Res. 66, 237.

3

PRINCIPLES OF JOINT TREATMENT

CLAIR HEBRON

CHAPTER CONTENTS

This chapter will focus on the treatments which are directed at joint and associated structures; however, it is essential to emphasize that joints should not be treated in isolation but within a holistic approach to person-centred care. A person is embodied and is influenced by not just psychosocial factors, but by that person's being in the world, with its historical, contextual and situational influences (Heidegger 1962). Thus treatment of people with musculoskeletal dysfunction should include consideration of the whole person and his or her embodied experience. The therapeutic value of communication in the therapeutic setting should not be underestimated and is considered further in Chapter 9. Treatment of joints may comprise one aspect of management; however consideration of health promotion is recognized as core to physiotherapy practice and therefore treatment of joints should be complemented by recommendations regarding physical activity, smoking, basic nutrition, stress, sleep hygiene and alcohol consumption. Readers are recommended to refer to literature on behaviour change techniques, such as Michie et al. (2011).

From a biomechanical perspective there is no pure treatment for joints, that is, treatment cannot be isolated to joints alone; it will always, to a greater or lesser extent, affect muscle and/or nerve tissues. Some sort of classification system for treatment is needed in order to have meaningful communication between clinicians and this text follows the traditional classification of joint, muscle and nerve treatment. In this text, a 'joint treatment' is defined as a 'treatment to effect a change in a joint'; that is, the intention of the clinician is to produce a change in a joint. Similarly, where a technique is used to effect a change in a muscle, it will be referred to as a 'muscle treatment' and where a technique is used to effect a change in nerve, it will be referred to as a 'nerve treatment'. Thus, techniques are classified according to which tissue the clinician is predominantly attempting to affect. An example may help to illustrate the impurity of a joint mobilization technique. A posteroanterior (PA) glide on the head of the fibula will move the superior tibiofibular joint, the lateral collateral ligament of the tibiofemoral joint, the common peroneal nerve, and soleus and biceps femoris muscles. A PA glide to the head of the fibula can therefore be applied to affect any of these structures. It may be used to affect the superior tibiofibular joint, in which case it would be described as a joint treatment, or it may

51

BOX 3.1
DESIRED EFFECT OF JOINT MOBILIZATION

Create an afferent barrage to initiate a neurophysiological response to reduce pain

Glide joint surface parallel to plane of joint or rotate joint surfaces

Move joint surface to lengthen periarticular tissues

Move joint to affect nerve or muscle tissue

Encourage normal patterns of movement

Reduce fear of movement

be used to affect the common peroneal nerve, in which case it is referred to as a nerve treatment. Similarly, physiological joint movements will move local joint, nerve and muscle tissues.

The possible desired effects of joint mobilization on joint, nerve and muscle tissue are summarized in Box 3.1. For example, active shoulder flexion moves the glenohumeral and scapulothoracic joints, involves muscle contraction of numerous shoulder and scapular muscles, while also applying mechanical stress to the nerves of the brachial plexus. Further information on the treatment of muscle and nerve tissue using joint mobilization and exercise can be found in Chapters 5 and 7. In this chapter it is assumed that joint mobilization or exercise treatment is being applied to affect joint tissues. The reader is reminded that there are a number of specific precautions and contraindications to joint mobilization treatment (Petty & Ryder 2017).

Joint treatments are normally applied with the aim of decreasing pain or improving the range or quality of movement. The research evidence supporting the possible effects of treatment will be explored. However, it should be acknowledged that most clinical trials report on mean responses and do not necessarily represent individual patients. Therefore the physiotherapist should monitor the response to treatment on an individual basis and use joint treatment within an evidence-based framework of practice which considers evidence from the patient, therapist and research.

This chapter will examine joint mobilizations and manipulation and discuss the role of exercise in joint treatment. Readers are advised to refer to Chapter 5 for further details on exercise.

JOINT MOBILIZATIONS

Types of Joint Mobilizations

Joint mobilizations are passive joint movements performed in such a way that at all times they are within the control of the patient, and within the physiological range of the joint. This is in contrast to joint manipulation, which involves a sudden movement or thrust at high speed, which cannot be controlled by the patient and often occurs at the end of joint range.

Having identified a dysfunction, treatment aims to restore normal joint function, whether by reducing pain or by restoration of movement (the rotation movement, the translation movement or a combination of the two). This method of treating joints can therefore be broadly divided into physiological movements (which emphasize rotation of the bone) and accessory movements (which emphasize translation of the bone), or a combination of the two (Fig. 3.1). The physiological movements can be further subdivided into passive or active physiological movements; accessory movements, by definition, will always be passive. Combinations of accessory and physiological movements are also possible. Details of these accessory and physiological movements are provided in the companion text (Petty & Ryder 2017).

Accessory Movements

Every accessory movement available at a joint can be used as a treatment technique. Having examined and identified a dysfunction of an accessory movement, the clinician can draw a movement diagram (described in Petty & Ryder 2017) and then choose a suitable treatment dose, described in the next section. The accessory movement can be carried out in any part of the physiological range of that joint; for example, an anteroposterior (AP) glide to the tibiofemoral joint can be applied with the knee in flexion, extension or tibial rotation. The chosen position depends on the desired effects of the treatment, discussed later in this chapter.

Physiological Movements

Every physiological movement available at a joint can be converted to a treatment technique and can be carried out actively by the patient or passively by the patient or clinician. Active repetitive movements of the spine have, for example, been advocated by McKenzie (1981,

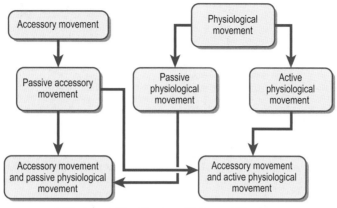

FIG. 3.1 ■ Classification of joint mobilizations.

1983, 1985). Having examined the passive physiological movement the clinician can then choose a suitable treatment dose, described in the next section.

The principles of applying passive physiological movement treatment are:

- The body part is fully supported.
- The movement is fully controlled by the clinician or patient, in terms of: where in the range the movement begins and ends, the amplitude, smoothness and speed of oscillations.
- The clinician constantly monitors symptoms during the application of the technique.
- In order to determine the immediate effects of the treatment the clinician reassesses the comparable signs.
- Normally treatment is converted to a home exercise which can be performed by the patient.

Passive Physiological Movement Combined With Accessory Movements

A physiological movement can be applied while also applying an accessory movement. Thus, the physiological movement and the accessory movement can both be oscillated at the same time; the physiological movement can be oscillated while the accessory movement is sustained; or the physiological movement can be sustained while the accessory movement is oscillated. For example, a longitudinal caudad and shoulder abduction can each be oscillated at the same time, the shoulder abduction can be oscillated while the longitudinal caudad is sustained, or the shoulder abduction can be

sustained while the longitudinal caudad is oscillated. These techniques can be applied in a variety of positions. For example, shoulder abduction with a longitudinal glide can be applied in sitting, lying or standing. Accessory mobilizations can also be applied during patients' functional aggravating movements. This may be limited by the ability of the therapist to apply force effectively, but it can help to contextualize the treatment for the patient and thus improve compliance with a home exercise programme.

Active Physiological Movement With Accessory Movement

As the patient performs an active physiological movement the clinician can apply an accessory movement, often called a mobilization with movement (MWM) when applied to a peripheral joint or a sustained natural apophyseal glide (SNAG) when applied to the spine (Hing et al. 2015). For example, the clinician can apply an AP glide to the talus and ask the patient to dorsiflex the foot actively. For the cervical spine, the clinician can apply a transverse glide to a spinous process and then ask the patient to flex the head laterally. When the physiological movement is performed actively by the patient, as opposed to passively by the clinician, this can sometimes enable the technique to be carried out in a more functional position. For example, it would be extremely difficult, if not impossible, to dorsiflex the foot passively while the patient is weight bearing. For further information on accessory movement with active physiological movements, see Hing et al. (2015), or the review by Hing et al. (2008), which proposes an algorithm by which MWMs may be incorporated into patient management.

As originally described, MWMs were applied as treatment if they resulted in a previously painful movement becoming painfree. However, clinicians might apply MWMs if they resulted in a reduction in symptoms or an increase in patients' confidence of movement. MWMs can often be applied by patients as a home exercise and can be performed during functional movements. Therefore they can be useful in empowering patients and helping them to gain control over their pain. Because they are encouraging movement in the painful direction they can also reduce fear avoidance, a factor that is associated with poor recovery (Wertli et al. 2014). Careful communication and use of language whilst the treatment technique is applied and during the whole patient encounter are essential in order to maximize the reduction of fear and empower patients (see Chapter 9).

Manipulation

In a joint manipulation, the joint is moved through its full passive range of motion towards the end of its anatomical range, or to the appropriate movement barrier. A commonly used form of manipulation is a high-velocity, low-amplitude (HVLA) thrust. The purpose of the high-velocity technique is to overcome the patient's protective reflex mechanism which might halt the movement. Manipulation is often (but not necessarily) associated with an audible pop sound.

Application of Joint Mobilizations

Dose

The term 'treatment dose' is often used by the medical profession when prescribing the quantity of a drug. The term is used here to describe the nature of the movement applied by the clinician or by the patient. The treatment dose incorporates quite a large number of factors, most of which have a number of variables; these variables are outlined in Table 3.1.

An example of treatment dose, which might be used and documented in the patient's notes, is:

In left side lie with arm back and pelvis rotated, did left rotation grade II in line of femur, slowly and smoothly, for 30 seconds, to partial reproduction of patient's back pain.

TABLE 3.1	
Aspects of Treatment Dose for Joint Mobilization	
Factors	**Variables**
Patient position	E.g. prone, side-lying, sitting, functional, aggravating
Movement	This may be a physiological movement, e.g. flexion, lateral rotation, or an accessory movement or a mixture of the two
Direction of force applied	E.g. anteroposterior, posteroanterior, medial, lateral, caudad, cephalad
Magnitude of force applied	Related to therapist's perception of resistance: grades I–V
Amplitude of oscillation	None: sustained (quasistatic) Small: grades I and IV Large: grades II and III
Speed	Slow or fast
Rhythm	Smooth or staccato
Time	Duration and number of repetitions
Symptom response	Short of symptom production Point of onset or increase in resting symptom Partial reproduction of symptom Full reproduction of symptom

This clinical note describes the patient in left side-lying, with the arm resting on the trunk and right hip and the knee flexed so that the knee rests on the couch, in front of the underlying leg. The clinician applied a slow and smooth passive physiological movement (grade II) to the pelvis, in the direction of the line of the femur, for 30 seconds, such that the patient felt only partial reproduction of the back pain.

Patient Position

This includes the general position of the patient, such as lying, sitting or standing, and the specific position of the body part; for example, the knee may be flexed or extended during the application of an AP glide on the tibia. For example, a patient with limitation of knee flexion due to resistance may be positioned in long sitting with the knee flexed to the end of the available range, while the clinician applies an AP glide to the tibia. The choice of general and specific positioning will depend on a number of factors, including:

- the comfort and support of the patient
- the comfort of the clinician applying the technique
- the desired effect of the treatment (e.g. decrease pain or increase range of movement)
- whether the joints are to be weight bearing or non-weight bearing
- to what extent the movement is to be functional
- to what extent symptoms are to be produced.

Direction of Movement

Choice of treatment direction is generally based on the clinician's assessment of passive accessory and physiological motion and symptom response, including knowledge of the normal direction of bone translation. Where a physiological movement is used, a description of the physiological movement and naming the joint will describe this aspect of the treatment dose. For example, knee flexion, hip lateral rotation or lumbar rotation to the left each identifies the direction of the movement and the joint complex. Where an accessory movement is used, the direction of the force and the joint will describe the movement. Examples include an AP to the tibiofemoral joint, a lateral glide of the glenohumeral joint or an AP to the talocrural joint. Again, each identifies the direction of the force and the joint complex. The general convention would assume that the force was applied to the distal bone of the joint – in the above examples, to the tibia, humerus and talus, respectively. Techniques, of course, can be applied to the proximal bone; when this occurs the bone needs to be identified in the written description. For example, the description may read 'AP to tibiofemoral joint, on femur'.

In the spine, where each spinal level consists of a number of joints, an additional descriptor is added for accessory movements. The point of application of the force needs to be identified. For example, a central PA on L3, a transverse glide to the left on T5, a unilateral PA on C5. In these examples, the word 'central' means that the force is applied over the spinous process, 'transverse' to the lateral aspect of the spinous process and 'unilateral' to the articular pillar or transverse process. Where the severity, irritability and nature of the condition allow, treatment is normally directed at the most symptomatic level and in the most symptomatic direction as from a biomechanical perspective

this suggests that it will be affecting the structure(s) at fault.

Magnitude of the Force/Grades of Movement

Whenever a clinician passively moves a joint, with either a physiological or accessory movement, the clinician is applying a force. Clearly, this has a certain magnitude and it is commonly described using a grade of movement (Magarey 1985, 1986; Hengeveld & Banks 2013). Grades of movement in this text are defined according to where the movement occurs, within joint resistance. The resistance to movement perceived by the clinician is depicted on a movement diagram (described in Petty & Ryder 2017). Grades of movement (I–IV+) are then defined according to the resistance curve. The grades of movement defined in this text (Fig. 3.2 and Table 3.2) are a modification of Magarey (1985, 1986). The modification allows every possible position in range to be described (Magarey 1985, 1986), and each grade to be distinct from one another (Hengeveld &

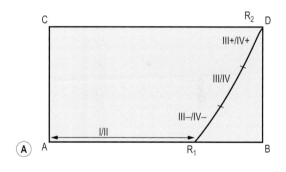

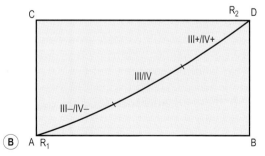

FIG. 3.2 ▪ Movement diagram with grades of movement for (A) a typical asymptomatic physiological movement, and (B) a typical asymptomatic accessory movement. The resistance is divided into thirds, so that a large-amplitude movement within the middle third will be a grade III.

TABLE 3.2 Grades of Movement	
Grade	**Definition**
I	Small-amplitude movement short of resistance
II	Large-amplitude movement short of resistance
III–	Large-amplitude movement in the first third of resistance
IV–	Small-amplitude movement in the first third of resistance
III	Large-amplitude movement in the middle third of resistance
IV	Small-amplitude movement in the middle third of resistance
III+	Large-amplitude movement in the last third of resistance
IV+	Small-amplitude movement in the last third of resistance
V	Manipulative thrust

Banks 2013). A grade V technique is a manipulative thrust.

With most physiological joint movements there is minimal resistance within the range of movement. For example, elbow flexion or knee extension will have little resistance in the early part of the range, and the clinician may mark the onset of resistance (R_1) somewhere towards the end of the movement (Fig. 3.2A). Grades of movement available for physiological movements include I, II, III–, IV–, III, IV, III+, IV+ (Fig. 3.2A). With accessory movements, however, resistance occurs at the beginning of range (Petty et al. 2002), that is, R_1 is at A on the movement diagram (Fig. 3.2B). Grades of movement available will be limited to grades III–, IV–, III, IV, III+ and IV+ (Fig. 3.2B); that is, a grade I and II may not be possible as these grades are defined as movements within a resistance-free range (Table 3.2). The grade of movement is defined according to where the maximum force is applied in resistance, and whether the clinician considers the movement to be large or small.

Studies investigating force of shoulder and elbow mobilizations suggest that higher treatment force may result in better outcomes (Vicenzino et al. 2001; McLean et al. 2002; Vermeulen et al. 2006) and in participants with chronic low-back pain higher lumbar mobilization treatment forces were associated with a greater increase in pressure pain thresholds and reduction in verbal rating of pain (Hebron 2014). Collectively these studies suggest that where pain allows using higher grades of treatment should be considered.

Amplitude of Oscillation

A movement can be a sustained or an oscillatory force. It is impossible for a truly sustained force to be applied – there will always be some variation in the force, albeit very small. For this reason, it is sometimes referred to as a quasistatic force. If the force is deliberately oscillated it is described as having a small or large amplitude. The amplitude is relative to the available range of any particular movement so it will vary quite dramatically between physiological and accessory movements. For example, small-amplitude accessory movements may be a few millimetres of movement, compared with a 40° arc of movement for a physiological movement. The amplitude of oscillatory movement is described within the definition of grades of movement: grades I and IV are small-amplitude movements and grades II and III are large-amplitude movements. It can be seen that grades of movement describe both the magnitude of force applied and the amplitude of oscillation. The choice of grade of movement is determined by the relationship of pain (or other symptom) and resistance through the range of movement; this is depicted on a movement diagram (Hengeveld & Banks 2013). Where resistance limits the range of movement (Fig. 3.3A), a grade III+ or IV+, provoking some pain, may be appropriate (pain would be 4 out of 10 or more in this example). The extent of pain reproduction can be altered according to what is acceptable to the patient and thus with some patients a grade III or IV might be used in this example. Where pain limits the range of movement (Fig. 3.3B), a grade III– or IV– that does not produce any pain may be appropriate.

There is little evidence to inform clinicians when deciding on the amplitude of mobilizations; theoretically increasing the amplitude will stimulate more mechanoreceptors and thus increase pain relief mediated via the pain gate mechanism (van Griensven 2005). However a study including asymptomatic participants did not find a difference in the hypoalgesic effect of different amplitudes of lumbar mobilization oscillations (Krouwel et al. 2010).

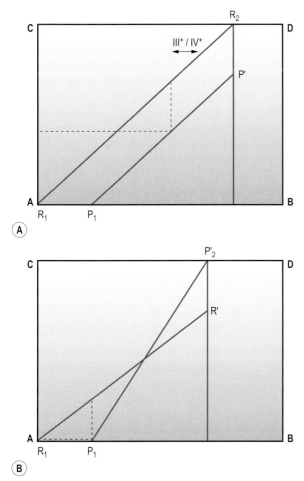

FIG. 3.3 ■ Grades of movement are determined by the relationship of pain and resistance through the range of movement; this is depicted on a movement diagram. (A) Resistance limiting movement. (B) Pain limiting movement.

Speed and Rhythm of Movement

The speed of the movement can be described as slow or fast, and the rhythm as smooth or staccato (jerky); of course, these descriptors will apply only to oscillatory forces. Speed and rhythm go hand in hand; movements will tend to be slow and smooth, fast and smooth or fast and staccato. A grade V manipulative thrust is often described as an HVLA thrust. The tissues around a joint are viscoelastic and, as such, are sensitive to the speed of the applied force. A force applied quickly will produce less movement, provoking a greater stiffness in the tissues; a force applied more slowly, on the

other hand, will cause more movement as the stiffness is relatively less (Noyes et al. 1974). The choice of rhythm may be influenced by patients' aggravating factors, for example, when activities such as running or jumping are aggravating staccato rhythms may be used, whereas in patients with pain in sustained positions such as sitting a quasistatic mobilization may be used.

There is a paucity of evidence regarding the influence of different speeds of mobilizations. Chiu and Wright (1996) reported greater changes in skin conductance (indicating sympathoexcitation) following mobilization at 2 Hz than those at 0.5 Hz, but no difference in the hypoalgesic effect of different speeds of mobilization was reported in asymptomatic participants (Willett et al. 2010).

Time

In terms of treatment dose, this relates to the duration for which a movement is carried out in a treatment session, the number of times this is repeated within a treatment session and the frequency of appointments. When applying MWMs or SNAGs the movement and associated pressure are normally applied five to seven times. In contrast, an HVLA thrust is often only applied once if cavitation is successful on the first attempt; otherwise it might be repeated on a further two occasions. When using mobilizations clinical practice typically involves up to three repetitions (sets) of a treatment technique, each lasting between 30 seconds and 1 minute – most research exploring the effects of joint mobilizations has used this time range. However, there is some evidence that longer treatment duration may have a greater treatment effect: in asymptomatic participants a greater increase in ankle range of movement was found with 2 minutes than with 30 seconds or 1 minute of mobilization treatment (Holland et al. 2015) and more treatment sets of lumbar mobilizations were found to have a greater hypoalgesic effect (Pentelka et al. 2012). An association between lumbar mobilization treatment duration and change in pressure pain threshold has been found in participants with chronic low-back pain, with significantly more participants responding to 6 minutes than to 1 minute of treatment (Hebron 2014).

The frequency of appointments is decided by the clinician and the patient and will depend on a number of factors. These factors include: the nature of the patient's condition, the severity and irritability of symptoms, the area of the symptoms, the functional limitations of the patient, the stage of the patient's condition, the prognosis, the available time the patient has to attend for treatment and the workload of the clinician.

Symptom Response

The clinician decides which symptom, and to what extent each symptom is to be provoked during treatment. Choices include:

- no provocation
- provocation to the point of onset, or increase, in resting symptoms
- partial reproduction
- total reproduction.

The decision as to what extent each symptom is provoked during treatment depends on the severity and irritability of the symptom(s) and the nature of the condition. If the symptoms are severe, that is, the patient is unable to tolerate the symptom being reproduced, the clinician would choose to apply treatment that did not provoke the symptoms. The clinician may also choose not to provoke symptoms if they are irritable; that is, once symptoms are provoked, they take some time to ease. If, however, the symptoms are not severe and not irritable, then the clinician is able to reproduce the patient's symptoms during treatment, and the extent to which the symptoms are provoked will depend on the tolerance of the patient. The nature of the condition may also limit the extent to which symptoms are produced, such as a recent traumatic injury, acute inflammatory state or central sensitization.

Choice of Treatment Dose

The best treatment is the one that improves the patient's signs and symptoms in the shortest period of time. Any physical test that reproduces or eases the patient's symptoms can be converted to a treatment technique by applying components of a treatment dose. Converting positive physical testing procedures to treatment techniques would seem the most logical approach to choosing treatment, as the clinician can be confident that the treatment is, somehow or other, affecting the structure at fault. Reproduction of the patient's symptoms

is a vital anchor from which to decide aspects of the treatment dose. Only when symptoms are produced can the clinician be sure that they are affecting, somehow or other, the structure(s) at fault. This may require some careful and time-consuming examination procedures, taking an attitude of the explorer, the researcher or the detective who must explore all possible avenues of investigation. For example, testing elbow flexion overpressure is fully explored only if variations of forearm pronation and supination and variations in direction of flexion medially and laterally are carried out. Similarly, when applying accessory movements, a wide variation in the direction of the force needs to be used before deciding that the accessory movement is not symptomatic.

Where a joint (which includes both intra- and periarticular tissues) is considered to be the source of the symptoms, the clinician may be able to link the findings of the active and passive physiological movements with the findings of the accessory movements. For example, limited range of wrist extension may be accompanied by limited PA glide of the radiocarpal joint; this would make sense because wrist extension at the radiocarpal joint involves a PA glide of the scaphoid and lunate on the radius. The clinician could choose a physiological wrist extension movement, a PA glide of the proximal carpal bones, or could choose to combine physiological wrist extension with a PA glide to the proximal carpal bones. In the same way, limited dorsiflexion of the ankle may be accompanied by limited AP glide of the talus because these two movements occur together. In this case the clinician could choose to apply a physiological ankle dorsiflexion movement, an AP glide to the talus, or combine physiological ankle dorsiflexion with an AP to the talus. In both examples, the choice would depend on the relative dysfunction of the physiological movement and the accessory movement.

Let us consider treatment to the wrist. If the movements (physiological and accessory) are limited in range by resistance, then the treatment dose will tend to be with the wrist in extension. In this position, the clinician might then apply an end-range sustained or oscillatory grade IV+ PA, to the radiocarpal joint, fast with a staccato rhythm, and continuing for three repetitions of 1 minute each, producing some ache in the wrist. These treatment doses are given in Table 3.3.

TABLE 3.3		
Variation in Treatment Dose Depending on Whether the Joint Movement Is Limited by Resistance or by Pain		
	Resistance Limiting Movement	Pain Limiting Movement
Limited radiocarpal extension and limited PA glide of radiocarpal joint	In wrist extension did IV+ PA radiocarpal joint fast and staccato ×3 (1 minute) with some ache	In wrist flexion did III-PA radiocarpal joint slowly and smoothly ×3 (1 minute) with no pain provoked

PA, posteroanterior.

At the other end of the spectrum, if the movements are limited in range by pain, then the treatment dose will tend to be applied with the wrist in a painfree position, such as wrist flexion. In this position, the clinician might apply an oscillatory PA to the radiocarpal joint, grade III-technique, slowly and smoothly, continuing for three repetitions of 1 minute each, with no production of symptoms. This example highlights how the treatment dose can be varied in terms of grade of movement, speed and rhythm.

The decision on the treatment of choice will be based on a number of factors, including the:

■ desired therapeutic effect, e.g. to decrease pain or increase range of movement
■ severity and irritability of the symptoms
■ most symptomatic findings on physical examination: these are normally converted to treatment
■ results of reassessment of the comparable signs within the assessment. For example if reassessment of active range of movement improves most after passive physiological intervertebral movement assessment, then passive physiological treatment might be the treatment of choice
■ patients' aggravating factors: the treatment position, rate and rhythm may be designed to replicate elements of aggravating movements or positions
■ nature of the condition: for example, the stage in the healing process postinjury or the predominant pain mechanism; for example, in patients with central sensitization, where possible, treatment would be painfree to avoid triggering more nociceptive barrage (Nijs & Van Houdenhove 2009)
■ aim of treatment, in terms of the patient's functional goals

■ patient's treatment preferences and expectations: there is some evidence to suggest that patients have better outcomes when they receive their preferred treatment (Kalauokalani et al. 2001)
■ patients' beliefs: where patients display fear-avoidant behaviour, treatment may centre on encouraging normal joint movement and reducing fear
■ what is feasible for patients to perform at home: in order to aid the transition into home exercise and help empower patients.

When choosing between manipulations and mobilizations, the particular treatment may be unimportant as studies have reported no difference in the effects of mobilization and manipulation (Gross et al. 2010, 2015; Leaver et al. 2010; Salom-Moreno et al. 2014; Young et al. 2014) or mobilizations and SNAGS (Ganesh et al. 2015). Furthermore, manual therapy treatment directed at an adjacent region may be equally effective, with studies reporting decreased neck pain following thoracic mobilizations (Cleland et al. 2005; Gross et al. 2015) and a similar pain-relieving effect of manipulation when applied to the painful lumbar levels or upper thoracic spine in patients with low-back pain (Fernando de Oliveira et al. 2013). A systematic review of treatment for epicondylalgia reported moderate evidence for manipulation of the cervical and thoracic spine (Hoogvliet et al. 2013). Clinically this may be useful in patients with central sensitization, or severe and irritable symptoms, where applying treatment to adjacent segments or joints may induce an analgesic effect whilst minimizing reproduction of symptoms.

Modification, Progression and Regression

The choice of treatment dose on second and subsequent treatment occasions needs to be informed by patients' response to the previous treatment (same, better, worse) as well as the level of presenting symptoms and irritability at the time. The decision may be to continue the initial treatment, to modify it in some way, to progress the treatment or to regress the treatment. For instance, if a quick improvement was expected but only some improvement occurred, the clinician may progress treatment. If the patient is worse after treatment the dose may be regressed in some way, and if the treatment made no difference at all then a more substantial modification may be made.

A treatment is progressed or regressed by altering appropriate aspects of the treatment dose in such a way that more or less treatment is applied to the tissues. The aspects of treatment dose that can be altered are outlined in Table 3.4. It may be important to modify only one or two components of the treatment technique at any one time to avoid excessively irritating symptoms and to be able to identify the treatment components that are having an effect. Treatment with joint mobilization should continue until the desired treatment goal is reached, or it is no longer having an effect, and ceased if it is having any adverse effect.

Specific examples of how a treatment dose may be progressed and regressed are provided in Table 3.5.

TABLE 3.4
Progression and Regression of Treatment Dose

Treatment Dose	Progression	Regression
Position	Joint towards end of available range/more pain provoking	Joint towards beginning of available range/less pain provoking
Direction of force	More provocative	Less provocative
Magnitude of force	Increased	Decreased
Amplitude of oscillation	Decreased	Increased
Rhythm	Staccato	Smoother
Time	Longer	Shorter
Speed	Slower or faster	Slower
Symptom response	Allowing more symptoms to be provoked	Allowing fewer symptoms to be provoked

TABLE 3.5
Examples of How a Treatment Dose Can Be Progressed and Regressed

Regression	Dose	Progression	Explanation
In cervical extension did central PA C4 IV ×3 (1 minute) slowly and smoothly to partial reproduction of patient's neck pain	In cervical neutral did central PA C4 IV ×3 (1 minute) slowly and smoothly to partial reproduction of patient's neck pain	In cervical flexion did central PA C4 IV ×3 (1 minute) slowly and smoothly to partial reproduction of patient's neck pain	The starting position has been altered. It might be assumed that extension is a position of ease and flexion a more provocative position
In 90° knee flexion did medial glide tibiofemoral joint III– ×3 (1 minute) slowly and smoothly short of P1	In 90° knee flexion did medial glide tibiofemoral joint III slowly and smoothly ×3 (1 minute) short of P1	In 90° knee flexion did medial glide tibiofemoral joint IIII+ ×3 (1 minute) slowly and smoothly short of P1	The grade of movement has been altered
Physiological plantarflexion II ×3 (1 minute) slowly and smoothly to full reproduction of ankle pain	Physiological plantarflexion III– ×3 (1 minute) slowly and smoothly to full reproduction of ankle pain	Physiological plantarflexion III+ ×3 (1 minute) fast and staccato to full reproduction of ankle pain	Grade has been altered as a regression. Grade, speed and rhythm have been altered as a progression

PA, posteroanterior.

Assessment of Outcome

The measurement of outcome is an important part of ensuring that the desired treatment effect is being achieved. In terms of joint mobilization, the typical outcome is likely to be a change in pain, and/or range of motion, which will be evaluated by reassessment of the subjective and physical asterisks. Measuring these variables before, during and after treatment is an appropriate way to assess the ongoing treatment effect. The clinician may choose a relevant joint movement (single plane, or a more functional combination, as relevant) and ask the patient to rate the pain while performing the movement on an 11-point numerical rating scale, an instrument found to be responsive in musculoskeletal pain (Bolton & Wilkinson 1998; Hefford et al. 2012). This same movement, and questioning regarding pain intensity, may be used between sets of joint mobilization to see if the pain level is changing. Equally the range of motion for a relevant movement may be measured using standard goniometry (Soames 2003), or a more functional measure, and this can be repeated at intervals before and after treatment. The importance of patient-based measures such as quality-of-life scales, return to work or sport, or satisfaction measures is an important component of measurement of the long-term effect of treatment.

Effect of Mobilizations

The underlying mechanisms by which joint mobilizations and manipulations can increase the range of movement and reduce pain can be broadly divided into mechanical effects and neurophysiological effects.

Mechanical Effects

It is recognized that mobilizations have a widespread mechanical effect, influencing other joints, subcutaneous tissues, muscles and local nerves. This is particularly evident in the spine where, for example, during the application of a central PA mobilization to the lumbar spine, movement occurs throughout the whole thoracolumbar region (Lee et al. 1996). This is made up of rotation of the pelvis and thoracic cage (Chansirinukor et al. 2001, 2003), compression of the skin and soft tissue (Lee et al. 1996; Lee & Evans 2000) and movement at local and distant spinal joints (Lee & Evans 1997; Powers et al. 2003; Kulig et al. 2004).

There is a mechanical effect on soft tissue; however if the aim of treatment is to elongate periarticular tissues permanently then this will require application of force of sufficient magnitude to produce microtrauma (Threlkeld 1992). The force needs to lie within the plastic zone of the force–displacement curve. A force of lesser magnitude, within the elastic zone, will result in only a temporary increase in length owing to creep and hysteresis (Panjabi & White 2001). A rough guide to the amount of force needed to cause a permanent change in length has been estimated to be between 224 and 1136 N (Threlkeld 1992). Forces used by clinicians during mobilization have been measured up to about 350 N in the lumbar spine (Harms & Bader 1997) and 70 N in the cervical spine (Snodgrass et al. 2009). It is as yet unknown whether clinically applied forces are able to cause a permanent increase in length. There has been some suggestion that manual forces applied are insufficient to produce microtrauma and that the clinically applied forces lie within the elastic range of the tissues (McQuade et al. 1999).

High intraarticular pressure can be caused by high levels of intraarticular fluid or increased muscle tension on the joint capsule (Levick 1979) and is considered to be partly responsible for the pain and limitation of movement in injured or arthritic joints (Ferrell et al. 1986). Repetitive active joint movements (Giovanelli-Blacker et al. 1985) and passive joint movements (Nade & Newbold 1983; Giovanelli-Blacker et al. 1985) have been found to cause a reduction in intraarticular pressure. A mechanical treatment effect specific to manipulation is cavitation, which causes an audible 'crack'. Cavitation is caused by the separation of the joint space creating a vacuum effect and a resulting collapse of microbubbles within the joint (Cascioli et al. 2003). An increase in joint space has been reported following manipulation of a metacarpophalangeal joint (Unsworth et al. 1971). However, contradictory evidence has been reported in zygapophyseal joints; Cramer et al. (2000) observed an increase in lumbar zygapophyseal joint space following lumbar manipulation (although this was not tested statistically), whereas Cascioli et al. (2003) reported non-significant changes in joint space following cervical manipulation. There is debate as to whether cavitation is important in creating a treatment effect. A number of studies have shown that the hypoalgesic effect of manipulation is independent of cavitation, suggesting that it is not therapeutically important (Flynn et al. 2006; Cleland et al. 2007b; Bialosky et al. 2010; Sillevis & Cleland 2011). However stretch reflex following manipulation was attenuated only when cavitation occurred (Clark et al. 2011).

MWM of peripheral joints has been shown to increase range of movement of the ankle joint (Nisha et al. 2014; Holland et al. 2015), shoulder (Teys et al. 2008; Delgado et al. 2015) and hip (Beselga et al. 2016). However, evidence of increased range of movement following mobilizations to the spine is inconclusive; a systematic review reported mobilization treatment had no effect on range of movement in the lumbar spine and sacroiliac joint and a small effect on cervical range of movement (Millan et al. 2012b). Most evidence demonstrates that mobilizations do not reduce spinal stiffness (Goodsell et al. 2000; Allison et al. 2001). Although Lee et al. (2005) reported a significant reduction in stiffness following lumbar PA mobilization treatment, this study did not include a placebo or control group and thus should be interpreted with caution.

Current thinking suggests that there is an interaction between the biomechanical and neurophysiological effects, whereby a mechanical stimulus initiates a neurophysiological response (Bialosky et al. 2009a; Pickar & Bolton 2012).

Neurophysiological Effects

A greater knowledge and understanding of the underlying neurophysiological effects of joint mobilization and manipulation have begun to emerge over the last few years. Both techniques cause activation of afferents in skin, joints, muscles and nerves and this biomechanical stimulus initiates a neurophysiological response, causing alteration of input to the central nervous system. An analgesic response is thought to occur through local effects (Teodorczyk-Injeyan et al. 2006; Molina-Ortega et al. 2014), through mechanisms at the level of the spinal cord (Boal & Gillette 2004; George et al. 2006; Bialosky et al. 2009a) and via supraspinal mechanisms (Wright 1995). It is likely that more than one of these mechanisms or an interaction between them results in analgesia induced by joint treatments.

Local Analgesic Mechanisms

Mobilizations and manipulation are thought to have an antiinflammatory effect as they have been found to result in an increase in the inflammatory mediator substance P (Brennan et al. 1991; Molina-Ortega et al. 2014) and reduction in proinflammatory cytokines (Teodorczyk-Injeyan et al. 2006). The increase in substance P observed by Molina-Ortega et al. (2014) was accompanied by hypoalgesia (measured by pressure pain thresholds), leading the authors to propose that substance P also has an influence on mediating pain.

Spinal Cord-Mediated Mechanisms

Manual therapy stimulates mechanosensitive, large-diameter joint afferents which, at the level of the spinal cord, cause inhibition of joint nociceptor activity (Wyke & Polacek 1975; Pickar & Bolton 2012) in accordance with the pain gate theory (Melzack & Wall 1965). This is based on the finding that type I mechanoreceptors in joints have been found to have an inhibitory effect, at the spinal cord, on type IV nociceptor afferent activity (Wyke & Polacek 1975). Central sensitization may be a factor in ongoing pain and dysfunction and it has been suggested that the afferent stimulus provided by manual therapy reduces central sensitization through depression of dorsal horn neurones (Boal & Gillette 2004). This is supported by studies that have measured temporal sensory summation, a phenomenon which occurs in central sensitization. An immediate reduction in temporal summation has been reported following spinal manipulation in healthy participants (George et al. 2006; Bishop et al. 2011) and participants with low-back pain (Bialosky et al. 2009b). This was found to occur in the lumbar but not in the cervical innervated regions, leading the authors to conclude pain was modulated at the dorsal horn of the spinal cord (George et al. 2006; Bialosky et al. 2009b). Conversely, Skyba et al. (2003) claimed that presynaptic or local inhibitor pathways are not involved as, in a rodent model, blockade of gamma-aminobutyric acid (GABA) receptors (found in the dorsal horn of the spinal cord) had no effect on the analgesic effects of knee mobilizations.

Supraspinal Mechanisms

Mobilizations and manipulations may reduce pain through the stimulation of supraspinal analgesic mechanisms. Wright (1995) proposed that mobilizations modulate pain-descending inhibition via the periaqueductal grey (PAG) area of the midbrain, an area important in the mediation of pain in both animals (Reynolds 1969) and humans (Hosobuchi et al. 1977). The PAG projects to the dorsal horn and has a descending control on nociception (Fig. 3.4). It also projects upwards to the medial thalamus and orbital frontal cortex, and so may have an ascending control of nociception (Fields & Basbaum 1999). The PAG has two distinct regions: the dorsolateral PAG (dPAG) and the ventrolateral PAG (vPAG). In the rat, stimulation of the dPAG causes mechanical analgesia and sympathoexcitation, whereas stimulation of the vPAG causes analgesia associated with thermal analgesia and sympathetic inhibition (Lovick 1991). The neurotransmitters used are noradrenaline (norepinephrine) from the dPAG and serotonin from the vPAG. The response to stimulation of the PAG in rats has been likened to the behaviour of animals under threat, which initially act with a defensive flight-or-fight response, followed by recuperation (Fanselow 1991; Lovick 1991); this is summarized in Fig. 3.5.

A number of research studies support the proposal of modulation of pain via the PAG, as they have reported concurrent sympathoexcitation and mechanical analgesia that mirror the effects of stimulation of the PAG in rats (Vicenzino 1995; Vicenzino et al. 1996, 1998; Sterling

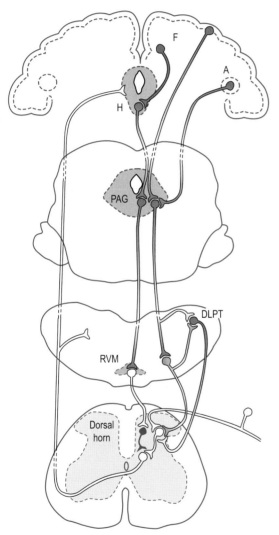

FIG. 3.4 ■ Pain-modulating pathway. Periaqueductal grey (*PAG*) receives input from the frontal lobe (*F*), the amygdala (*A*) and the hypothalamus (*H*). Afferents from PAG travel to the rostral ventromedial medulla (*RVM*) and the dorsolateral pontomesencephalic tegmentum (*DLPT*) and on to the dorsal horn. The RVM has bidirectional control of nociceptive transmission. There are inhibitory (filled) and excitatory (unfilled) interneurones. *(From Fields & Basbaum 1999, with permission.)*

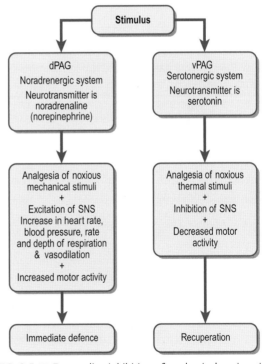

FIG. 3.5 ■ Descending inhibition of mechanical nociception from the dorsolateral periaqueductal grey (*dPAG*: noradrenergic system), and thermal nociception from the ventrolateral periaqueductal grey (*vPAG*: serotonergic system). *SNS*, sympathetic nervous system.

et al. 2001). Furthermore, systematic reviews support the sympathoexcitatory effects of mobilizations (Kingston et al. 2014) and an increase in pressure pain threshold at local and remote sites (Coronado et al. 2012; Lascurain-Aguirrebena et al. 2016), although other reviews have reported local increases in pressure pain threshold following intervention but inconsistent effects at more remote locations (Millan et al. 2012a; Voogt et al. 2015).

Skyba et al. (2003) provided further support for involvement of the PAG using pharmacological manipulation of neurotransmitters, as in rats with experimental-induced ankle inflammation, the analgesic effects of 9 minutes of knee mobilization were reversed by serotonin and noradrenaline antagonists. However, this was an animal model and it employed 9 minutes of mobilization as opposed to the commonly applied 3 minutes of mobilization; furthermore, treatment was targeted at an adjacent joint. Preliminary studies have used functional magnetic resonance imaging to observe activity in the areas of the brain associated with pain relief. Although the findings were not significant, a trend towards decreased activation of the brain areas associated with pain was found following knee mobilization in rats with experimentally induced ankle inflammation (Malisza et al. 2003). Furthermore, changes in functional connectivity in the insular cortex, somatosensory cortices and PAG were observed post manual therapy (in groups receiving mobilization, manipulation and therapeutic touch) in human participants with exercise-induced back pain (Gay et al. 2014). However this was not compared to a control intervention and thus changes could result from natural history.

Effect of Manual Therapy on Motor Activity

There is some evidence to suggest that joint treatment influences motor control and proprioception, thought to be factors in ongoing pain and dysfunction. Manual therapy may also reduce pain through interruption of the pain–muscle spasm–pain cycle. Zusman (1986) proposed a theory for the relief of pain with passive end-range joint movement through inhibiting reflex muscle contraction and reducing the level of joint afferent activity (Fig. 3.6). A number of studies investigating articular neurology have demonstrated that end-of-range passive joint movements cause a reduction in local and distant reflex muscle contraction (Freeman

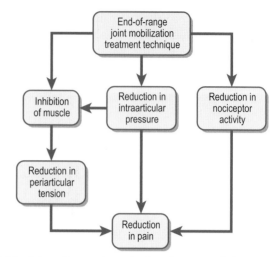

FIG. 3.6 ■ Proposed mechanism for pain relief following end-of-range joint mobilization treatment. *(From Zusman 1986.)*

& Wyke 1967; Baxendale & Ferrell 1981; Taylor et al. 1994) and reduction in muscle tension at the limits of joint movement (Lundberg et al. 1978). This reduction in muscle contraction is thought to reduce ischaemic muscle pain (Freeman & Wyke 1967) and to reduce muscle tension on periarticular and aponeurotic structures, with a subsequent reduction in the peripheral afferent activity (Millar 1973; Grigg 1976). Greater inhibition of muscle has been shown to occur with mechanical stimulation of joint afferents than with cutaneous or muscle stimulation, albeit in decerebrate cats (Baxendale & Ferrell 1981). Another theory to explain the inhibition of muscle was proposed by Korr (1975), who believed that mobilizations could reset gamma activity by directly affecting muscle spindles.

The majority of studies directly investigating the effects of manual therapy on motor activity have focused on manipulation and have reported contradictory findings. Those using electromyography (EMG) to determine muscle response to manipulation provide some evidence that motor activity may be facilitated in response to manipulation (Herzog 1999; Colloca & Keller 2001; Colloca et al. 2003); however, the lack of control groups and low participant numbers in these studies cast doubt over the strength of this evidence. A stronger randomized controlled trial using patients with low-back pain reported similar results of an increase in EMG output during trunk extension in prone after manipulation; this was not observed in the control or sham manipulation groups (Keller & Colloca 2000). In agreement with EMG studies, a study using transcranial magnetic stimulation reported postsynaptic facilitation of alpha and cortical motoneurons following manipulation (Dishman et al. 2002). In contrast, studies measuring the H-reflex have found that manipulation results in a transient suppression of motor neurone excitability (Dishman & Bulbulian 2000; Dishman & Burke 2003). Dishman and Burke (2003) proposed that this may be due to presynaptic inhibition of Ia fibres in the dorsal horn or changes in segmental and descending pathways mediating postsynaptic inhibition of motor neurons.

Pain can result in altered sensorimotor input, the process that coordinates afferent information and resultant control of the motor system. The afferent input from manipulation has been shown to alter somatomotor information by changing the way in which the somatosensory cortex responds to subsequent input (Haavik-Taylor & Murphy 2007, 2008, 2009; Haavik & Murphy 2012). For example, manipulation of the cervical spine in people with subclinical neck pain has been shown to improve suppression of somatosensory evoked potential indicating changes in cortical excitability (Haavik-Taylor & Murphy 2007, 2008). In a later study the same research group found that manipulation in participants with subclinical neck pain resulted in cerebellar modulation which normalized sensorimotor integration and motor output in a subsequent motor task (Daligadu et al. 2013).

Studies investigating the effects of mobilizations on motor activity consistently report a reduction in motor activity following treatment, both at rest and during active movements. Gross et al. (2012) reported side-to-side differences in short-latency stretch reflexes of erector spinae in patients with chronic low-back pain which were normalized following mobilizations. This was proposed to be due to downregulation of the stretch reflex response in muscle spindles. A significant reduction in EMG activity has been reported in the superficial neck muscles following cervical spine mobilizations in patients with neck pain (Sterling et al. 2001), the erector spinae following lumbar mobilizations in an asymptomatic population (Krekoukias et al. 2009) and the masseter muscle following temporomandibular joint mobilization (Taylor et al. 1994). The effect in masseter muscle remained evident for 15 minutes post treatment and was apparent both at rest and during active movement (Taylor et al. 1994). Similarly reduced EMG activity during trunk extension has been found following mobilization of the thoracic spine (Pecos-Martin et al. 2015).

Placebo Effect

There is little doubt that the therapeutic relationship between the clinician and patient forms as much a part of the treatment as the manual therapy itself. A number of studies have shown that manual contact alone, without joint mobilization, can have a demonstrable physiological effect (Petersen et al. 1993; Sterling et al. 2001; Moulson & Watson 2006). Moreover, a general expectation of beneficial treatment has been found to have an influence on clinical outcome in patients with neck pain (Bishop et al. 2013). There may be additional benefit from providing patients with their treatment of choice, as it has been shown that patient preferences may have a positive influence on treatment outcome in patients with low-back pain (Kalauokalani et al. 2001) and matching the patients' beliefs with a manipulation added to the perception of a successful treatment (Bishop et al. 2013). Allowing patient preference and beliefs to influence the treatment of choice sits within a framework of evidence-based practice (Sackett et al. 1996). Patients' expectations and beliefs are often related to their previous experience (Thompson & Sunol 1995) and therefore listening to patients' experience of previous treatment may influence treatment choice. Furthermore, activating and taking advantage of the additional placebo effects of treatment, by maximizing the therapeutic alliance and explaining the beneficial effects of treatment, can enhance clinical outcomes (Bystad et al. 2015).

Evidence Base for Joint Mobilizations

As discussed above, there is a large amount of basic science research to support the therapeutic effects of joint mobilizations. However, it is also important to know that these effects translate to an improvement in clinical outcomes for patients. There are numerous systematic reviews and meta-analyses examining the effectiveness of joint mobilizations.

In spinal joint dysfunction, there is evidence from systematic reviews of moderate benefit for spinal manual therapy in neck disorders (Bronfort et al. 2004; Gross et al. 2004, 2015; Sarigiovannis & Hollins 2005), cervicogenic headache (Bronfort et al. 2001) and acute low-back pain (Hettinga et al. 2008). The outcomes in chronic low-back pain have been variable, with some trials finding that manual therapy is an effective treatment (UK BEAM Trial 2004) while others have found it not superior to other advocated treatments (Assendelft et al. 2004; Goldby et al. 2006; Goertz et al. 2012). In trials considering spinal care, the separation of the manual therapy component from other aspects of physiotherapy care such as exercise and advice is often not achieved.

In the case of peripheral disorders, there is also a moderate level of evidence from systematic reviews for the use of joint mobilizations in lower-limb joint dysfunction (Brantingham et al. 2009), upper-limb joint injury (Michlovitz et al. 2004), adhesive capsulitis of the shoulder (Noten et al. 2016), lateral epicondylalgia (Herd & Meserve 2008; Heiser et al. 2013) and ankle sprain (van der Wees et al. 2006; Loudon et al. 2014) and for the use of MWMs in a variety of peripheral disorders (Hing et al. 2008). Equally, there have been trials that suggest that adding joint mobilizations to a standard physiotherapy programme of exercise and advice does not improve outcomes in peripheral disorders such as radial fractures (Kay et al. 2000), shoulder pain (Chen et al. 2009) and ankle fractures (Lin et al. 2008). As low-back pain is not a homogeneous disorder, many authors support the notion of subclassification of patients with spinal disorders, in order to determine those who may be best managed with specific treatments (Hancock et al. 2009). Using a single-arm trial, Flynn et al. (2002) developed a clinical prediction rule to identify patients who respond best to spinal manipulation, i.e. those with recent onset of non-radicular back pain, with low fear avoidance and hip and local spinal hypomobility. This was validated in a randomized controlled trial (Childs et al. 2004). Similar clinical prediction rules have been proposed for the use of cervical (Tseng et al. 2006) and thoracic (Cleland et al. 2007a) manipulation and for mobilization and exercise treatment for lateral epicondylalgia (Vicenzino et al. 2009). Although there is preliminary evidence that subgroup-specific manual therapy may be more effective (Slater et al. 2012), further research is needed to ensure that these predictors are not due to chance association

or indicative of overall prognosis and confirm that they are treatment effect modifiers (Haskins et al. 2012).

There is widespread concordance that the quality of randomized control trials examining the effect of joint mobilizations needs to be improved, particularly in terms of subject numbers, description of intervention, blinding and length of follow-up (Koes et al. 1996; Bronfort et al. 2004). There is also a move towards pragmatic and multimodal trials that better reflect physiotherapy practice and therefore have better external validity. An increase in mixed-method and qualitative studies is an important direction for future studies as developing an understanding of the expectations, beliefs and experience of people receiving treatment and the clinical reasoning of those providing treatment will help to provide a more complete picture of joint treatment within the broader therapeutic encounter.

EXERCISE FOR JOINT DYSFUNCTION

Physical activity and exercise play an essential and distinct role in the maintenance of health. Physiotherapists have prolonged contact with patients and therefore have an important role in health education. With the roots of physiotherapy in exercise, physiotherapists are well placed to employ behavioural change techniques and empower patients to become more physically active and take more exercise. A holistic, person-centred approach recognizes the embodied experience of people in pain and the importance of exercise in health should not be underestimated; for example, a recent metaanalysis found strong evidence that exercise was effective in the treatment of depression (Schuch et al. 2016) and a reciprocal relationship between increased physical activity and improved sleep has been reported in patients with chronic pain (Tang & Sanborn 2014). Furthermore exercise is important in primary and secondary disease prevention.

From a biomechanical perspective, therapeutic exercise has been widely reported to reduce and prevent the incidence of spinal and peripheral pathology as well as influence the rate of healing (Hertling & Kessler 2006a). The beneficial effects of exercise on pain and function in patients with osteoarthritis are proposed to result from increased leg muscle strength, and improvement in proprioception (Runhaar et al. 2015). Research supports the theory that exercise can help in improving the strength, integrity and organization of collagen, an important substance in the healing process (Taunton et al. 1998; Hertling & Kessler 2006a). Furthermore, physical activity can help increase tensile strength in injured tendons and ligaments, and has been shown to be superior to rest in relation to time taken to return to activity (Hertling & Kessler 2006a). It is believed that early movement is crucial from the proliferative stage of ligament injury, owing to the profound effect it has on healing tissue (Taunton et al. 1998). Mobilizing exercises, whether passive, active or a combination of both, in these early stages post ligamentous or muscular injury, influence the alignment and orientation of collagen, increase the tensile strength of repair and enhance the proliferative stage of healing as well as the next stage of remodelling (Taunton et al. 1998; Hassenkamp 2005). This emphasizes the necessity for early mobilization of periarticular structures postinjury (Jarvinen & Kaariainen 2007), but mobilization is also vital for maintenance of healthy intraarticular structures.

Several types of exercise are utilized in rehabilitation, including strengthening, agility, power training, stabilization, proprioception and balance exercises, flexibility drills, aerobic exercise and endurance training. With regard to joint dysfunction, the aim of exercise is to restore previous function, while remaining cognizant of adequate tissue healing and pain control in the acute stages of healing. In the presence of chronic pain and dysfunction the use of graded exposure and pacing techniques is important, as are more gentle exercise approaches such as yoga and tai chi, which have been shown to improve balance, mobility and mood (Carson et al. 2010; Wang 2012).

The benefits of exercise are:

- reduction in pain (Frank et al. 1984; Hertling & Kessler 2006b)
- reduced need for analgesia
- promotion of healing through circulatory effects and effects on collagen
- maintenance of muscle length and strength
- enhanced healing process due to increased protein synthesis
- improved psychological well-being
- improved sleep
- primary and secondary disease prevention.

Degenerative Joint Disease

Changes in joint and associated structures, such as facet degeneration, disc degeneration and disc bulges, are associated with normal ageing and the prevalence of these findings increases in an asymptomatic population with each subsequent decade of life (for example, disc degeneration is present in 53% of asymptomatic individuals in their third decade, 68% in their fourth decade and 80% in the fifth decade (Brinjikji et al. 2015). Although these findings may be asymptomatic, they may disrupt the afferent feedback loop of the sensorimotor system, causing subsequent loss of muscle activation and/or altered neuromuscular control with subsequent reduction in proprioception (Hurley 1997; Myers & Lephart 2000; Jackson et al. 2004; Cuomo et al. 2005) and thus strengthening and balance exercises are the mainstay of treatment. Specific joint treatments may be applied depending on the findings on examination in line with the guidance in this chapter.

KEY POINTS AND SUMMARY

Management of people with joint dysfunction should, where possible, restore and encourage normal movement while addressing people's beliefs and expectations, and listening to and acknowledging their lived experience.

- Treatments aimed at joints can be incorporated within a holistic approach to management of people with musculoskeletal pain and dysfunction.
- The physiotherapist should treat joints alongside addressing inappropriate pain beliefs and behaviours.
- Joint treatment should be complemented by recommendations regarding physical activity, smoking, basic nutrition, stress, sleep hygiene and alcohol consumption.
- Joint mobilizations and exercise both form components of evidence-based treatment of joint dysfunction.
- The choice and application of joint mobilizations are dependent on thorough and ongoing assessment of the patient's symptoms and signs, with the need for appropriate modification as required.
- Treatment in functional positions should be considered.

- The effect of joint mobilizations is both mechanical and neurophysiological, occurring at local, spinal and supraspinal levels.
- In joint dysfunction, exercise aims to restore function in terms of range and quality of motion and proprioceptive control, while helping to manage pain and enhance tissue healing.

REFERENCES

Allison, G., Edmonston, S., Kiviniemi, K., et al., 2001. Influence of standardized mobilization on the posteroanterior stiffness of the lumbar spine in asymptomatic subjects. Physiother. Res. Int. 6, 145–156.

Assendelft, W.J., Morton, S.C., Yu, E.I., et al., 2004. Spinal manipulative therapy for low back pain. Cochrane Database Syst. Rev. (1), CD000447.

Baxendale, R.H., Ferrell, W.R., 1981. The effect of knee joint afferent discharge on transmission in flexion reflex pathways in decerebrate cats. J. Physiol. 315, 231–242.

Beselga, C., Neto, F., Alburquerque-Sendin, F., et al., 2016. Immediate effects of hip mobilisation with movement in patients with hip osteoarthritis: a randomized controlled trial. Man. Ther. 22, 80–85.

Bialosky, J., Bishop, M., Price, D., et al., 2009a. The mechanism of manual therapy in the treatment of musculoskeletal pain: a comprehensive model. Man. Ther. 14, 531–538.

Bialosky, J., Bishop, M., Robinson, M., et al., 2009b. Spinal manipulative therapy has an immediate effect on thermal pain sensitivity in people with low back pain: a randomized controlled trial. Phys. Ther. 89, 1292–1303.

Bialosky, J., Bishop, M., Robinson, M., et al., 2010. The relationship of the audible pop to hypoalgesia associated with high-velocity, low-amplitude thrust manipulation: a secondary analysis of an experimental study in pain-free participants. J. Manipulative Physiol. Ther. 33, 117–124.

Bishop, M., Beneciuk, J., George, S., 2011. Immediate reduction in temporal sensory summation after thoracic spinal manipulation. Spine J. 11, 440–446.

Bishop, M., Mintken, P., Bialosky, J., et al., 2013. Patient expectation of benefit from intervention for neck pain and resulting influence on outcomes. J. Orthop. Sports Phys. Ther. 43, 457–465.

Boal, R., Gillette, R., 2004. Central neuronal plasticity, low back pain and spinal manipulative therapy. J. Manipulative Physiol. Ther. 27, 314–326.

Bolton, J.E., Wilkinson, R.C., 1998. Responsiveness of pain scales: a comparison of three pain intensity measures in chiropractic patients. J. Manipulative Physiol. Ther. 21, 1–7.

Brantingham, J.W., Globe, G., Pollard, H., et al., 2009. Manipulative therapy for lower extremity conditions: expansion of literature review. J. Manipulative Physiol. Ther. 32, 53–71.

Brennan, P., Kokjohn, K., Kaltinger, C., et al., 1991. Enhanced phagocytic cell respiratory burst induced by spinal manipulation: potential role of substance P. J. Manipulative Physiol. Ther. 14, 399–408.

Brinjikji, W., Luetmer, P., Comstock, B., et al., 2015. Systematic literature review of imaging features of spinal degeneration in asymptomatic populations. AJNR Am. J. Neuroradiol. 36, 598–602.

Bronfort, G., Assendelft, W.J., Evans, R., et al., 2001. Efficacy of spinal manipulation for chronic headache: a systematic review. J. Manipulative Physiol. Ther. 24, 457–466.

Bronfort, G., Haas, M., Evans, R., et al., 2004. Efficacy of spinal manipulation and mobilisation for low back pain and neck pain: a systematic review and best evidence synthesis. Spine J. 4, 335–356.

Bystad, M., Bystad, C., Wynn, R., 2015. How can placebo effects best be applied in clinical practice? A narrative review. Psychol. Res. Behav. Manag. 8, 41–45.

Carson, J., Carson, K., Jones, K., et al., 2010. A pilot randomized controlled trial of the yoga of awareness program in the management of fibromyalgia. Pain 151, 530–539.

Cascioli, V., Corr, P., Till, T., 2003. An investigation into the production of intra-articular gas bubbles and increase in joint space in the zygapophyseal joints of the cervical spine in asymptomatic subjects after spinal manipulation. J. Manipulative Physiol. Ther. 26, 356–364.

Chansirinukor, W., Lee, M., Latimer, J., 2001. Contribution of pelvic rotation to lumbar posteroanterior movement. Man. Ther. 6, 242–249.

Chansirinukor, W., Lee, M., Latimer, J., 2003. Contribution of ribcage movement to thoracolumbar posteroanterior stiffness. J. Manipulative Physiol. Ther. 26, 176–183.

Chen, J.F., Ginn, K.A., Herbert, R.D., 2009. Passive mobilisation of shoulder region joints plus advice and exercise does not reduce pain and disability more than advice and exercise alone: a randomised trial. Aust. J. Physiother. 55, 17–23.

Childs, J., Fritz, J., Flynn, T., et al., 2004. A clinical prediction rule to identify patients with low back pain most likely to benefit from spinal manipulation: a validation study. Ann. Intern. Med. 141, 920–930.

Chiu, T.W., Wright, A., 1996. To compare the effects of different rates of application of a cervical mobilisation technique on sympathetic outflow to the upper limb in normal subjects. Man. Ther. 1, 198–203.

Clark, B., Gross, D., Walkoski, S., et al., 2011. Neurophysiologic effects of spinal manipulation in patients with chronic low back pain. BMC Musculoskelet. Disord. 12, 170.

Cleland, J.A., Childs, J.D., McRae, M., et al., 2005. Immediate effects of thoracic manipulation in patients with neck pain: a randomized clinical trial. Man. Ther. 10, 127–135.

Cleland, J.A., Childs, J.D., Fritz, J.M., et al., 2007a. Development of a clinical prediction rule for guiding treatment of a subgroup of patients with neck pain: use of thoracic spine manipulation, exercise, and patient education. Phys. Ther. 87, 9–23.

Cleland, J.A., Flynn, T., Childs, J.D., et al., 2007b. The audible pop from thoracic spine thrust manipulation and its relation to short-term outcomes in patients with neck pain. J. Manipulative Physiol. Ther. 15, 143–154.

Coronado, R., Gay, C., Bialosky, J., et al., 2012. Changes in pain sensitivity following manipulation: a systematic review and meta-analysis. J. Electromyogr. Kinesiol. 22, 752–756.

Colloca, C., Keller, T., 2001. Stiffness and neuromuscular reflex response of the human spine to posteroanterior manipulative thrusts in patients with low back pain. J. Manipulative Physiol. Ther. 24, 489–500.

Colloca, C., Keller, T., Gunzburg, R., 2003. Neuromechanical characterization of in vivo lumbar spinal manipulation. Part II. Neurophysiological response. J. Manipulative Physiol. Ther. 26, 579–591.

Cramer, G., Tuck, N., Knudsen, T., et al., 2000. Effects of side-posture positioning and side-posture adjusting on the lumbar zygapophyseal joints as evaluated by magnetic resonance imaging: a before and after study with randomization. J. Manipulative Physiol. Ther. 23, 380–394.

Cuomo, F., Birdzell, M.G., Zuckerman, J.D., 2005. The effect of degenerative arthritis and prosthetic arthroplasty on shoulder proprioception. J. Shoulder Elbow Surg. 14, 345–348.

Daligadu, J., Haavik-Taylor, H., Yielder, P., et al., 2013. Alteration in cortical and cerebellar motor processing in subclinical neck pain patients following spinal manipulation. J. Manipulative Physiol. Ther. 36, 527–537.

Delgado, J., Prado-Robles, E., Rodrigues-de-Souza, D., et al., 2015. Effects of mobilisation with movement on pain and range of motion in patients with unilateral shoulder impingement syndrome: a randomized controlled trial. J. Manipulative Physiol. Ther. 38, 245–252.

Dishman, J.D., Ball, K.A., Burke, J., 2002. Central motor excitability changes after spinal manipulation: a transcranial magnetic stimulation study. J. Manipulative Physiol. Ther. 25, 1–9.

Dishman, J., Bulbulian, R., 2000. Spinal reflex attenuation associated with spinal manipulation. Spine 25, 2519–2525.

Dishman, J., Burke, J., 2003. Spinal reflex excitability changes after cervical and lumbar spinal manipulation: a comparative study. Spine J. 3, 204–212.

Fanselow, M.S., 1991. The midbrain periaqueductal gray as a coordinator of action in response to fear and anxiety. In: Depaulis, A., Bandler, R. (Eds.), The midbrain periaqueductal gray matter. Plenum Press, New York, pp. 151–173.

Fernando de Oliveira, R., Eloin Liebano, R., de Cunha Menezes Costa, L., et al., 2013. Immediate effects of region-specific and non-region specific spinal manipulative therapy on patients with chronic low back pain: a randomized controlled trial. Phys. Ther. 93, 748–756.

Ferrell, W.R., Nade, S., Newbold, P.J., 1986. The interrelation of neural discharge, intra-articular pressure, and joint angle in the knee of the dog. J. Physiol. 373, 353–365.

Fields, H.L., Basbaum, A.I., 1999. Central nervous system mechanisms of pain modulation. In: Wall, P.D., Melzack, R. (Eds.), Textbook of pain, fourth ed. Churchill Livingstone, Edinburgh, pp. 309–329.

Flynn, T., Childs, J., Fritz, J., 2006. The audible pop from high-velocity thrust manipulation and outcome in individuals with low back pain. J. Manipulative Physiol. Ther. 29, 40–45.

Flynn, T., Fritz, J., Whitman, J., 2002. A clinical prediction rule for classifying patients with low back pain who demonstrate short-term improvement with spinal manipulation. Spine 27, 2835–2843.

Frank, C., Akesan, W., Woo, S.L.Y., et al., 1984. Physiology and therapeutic value of passive joint motion. Clin. Orthop. Relat. Res. 185, 113–125.

Freeman, M.A.R., Wyke, B.D., 1967. Articular reflexes at the ankle joint: an electromyographic study of normal and abnormal influences of ankle-joint mechanoreceptors upon reflex activity in the leg muscles. Br. J. Surg. 54, 990–1001.

Ganesh, S., Mohanty, P., Pattnaik, M., et al., 2015. Effectiveness of mobilization therapy and exercise in mechanical neck pain. Physiother. Theory Pract. 31, 99–106.

Gay, C., Robinson, M., George, S., et al., 2014. Immediate changes after manual therapy in resting-state functional connectivity as measured by functional magnetic resonance imaging in participants with induced low back pain. J. Manipulative Physiol. Ther. 37, 615–627.

George, S., Bishop, M., Bialosky, J., et al., 2006. Immediate effects of spinal manipulation on thermal pain sensitivity: an experimental study. BMC Musculoskelet. Disord. 7, 1–10.

Giovanelli-Blacker, B., Elvey, R., Thompson, E., 1985. The clinical significance of measured lumbar zygapophyseal intracapsular pressure variation. Proceedings of the Manipulative Therapists Association of Australia 4th Biennial Conference, Brisbane, Queensland, pp. 122–139.

Goertz, C., Pohlman, K., Vining, R., et al., 2012. Patient-centered outcomes of high velocity, low amplitude spinal manipulation for low back pain: a systematic review. J. Electromyogr. Kinesiol. 22, 670–691.

Goldby, L.J., Moore, A.P., Doust, J., et al., 2006. A randomized control trial investigating the efficiency of musculoskeletal physiotherapy on chronic back pain disorder. Spine 31, 1083–1093.

Goodsell, M., Lee, M., Latimer, J., 2000. Short-term effects of lumbar posteroanterior mobilization in individuals with low-back pain. J. Manipulative Physiol. Ther. 23, 332–342.

Grigg, P., 1976. Response of joint afferent neurons in cat medial articular nerve to active and passive movements of the knee. Brain Res. 118, 482–485.

Gross, A., Hoving, J.L., Haines, T., et al., 2004. Manipulation and mobilisation for mechanical neck disorders. Cochrane Database Syst. Rev. (1), CD004249.

Gross, A., Langevin, P., Burnie, S., et al., 2015. Manipulation and mobilisation for neck pain contrasted against inactive control or another active treatment. Cochrane Database Syst. Rev. (9), CD004249.

Gross, A., Miller, J., D'Sylva, J., et al., 2010. Manipulation and mobilisation for neck pain. Man. Ther. 15, 315–333.

Gross, D., Thomas, J., Walkowski, S., et al., 2012. Non-thrust manual therapy reduces erector spinae short-latency stretch reflex asymmetries I patients with chronic low back pain. J. Electryomyogr. Kinesiol. 22, 663–669.

Haavik, H., Murphy, B., 2012. The role of spinal manipulation in addressing disordered sensorimotor integration and altered motor control. J. Electromyogr. Kinesiol. 22, 768–776.

Haavik-Taylor, H., Murphy, B., 2007. Cervical spine manipulation alters somatosensory integration: a somatosensory evoked potential study. Clin. Neurophysiol. 118, 391–402.

Haavik-Taylor, H., Murphy, B., 2008. Altered central integration of dual somatosensory input after cervical spine manipulation. J. Manipulative Physiol. Ther. 33, 178–188.

Haavik-Taylor, H., Murphy, B., 2009. The effects of spinal manipulation on central integration of dual somatosensory input observed after motor training: a crossover study. J. Manipulative Physiol. Ther. 33, 261–272.

Hancock, M., Maher, C., Latimer, J., et al., 2009. Can rate of recovery be predicted in patients with acute low back pain? Development of a clinical prediction rule. Eur. J. Pain 13, 51–55.

Harms, M.C., Bader, D.L., 1997. Variability of forces applied by experienced therapists during spinal mobilization. Clin. Biomech. (Bristol, Avon) 12, 393–399.

Haskins, R., Rivett, D., Osmotherly, P., 2012. Clinical prediction rules in the physiotherapy management of low back pain: a systematic review. Man. Ther. 17, 9–21.

Hassenkamp, A., 2005. Soft tissue injuries. In: Atkinson, K., Coutts, F., Hassenkamp, A. (Eds.), Physiotherapy in orthopaedics, second ed. Elsevier Churchill Livingstone, London.

Hebron, C., 2014. The biomechanical and analgesic effects of lumbar mobilisations. Doctoral thesis, University of Brighton.

Hefford, C., Haxby-Abbott, J., Arnold, R., et al., 2012. The patient-specific functional scale: validity, reliability, and responsiveness in patients with upper extremity musculoskeletal problems. J. Orthop. Sports Phys. Ther. 42, 56–65.

Heidegger, M., 1962. Being and time (J. Maquarrie and E. Robinson, Trans.). Blackwell, Oxford.

Heiser, R., O'Brien, V., Schwartz, D., 2013. The use of joint mobilization to improve clinical outcomes in hand therapy: a systematic review of the literature. J. Hand Ther. 26, 297–311.

Hengeveld, E., Banks, K., 2013. Maitland's vertebral manipulation, eighth ed. Churchill Livingstone, Edinburgh.

Herd, C.R., Meserve, B.B., 2008. Systematic review of the effectiveness of manipulative therapy in treating lateral epicondylalgia. J. Man. Manip. Ther. 16, 225–237.

Hertling, D., Kessler, R., 2006a. Introduction to manual therapy. In: Hertling, D., Kessler, R. (Eds.), Management of common musculoskeletal disorders: physical therapy principles and methods. Lippincott, Williams and Wilkins, Philadelphia.

Hertling, D., Kessler, R.M., 2006b. Shoulder and shoulder girdle. In: Hertling, D., Kessler, R.M. (Eds.), Management of common musculoskeletal disorders: physical therapy principles and methods. Lippincott, Williams and Wilkins, Philadelphia.

Herzog, W., 1999. Electromyographic responses of back and limb muscles associated with spinal manipulative therapy. Spine 24, 146–153.

Hettinga, D.M., Hurley, D.A., Jackson, A., et al., 2008. Assessing the effect of sample size, methodological quality and statistical rigour on outcomes of randomised controlled trials on mobilisation, manipulation and massage for low back pain of at least 6 weeks duration. Physiotherapy 94, 97–104.

Hing, W., Bigelow, R., Bremner, T., 2008. Mulligan's mobilisation with movement: a review of the tenets and prescription of MWMs. New Zealand Journal of Physiotherapy 36, 144–164.

Hing, W., Hallm, T., Rivett, D., et al., 2015. The Mulligan concept of manual therapy. Churchill Livingstone, Edinburgh.

Holland, C., Campbell, K., Hunt, K., 2015. Increased treatment duration lead to greater improvements in non-weight bearing dorsiflexion range of motion for asymptomatic individuals immediately following an anteroposterior grade IV mobilisation of the talus. Man. Ther. 20, 598–602.

Hoogvliet, P., Randsdorp, M., Dingemanse, R., et al., 2013. Does effectiveness of exercise therapy and mobilisation technique offer guidance for the treatment of lateral and medial epicondylitis? A systematic review. Br. J. Sports Med. 47, 1112–1119.

Hosobuchi, Y., Adams, J., Linchitz, R., 1977. Pain relief by electrical stimulation of the central gray matter in humans and its reversal by naloxone. Science 197, 183–186.

Hurley, M.V., 1997. The effect of joint damage on muscle function, proprioception and rehabilitation. Man. Ther. 2, 11–17.

Jackson, B.D., Wluka, A.E., Teichtahl, A.J., et al., 2004. Reviewing knee osteoarthritis – a biomechanical perspective. J. Sci. Med. Sport 7, 347–357.

Jarvinen, T., Kaariainen, M., 2007. Muscle injuries: optimising recovery. Best Pract. Res. Clin. Rheumatol. 21, 317–331.

Kalauokalani, D., Cherkin, D., Sherman, K., et al., 2001. Lessons from a trial of acupuncture and massage for low back pain. Spine 26, 1418–1424.

Kay, S., Haensel, N., Stiller, K., 2000. The effect of passive mobilisation following fractures involving the distal radius: a randomised study. Australian Journal of Physiotherapy 46, 93–101.

Keller, T., Colloca, C., 2000. Mechanical force spinal manipulation increases trunk muscle strength assessed by electromyography: a comparative clinical trial. J. Manipulative Physiol. Ther. 23, 585–595.

Kingston, L., Claydon, L., Tumilty, S., 2014. The effects of spinal mobilization on the sympathetic nervous system: a systematic review. Man. Ther. 19, 281–287.

Koes, B., Assendelft, W.J., Van der Heijden, G.J.M., et al., 1996. Spinal manipulation for low back pain: an updated systematic review of randomized clinical trials. Spine 21, 2860–2871.

Korr, I., 1975. Proproiception and somatic dysfunction. J. Am. Osteopath. Assoc. 74, 638–650.

Krekoukias, G., Petty, N., Cheek, L., 2009. Comparison of surface electromyographic activity of erector spinae before and after the application of central posteroanterior mobilisation on the lumbar spine. J. Electromyogr. Kinesiol. 19, 39–45.

Krouwel, O., Hebron, C., Willett, E., 2010. An investigation into the potential hypoalgesic effects of different amplitudes of PA mobilisations on the lumbar spine as measured by pressure pain thresholds (PPT). Man. Ther. 15, 7–12.

Kulig, K., Landel, R., Powers, C., 2004. Assessment of lumbar spine kinematics using dynamic MRI: a proposed mechanism of sagittal plane motion induced by manual posterior-to-anterior mobilisation. J. Orthop. Sports Phys. Ther. 34, 57–64.

Lascurain-Aguirrebena, I., Newham, D., Critchley, D., 2016. Mechanism of action of spinal mobilizations: a systematic review. Spine 41, 159–172.

Leaver, A., Maher, C., Herbert, R., et al., 2010. A randomized controlled trial comparing manipulation with mobilisation for recent onset neck pain. Arch. Phys. Med. Rehabil. 91, 1313–1318.

Lee, R., Evans, J., 1997. An in vivo study of the intervertebral movements produced by posteroanterior mobilization. Clin. Biomech. (Bristol, Avon) 12, 400–408.

Lee, R., Evans, J., 2000. The role of spinal tissues in resisting poster-oanterior forces applied to the lumbar spine. J. Manipulative Physiol. Ther. 23, 551–555.

Lee, M., Steven, G., Crosbie, R., 1996. Towards a theory of lumbar mobilisations – the relationship between applied manual force and movements of the spine. Man. Ther. 2, 67–75.

Lee, R., Tsung, B., Tong, P., et al., 2005. Posteroanterior mobilisation reduces the bending stiffness and pain response of the lumbar spine. Paper presented at Second International Conference on Movement Dysfunction. Edinburgh, UK.

Levick, J.R., 1979. An investigation into the validity of subatmospheric pressure recordings from synovial fluid and their dependence on joint angle. J. Physiol. 289, 55–67.

Lin, C.W., Moseley, A.M., Haas, M., et al., 2008. Manual therapy in addition to physiotherapy does not improve clinical or economic outcomes after ankle fracture. J. Rehabil. Med. 40, 433–439.

Loudon, J., Reiman, M., Sylvain, J., 2014. The efficacy of manual joint mobilisation / manipulation in treatment of lateral ankle sprains: a systematic review. Br. J. Sports Med. 48, 365–379.

Lovick, T.A., 1991. Interactions between descending pathways from the dorsal and ventrolateral periaqueductal gray matter in the rat. In: Depaulis, A., Bandler, R. (Eds.), The midbrain periaqueductal gray matter. Plenum Press, New York, pp. 101–120.

Lundberg, A., Malmgren, K., Schomburg, E.D., 1978. Role of joint afferents in motor control exemplified by effects on reflex pathways from 1b afferents. J. Physiol. 284, 327–343.

Magarey, M.E., 1985. Selection of passive treatment techniques. Proceedings of the Manipulative Therapists Association of Australia 4th Biennial Conference, Brisbane, pp. 298–320.

Magarey, M.E., 1986. Examination and assessment in spinal joint dysfunction. In: Grieve, G.P. (Ed.), Modern manual therapy of the vertebral column. Churchill Livingstone, Edinburgh, pp. 481–497.

Malisza, K., Gregorash, L., Turner, A., et al., 2003. Functional MRI involving painful stimulation of the ankle and the effect of physiotherapy joint mobilization. Magn. Reson. Imaging 21, 489–496.

McKenzie, R., 1981. The lumbar spine, mechanical diagnosis and therapy. Spinal Publications, New Zealand.

McKenzie, R., 1983. Treat your own neck. Spinal Publications, New Zealand.

McKenzie, R., 1985. Treat your own back. Spinal Publications, New Zealand.

McLean, S., Naish, R., Reed, L., et al., 2002. A pilot study of the manual force levels required to produce manipulation induced hypoalgesia. Clin. Biomech. (Bristol, Avon) 17, 304–308.

McQuade, K.J., Shelley, I., Cvitkovic, J., 1999. Patterns of stiffness during clinical examination of the glenohumeral joint. Clin. Biomech. (Bristol, Avon) 14, 620–627.

Melzack, R., Wall, P.D., 1965. Pain mechanisms: a new theory. Science 150, 971–979.

Michie, S., van Stralen, M., West, R., 2011. The behavioural change wheel: a new method for characterizing and designing behavior change interventions. Implement. Sci. 6, 42.

Michlovitz, S., Harris, B.A., Watkins, M.P., 2004. Therapy interventions for improving joint range of motion: a systematic review. J. Hand Ther. 17, 118–131.

Millan, M., Leboeuf-Yde, C., Budgell, B., et al., 2012a. The effects of spinal manipulative therapy on experimentally induced pain: a systematic literature review. Chiropr. Man. Therap. 20, 1–22.

Millan, M., Leboeuf-Yde, C., Budgell, B., et al., 2012b. The effects of spinal manipulative therapy on spinal range of movement: a systematic literature review. Chiropr. Man. Therap. 20, 1–18.

Millar, J., 1973. Joint afferent fibres responding to muscle stretch, vibration and contraction. Brain Res. 63, 380–383.

Molina-Ortega, F., Lomas-Vega, R., Hita-Contreras, F., et al., 2014. Immediate effects of spinal manipulation on nitric oxide, substance P and pain perception. Man. Ther. 19, 411–417.

Moulson, A., Watson, T., 2006. A preliminary investigation into the relationship between cervical snags and sympathetic nervous system activity in the upper limbs of an asymptomatic population. Man. Ther. 11, 214–224.

Myers, J.B., Lephart, S.M., 2000. The role of the sensorimotor system in the athletic shoulder. J. Athl. Train. 35, 351–363.

Nade, J.S., Newbold, P.J., 1983. Factors determining the level and changes in intra-articular pressure in the knee joint of the dog. J. Physiol. 338, 21–36.

Nijs, J., Van Houdenhove, B., 2009. From acute musculoskeletal pain to chronic widespread pain and fibromyalgia: application of pain neurophysiology in manual therapy practice. Man. Ther. 14, 3–12.

Nisha, K., Megha, N., Paresh, P., 2014. Efficacy of weight bearing distal tibiofibular joint mobilisation with movement (MWM) in improving pain, dorsiflexion range and function in patients with postacute lateral ankle sprain. International Journal of Physiotherapy Research 2, 542–548.

Noten, S., Meeus, M., Stassijns, G., et al., 2016. Efficacy of different types of mobilization techniques in patients with primary adhesive capsulitis of the shoulder: a systematic review. Arch. Phys. Med. Rehabil. 97, 815–825.

Noyes, F.R., DeLucas, J.L., Torvik, P.J., 1974. Biomechanics of anterior cruciate ligament failure: an analysis of strain-rate sensitivity and mechanisms of failure in primates. J. Bone Joint Surg. Am. 56A, 236–253.

Panjabi, M.M., White, A.A., 2001. Biomechanics in the musculoskeletal system. Churchill Livingstone, New York.

Pecos-Martin, D., de Melo Aroeira, A., Veras Sila, R., et al., 2015. Immediate effects of thoracic mobilisation on erector spinae muscle activity and pain in patients with thoracic spine pain: a preliminary randomized controlled trial. Physiotherapy pii: S0031-9406(15)03859-6.

Pentelka, L., Hebron, C., Shapleski, R., et al., 2012. The effect of increasing sets (within one treatment session) and different set durations (between treatment sessions) of lumbar spine poster-oanterior mobilisations on pressure pain thresholds. Man. Ther. 17, 526–530.

Petersen, N., Vicenzino, B., Wright, A., 1993. The effects of a cervical mobilisation technique on sympathetic outflow to the upper limb in normal subjects. Physiother. Theory Pract. 9, 149–156.

Petty, N.J., Maher, C., Latimer, J., et al., 2002. Manual examination of accessory movements – seeking R1. Man. Ther. 7, 39–43.

Petty, N.J., Ryder, D., 2017. Musculoskeletal examination and assessment: a handbook for therapists, fourth ed. Churchill Livingstone, Edinburgh.

Pickar, J.G., Bolton, P., 2012. Spinal manipulative therapy and somatosensory activation. J. Electromyogr. Kinesiol. 22, 785–794.

Powers, C., Kulig, K., Harrison, J., et al., 2003. Segmental mobility of the lumbar spine during a posterior to anterior mobilization: assessment using dynamic MRI. Clin. Biomech. (Bristol, Avon) 18, 80–83.

Reynolds, D., 1969. Surgery in the rat during electrical analgesia induced by focal brain stimulation. Science 164, 444–445.

Runhaar, J., Luijsterburg, P., Dekker, J., et al., 2015. Identifying potential mechanisms behind the positive effects of exercise therapy on pain and function in osteoarthritis; a systematic review. Osteoarthritis Cartilage 23, 1071–1082.

Sackett, D., Rosenberg, W., Gray, J., 1996. Evidence based medicine: what it is and what it isn't – it's about integrating clinical expertise and best external evidence. Br. Med. J. 312, 71–72.

Salom-Moreno, R., Ortega-Santiago, R., Cleland, J., et al., 2014. Immediate changes in neck pain intensity and widespread pressure pain sensitivity in patients with bilateral chronic mechanical neck pain: a randomized controlled trial of thoracic thrust manipulation vs non-thrust mobilization. J. Manipulative Physiol. Ther. 37, 312–319.

Sarigiovannis, P., Hollins, B., 2005. Effectiveness of manual therapy in the treatment of non-specific neck pain: a review. Physical Therapy Review 10, 35–50.

Schuch, F., Vancampfort, D., Richards, J., et al., 2016. Exercise as a treatment for depression: a meta-analysis adjusting for publication bias. J. Psychiatr. Res. 77, 42–51.

Sillevis, R., Cleland, J., 2011. Immediate effects of the audible pop from a thoracic spine thrust manipulation on the autonomic nervous system and pain: a secondary analysis of a randomized controlled trial. J. Manipulative Physiol. Ther. 34, 37–45.

Skyba, D., Radhakrishnan, R., Rohlwing, J., et al., 2003. Joint manipulation reduces hyperalgesia by activation of monoamine receptors but not opioid or GABA receptors in the spinal cord. Pain 106, 159–168.

Slater, S., Ford, J., Richards, M., et al., 2012. The effectiveness of sub-group specific manual therapy for low back pain: a systematic review. Man. Ther. 17, 201–212.

Snodgrass, S., Rivett, D., Robertson, V., et al., 2009. Cervical spine mobilisation forces applied by physiotherapy students. Physiotherapy 96, 120–129.

Soames, R., 2003. Joint motion: clinical measurement and evaluation. Churchill Livingstone, Edinburgh.

Sterling, M., Jull, G., Wright, A., 2001. Cervical mobilisation: concurrent effects on pain, sympathetic nervous system activity and motor activity. Man. Ther. 6, 72–81.

Tang, N., Sanborn, A., 2014. Better quality sleep promotes daytime physical activity in patients with chronic pain? A multilevel analysis of the within-person relationship. PLoS ONE 9, e92158.

Taunton, J., Robertson Lloyd-Smith, D., Fricker, P., 1998. The ankle. In: Harries, M., Williams, C., Stanish, W. (Eds.), Oxford textbook of sports medicine, second ed. Oxford University Press, Oxford.

Taylor, M., Suvinen, T., Reade, P., 1994. The effect of grade IV distraction mobilisation on patients with temporomandibular pain-dysfunction disorder. Physiother. Theory Pract. 10, 129–136.

Teodorczyk-Injeyan, J., Injeyan, S., Ruegg, R., 2006. Spinal manipulative therapy reduces inflammatory cytokines but not substance P production in normal subjects. J. Manipulative Physiol. Ther. 29, 14–21.

Teys, P., Bisset, L., Vicenzino, B., 2008. The initial effects of a Mulligan's mobilisation with movement technique on range of movement and pressure pain threshold in pain-limited shoulders. Man. Ther. 13, 37–42.

Thompson, A., Sunol, R., 1995. Expectations as determinants of patient satisfaction: concepts, theory and evidence. Int. J. Qual. Health Care 7, 127–141.

Threlkeld, A.J., 1992. The effects of manual therapy on connective tissue. Phys. Ther. 72, 893–902.

Tseng, Y.L., Wang, W.T.J., Chen, W.Y., et al., 2006. Predictors for the immediate responders to cervical manipulation in patients with neck pain. Man. Ther. 11, 306–315.

UK BEAM Trial, 2004. United Kingdom Back Pain Exercise and Manipulation (UK BEAM) randomised trial: effectiveness of physical treatments for back pain in primary care. Br. Med. J. doi:10.1136/bmj.38282.669225.AE. Available online at: http://bmj.com. published 29 November 2004.

Unsworth, A., Dowson, D., Wright, V., 1971. Cracking joints': a bioengineering study of cavitation in the metacarpophalangeal joint. Ann. Rheum. Dis. 30, 348–358.

van der Wees, P.J., Lenssen, A.F., Hendriks, E.J.M., et al., 2006. Effectiveness of exercise therapy and manual mobilisation in acute ankle sprain and functional instability: a systematic review. Aust. J. Physiother. 52, 27–37.

van Griensven, H., 2005. Pain in practice: theory and treatment strategies for manual therapists. Butterworth Heinemann, Elsevier, London.

Vermeulen, H., Rozing, P.M., Obermann, W.R., et al., 2006. Comparison of high-grade and low-grade mobilization techniques in the management of adhesive capsulitis of the shoulder: randomized controlled trial. Phys. Ther. 86, 355–368.

Vicenzino, B., 1995. An investigation of the effects of spinal manual therapy on forequater pressure and thermal pain thresholds and sympathetic nervous system activity in asymptomatic subjects: a preliminary report. In: Shacklock, M.O. (Ed.), Moving in on pain. Butterworth-Heinemann, Australia, pp. 185–193.

Vicenzino, B., Collins, D., Wright, A., 1996. The initial effects of a cervical spine manipulative physiotherapy treatment on the pain and dysfunction of lateral epicondylalgia. Pain 68, 69–74.

Vicenzino, B., Collins, D., Benson, H., et al., 1998. An investigation of the interrelationship between manipulative therapy-induced hypoalgesia and sympathoexcitation. J. Manipulative Physiol. Ther. 21, 448–453.

Vicenzino, B., McLean, S., Naish, R., 2001. Preliminary evidence of a force threshold required to produce manipulation inducted hypoalgesia. Procceedings of the 12th Biennial Conference Musculoskeletal Physiotherapy Australia, November.

Vicenzino, B., Smith, D., Cleland, J., et al., 2009. Development of a clinical prediction rule to identify initial responders to mobilisation with movement and exercise for lateral epicondylalgia. Man. Ther. 14, 550–554.

Voogt, L., de Vries, J., Meeus, M., et al., 2015. Analgesic effects of manual therapy in patients with musculoskeletal pain: a systematic review. Man. Ther. 20, 250–256.

Wang, C., 2012. Role of tai chi in the treatment of rheumatologic diseases. Curr. Rheumatol. Rep. 14, 598–603.

Wertli, M., Rasmussen-Barr, E., Held, U., 2014. Fear-avoidance beliefs – a moderator of treatment efficacy in patients with low back pain: a systematic review. Spine J. 14, 2658–2678.

Willett, E., Hebron, C., Krouwel, O., 2010. The initial effects of different rates of lumbar mobilisations on pressure pain thresholds in asymptomatic subjects. Man. Ther. 15, 173–178.

Wright, A., 1995. Hypoalgesia post-manipulative therapy: a review of a potential neurophysiological mechanism. Man. Ther. 1, 11–16.

Wyke, B.D., Polacek, P., 1975. Articular neurology: the present position. J. Joint Bone Surg. 57B, 401.

Young, J.L., Walker, D., Snyder, S., et al., 2014. Thoracic manipulation versus mobilization in patients with mechanical neck pain: a systematic review. J. Man. Manip. Ther. 22, 141–153.

Zusman, M., 1986. Spinal manipulative therapy: review of some proposed mechanisms, and a new hypothesis. Australian Journal of Physiotherapy 32, 89–99.

4

FUNCTION AND DYSFUNCTION OF MUSCLE AND TENDON

PAUL COMFORT ▪ LEE HERRINGTON

CHAPTER CONTENTS

The function of the neuromusculoskeletal system is to produce movement and this is dependent on optimal functioning of each component – muscles, tendons, joints and nerves (Fig. 4.1) – which was originally devised to describe the stability of the spine (Panjabi 1992) but is applicable to the function of the whole neuromusculoskeletal system. This interrelationship has been described in relation to the knee as 'a complex systematic sensory–motor synergy, which includes the ligaments, antagonistic muscle pairs (flexors and extensors), bones, and sensory mechanoreceptors in the ligaments, joint capsule, and associated muscles' (Solomonow et al. 1987). Once again, this description could equally be applied to the entire neuromusculoskeletal system. Therefore, although this chapter is concerned with the function of muscle, it is important to stress that muscles do not function in isolation but in a highly interdependent way with joints and nerves. For a muscle to function normally there must be normal functioning of the relevant joints and nerves.

Muscles contribute to the stability of a joint by contributing to joint stiffness. In the human knee, antagonistic actions of the quadriceps and the hamstring muscles can substantially increase joint stiffness (Louie & Mote 1987; Zhang et al. 1998), with increases of 200–300% for quadriceps and 100–250% for hamstrings (Louie & Mote 1987). Additionally, it has been estimated that co-contraction of the quadriceps and hamstring muscle groups can reduce knee joint laxity by about 70% (Louie & Mote 1987). As the hamstring muscles are an agonist for the anterior cruciate ligament (ACL), co-contraction of the hamstrings can reduce the strain on the ACL (Renstrom et al. 1986). Antagonistic quadriceps and hamstring muscle actions enhance joint stability.

Muscle also enhances joint stability during joint movement (McGill & Norman 1986; Hortobagyi & DeVita 2000). For example, in the upper limb, isometric action of the elbow flexors or extensors at 45, 90 and 135° elbow flexion is coupled with activity in the

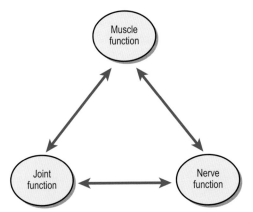

FIG. 4.1 ■ Interdependence of the function of muscle, joint and nerve for normal movement. Normal function of the neuromusculoskeletal system requires normal function of muscle, joint and nerve. *(After Panjabi 1992, with permission.)*

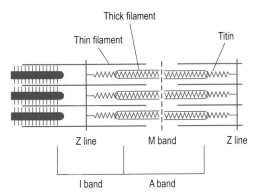

FIG. 4.2 ■ The basic contractile unit of muscle, the sarcomere, formed by thin actin and thick myosin filaments. *(From Herzog & Gal 1999, with permission.)*

antagonistic triceps or biceps muscle, which varies with joint angle; and the pattern of activity of the antagonistic muscle suggests that it regulates the joint torque, thus enhancing elbow joint stability (Solomonow et al. 1986). In the lumbar spine, during flexion and extension movements, muscles have been shown to affect segmental stability (Panjabi et al. 1989; Wilke et al. 1995). The posterior layer of thoracolumbar fascia is considered to act as an accessory ligament, helping to stabilize the lumbar spine during movement (Bogduk & MacIntosh 1984).

SKELETAL MUSCLE FUNCTION

The following aspects of joint function will be considered:

- anatomy, biomechanics and physiology of muscle
- nerve supply of muscle
- muscle action
- muscle strength, power, endurance and motor control and muscle length
- simple classification of muscle.

Anatomy, Biomechanics and Physiology of Muscle

Muscle constitutes approximately 40% of total body weight and is regarded as 'the most efficient and adaptable *machine* known to man'. A muscle (that is, muscle

and its tendons) can be divided grossly into contractile tissue and non-contractile tissue. The non-contractile tissue includes the connective tissue layers within muscle and the tendons.

Contractile Tissue of Muscle

The smallest unit of muscle is the myofibril, made up of thin actin and thick myosin filaments, giving a striated appearance under the microscope (Fig. 4.2). The myosin filaments produce the dark A band, and the actin filaments produce the light I band. In addition, elastic titin filaments lie between the myosin filaments. The titin filaments act like a spring, with increased tension when the sarcomere is lengthened, thus enabling it to return to its resting length when the tension is removed; this is also thought to keep the myosin in the centre of the sarcomere when there is an asymmetrical pull (Horowits et al. 1989). The Z line demarcates the sarcomere, which is the basic contractile unit of muscle.

Individual muscle fibres (or cells) are covered in a membrane called the sarcolemma and by a connective tissue sheath called the endomysium (Fig. 4.3). The individual muscle fibres are collected into bundles (or fascicles) by a connective tissue sheath called the perimysium. Numbers of muscle bundles constitute the muscle and are surrounded by a connective tissue sheath called the epimysium and by an outer layer of fascia. These muscle fibres are known as extrafusal fibres, compared with intrafusal fibres, which lie within the muscle spindle (discussed later under nerve supply).

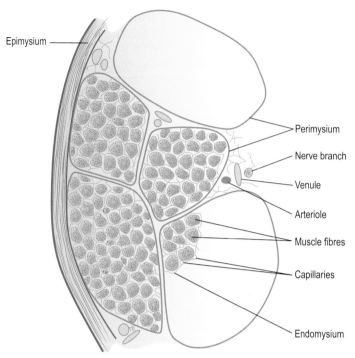

Epimysium

Perimysium

Nerve branch

Venule

Arteriole

Muscle fibres

Capillaries

Endomysium

FIG. 4.3 ■ Schematic illustration of the cross-sectional structure of muscle. *(From McComas 1996, with permission.)*

Non-Contractile Tissue of Muscle

Connective tissue is found in layers within the muscle and tendons and consists of collagen fibres, and some elastin fibres. The elastin fibres enable muscle to regain its shape, following both shortening and lengthening. Connective tissue makes up 30% of muscle mass (Alter 1996) and is vital for normal muscle function.

Connective tissue forms a sheath around each muscle fibre (endomysium), around bundles of muscle fibres (perimysium) and around the whole muscle (epimysium), as shown in Fig. 4.3. The connective tissue, along with the nerves and blood vessels, forms the non-contractile element of the muscle belly. The outer layer of connective tissue enables identification of particular muscles, for example, semitendinosus muscle in the thigh, and allows sliding of muscle on adjacent tissues, for example, movement of semitendinosus on the biceps femoris and the sciatic nerve. The perimysium around a bundle of muscle fibres provides a channel for blood vessels and nerves. The endomysium, perimysium and epimysium join to form the tendon or aponeurosis that attaches the muscle to bone.

Connective tissue is also the major constituent of fascia, which is divided into superficial and deep. Superficial fascia lies just below the skin and allows skin movement; it is thick on the plantar aspect of the hands and thin on the dorsum of the hands and feet. Deep fascia acts as retinacula, intermuscular septa, intermuscular aponeurosis and attachment for muscle. In the thoracic and abdominal cavities deep fascia covers and supports the viscera, for example, the pleura, pericardium and peritoneum. The flexor and extensor retinacula of the wrist and foot are deep fascia arranged as a transverse thickening to retain tendons deep to it. The intermuscular septa pass between groups of muscles and attach to bone. Muscles can take attachment from the intermuscular septa, which may then be better named intermuscular aponeurosis, for example, the rectal sheath. The deep fascia can be a point of attachment for muscle to bone and from muscle to muscle. For example, the tensor fasciae latae and gluteus maximus attach to the iliotibial tract (fascia), which then passes down the leg and attaches to the tibia. Deep fascia in the lower leg connects the peroneus longus to the biceps femoris, and, in the upper arm, pectoralis minor to the short head of biceps.

Musculotendinous (or Myotendinous) Junction

This is the junction between the muscle and the tendon. The contact area is characterized by the muscle cells forming finger-like projections in which the collagen fibres of the tendon insert (Fig. 4.4). This arrangement increases the surface area of the contact region and so reduces the tensile force applied to the tissue (Kvist et al. 1991). Interestingly, this is reflected in differences in surface area between type I and type II muscle fibres. The area is greater for type II fibres, which are involved in powerful voluntary movements, than for type I fibres, which generate lower forces and are largely involved in postural control (Kvist et al. 1991). Despite this arrangement, the region is the weakest part of the tendon–muscle unit and is susceptible to strain injuries (Garrett 1990; Tidball 1991).

Osteotendinous Junctions

This is where tendon attaches to bone. Tendons usually attach directly to bone, that is, there is an abrupt, well-defined area of attachment with a clear demarcation of tendon and bone; examples include supraspinatus, where it attaches to the superior facet on the greater tuberosity of the humerus, and the medial collateral ligament to the medial condyle of the femur (Woo et al. 1988). Tendons with direct attachments have a superficial layer which blends with periosteum, and a larger deep layer which inserts directly into bone via a thin layer of fibrocartilage (Woo et al. 1988). Sometimes tendons attach indirectly, such that there is a more gradual and less distinct area of attachment; the superficial layer in this case provides the predominant attachment, blending with the periosteum and bone via Sharpey's fibres, while the deep layer attaches directly to the bone (Woo et al. 1988).

Tendons

Tendons are designed to transmit high tensile force from muscle to bone. They are made up of approximately 70% of longitudinally arranged collagen tissue, with some elastin tissue (Hess et al. 1989) and are therefore flexible, relatively inextensible and able to withstand large tensile forces (Jozsa & Kannus 1997). They have a sparse blood supply, with this avascular nature decreasing the rate of adaptation and increasing the timescales for rehabilitation.

Tendons sometimes contain a sesamoid bone which increases the mechanical advantage of the muscle and decreases friction between adjacent tissues. They are

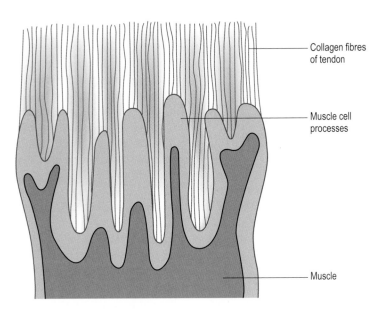

Collagen fibres of tendon

Muscle cell processes

Muscle

FIG. 4.4 ■ Schematic figure of musculotendinous junction. *(After Jozsa & Kannus 1997, with permission.)*

covered with hyaline cartilage. Examples include the pisiform bone within the flexor carpi ulnaris tendon, the patella within the quadriceps tendon and the sesamoid bone within the flexor hallucis brevis tendon. The existence and shape of sesamoid bones vary between individuals (McBryde & Anderson 1988).

During a concentric action of a muscle, tendon moves on adjacent tissue; the frictional resistance to this movement is minimized by bursae and sheaths which can be classified as fibrous, synovial and paratenon sheaths.

- A bursa may lie adjacent to tendon to aid gliding movement of the tendon on adjacent tissue.
- A fibrous sheath may surround a tendon, as in the tendons around the ankle. Bony grooves and notches contain a layer of fibrocartilage, and superficially the tendon is held in place by retinaculum.
- A synovial sheath may surround a tendon where ease of movement with adjacent tissue is of paramount importance, as in the tendons of the hands and feet. Synovial sheaths are composed of an outer fibrotic sheath and an inner synovial sheath. A thin film of synovial fluid, rich in hyaluronic acid, fills the space between the sheaths and acts as a lubricant reducing frictional resistance (Jozsa & Kannus 1997).
- A paratenon sheath (or peritendinous sheet) may surround a tendon – for example, the tendocalcaneus tendon. The paratenon is made up of collagen fibres, elastic fibrils and synovial cells, and acts as an elastic sleeve, facilitating movement between the tendon and its surrounding tissues (Hess et al. 1989; Jozsa & Kannus 1997). The paratenon and epitenon are sometimes referred to as the peritendon.

Tendon tissue is plastic and will alter its composition and construction according to the physical demands placed upon it (Pearson & Hussain 2014). For example, with exercise, there is an increase in tendon thickness and strength (Brumitt & Cuddeford 2015). The stimulus for tendon growth is the tension that is applied and is therefore correlated with the strength of the muscle (Muraoka et al. 2005).

Tendons have viscoelastic properties; the load–displacement curve for a tendon is shown in Fig. 4.5.

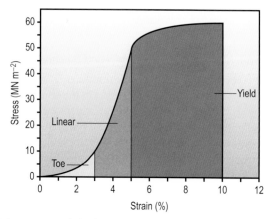

FIG. 4.5 ■ Load–displacement (stress–strain) curve for tendon. *(From Herzog & Gal 2007, with permission.)*

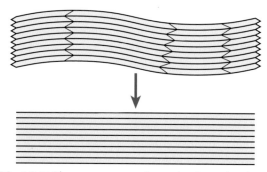

FIG. 4.6 ■ The wavy pattern of a tendon in a relaxed state straightens out when it is stretched. *(From Jozsa & Kannus 1997, with permission.)*

The toe region is concave and is considered to reflect the straightening of the wavy collagen fibres shown in Fig. 4.6 (Hirsch 1974). Little force is required to lengthen the tendon in this region. This region is considered to be responsible for the ability of tendon to absorb shock (T.O. Wood et al. 1988). With continued lengthening, the wave pattern straightens and the tendon behaves like a stiff spring; this occurs with about 3% elongation (Herzog & Gal 2007). As the force increases, there is an increase in the stiffness of the tendon, producing the linear part of the curve; this occurs at about 4% elongation (Wainwright et al. 1982). Both toe and linear regions are temporary and, on removal of the force, the tendon will return to its resting length. During normal everyday activities, tensile forces on tendon are thought to lie within the toe and linear region and are thought to be less than 4% strain (Fung 1993). If the force continues to elongate beyond this there is a permanent deformation in the yield region of the curve, up to a maximum of approximately 8–15% elongation, where failure occurs (Fung 1993). During the yield region, a relatively small increase in force will produce a relatively large increase in displacement. The stiffness of tendon is not the same throughout its length (Kolz et al. 2015). Tendon is stiffest in the middle of its length and least stiff at its insertion, so when a tendon is lengthened there is greatest displacement at the insertion region (Woo et al. 1988; Kolz et al. 2015).

Blood Supply of Tendon. Tendons receive their blood supply at the osteotendinous junction, from vessels within bone and periosteum. At the musculotendinous junction tendon receives blood from vessels within muscle and from the surrounding vessels within the paratenon, mesotenon and synovial sheath. The blood supply at the osteotendinous junction is fairly sparse and is limited to where the tendon attaches to bone. Blood vessels are present only in the distal third of the tendon (Jozsa & Kannus 1997).

Biomechanics of the Muscle–Tendon Unit

It is useful to consider the biomechanical behaviour of the muscle–tendon unit as a single unit. The strength of the muscle–tendon unit with respect to tensile loading can be depicted on a force–displacement curve (Fig. 4.7); this curve was obtained from the whole tibialis anterior muscle–tendon unit of a rabbit (Taylor et al. 1990). Force is plotted against the stretch or deformation. The slope of the curve is the modulus of elasticity, measured in Pa or N/m², and is a measure of the 'stiffness' of the muscle–tendon unit (Panjabi & White 2001). Only a little force is initially required to deform the muscle–tendon unit, a region referred to as the 'toe' region (Threlkeld 1992) or 'neutral zone' (Panjabi & White 2001). Stiffness then increases, so that greater force is required to deform the muscle–tendon unit; this region is referred to as the elastic zone. Forces within the elastic zone will result in no permanent change in length; as soon as the force is released the muscle–tendon unit will return to its preload shape and size (Panjabi & White 2001). The neutral zone and elastic zone fall within the normal physiological range of forces and deformation on the muscle–tendon unit during everyday activities (Nordin & Frankel 1989). The strength of a muscle or tendon is measured by stress (force per unit area, measured in Pa or N/m²) and strain (percentage change in length, from the resting length). The stress–strain properties of muscle and tendon are compared with those of bone, cartilage, ligament and nerve in Table 4.1. The ability of muscle to resist lengthening reduces with age (Panjabi & White 2001).

The muscle–tendon unit will elongate on loading and is dependent on the rate of loading. When the muscle–tendon unit of tibialis anterior is loaded quickly it will be stiffer and deform less than when it is loaded more slowly (Fig. 4.8). This is relevant when applying therapeutic force, as a slower rate will result in less resistance and more movement. An additional effect is that the failure point of the muscle–tendon unit will be higher with a higher loading rate; in other words, it will be stronger and less likely to rupture when the force is applied at a faster rate.

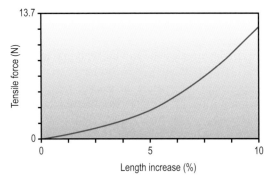

FIG. 4.7 ■ Force-displacement curve of the muscle-tendon unit. (*After Taylor et al. 1990, with permission.*)

TABLE 4.1		
Tensile Properties of Muscle and Tendon Compared With Bone, Cartilage, Ligament and Nerve (Panjabi & White 2001)		
Tissue	**Stress at Failure (MPa)**	**Strain at Failure (%)**
Muscle (passive)	0.17	60
Tendon	55	9–10
Cortical bone	100–200	1–3
Cancellous bone	10	5–7
Cartilage	10–15	80–120
Ligament	10–40	30–45
Nerve roots	15	19

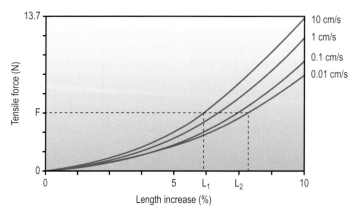

FIG. 4.8 ▪ The muscle–tendon unit and rate of loading. When it is loaded quickly it will be stiffer and will sustain a higher force before breaking than when it is loaded more slowly. For example, a given force, if applied at 10 cm/s, will cause a displacement L_1, but if applied more slowly, at 0.01 cm/s, will cause a greater displacement to L_2. These data are from the tibialis anterior muscle–tendon unit from New Zealand white rabbits. *(After Taylor et al. 1990, with permission.)*

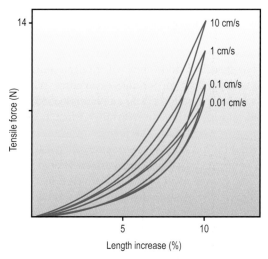

FIG. 4.9 ▪ The muscle–tendon unit demonstrates the phenomenon of hysteresis. The graph was produced from the tibialis anterior muscle–tendon unit of New Zealand white rabbits. The loading rate used was 0.01, 0.1, 1 and 10 cm/s. *(From Taylor et al. 1990, with permission.)*

The muscle–tendon unit demonstrates the phenomenon of hysteresis, which is the energy loss during loading and unloading (Fig. 4.9) (Taylor et al. 1990). The unloading curve lies below the loading curve and reflects a greater energy expenditure on loading than the energy regained during unloading. In contrast, the muscle belly is less stiff than the tendon, so when a muscle is passively lengthened most of the length change

TABLE 4.2			
Classification of Muscle Fibre Types (Staron 1997; Scott et al. 2001)			
Myosin ATPase	**Myosin ATPase Hydrolysis Rate**	**Myosin Heavy Chain (MHC)**	**Biochemical Identification of Metabolic Enzymes**
I	I	MHCI	Slow-twitch oxidative
	IC	MHCI and MHCIIa	
	IIC	MHCI and MHCIIa	
	IIAC	MHCI and MHCIIa	
IIA	IIA	MHCIIa	? Fast-twitch oxidative[a]
	IIAB	MHCIIa and MHCIIb	
IIB	IIB	MHCIIb	? Fast-twitch glycolytic[a]

[a]The question mark beside fast-twitch oxidative and fast-twitch glycolytic indicates that muscle fibre types IIA and IIB do not always rely on aerobic/oxidative and anaerobic/glycolytic metabolism (McComas 1996).

occurs in the muscle belly and the tendon is minimally affected (Jami 1992). In fact the primary aim of stretching is to lengthen/elongate the muscle to increase the range of motion around the joint and not to lengthen the tendons.

Types of Muscle Fibre

Muscle fibres can be classified in various ways (Table 4.2). Initially, muscle fibres were described according to the speed of shortening and were identified by staining for myoglobin concentration (myoglobin binds oxygen). Muscles were divided into: (1) slow muscles (type I), which stained red owing to a high concentration of myoglobin enabling aerobic energy metabolism, and (2) fast muscles (type II), which stained white owing to a low concentration of myoglobin enabling anaerobic energy metabolism (Pette & Staron 1990). Fast-twitch fibres (type II) contract more quickly, generate higher forces but fatigue more quickly than slow-twitch (type I) fibres (Table 4.3).

An alternative classification system identified type I and type II myofibrillar actomyosin adenosine triphosphate (ATP) which related to different contractile properties (Pette & Staron 1990). When this classification was combined with the myoglobin classification a metabolic enzyme-based classification was developed (Table 4.2). This classification describes three types of muscle fibre: slow-twitch oxidative (SO), fast-twitch oxidative (FOG) and fast-twitch glycolytic (FG) (Pette & Staron 1990; McComas 1996). Fibres that fall between slow-twitch (type I) and fast-twitch (type IIb) are termed intermediate (type IIa) (Pette et al. 1999), but adapt due to activity to become more like either the FG or

SO fibres dependent on the nature of the activity. The characteristics of these types of muscle fibre are summarized in Table 4.3.

Although it is convenient to classify muscle fibres into three types, the reality is more of a continuum between fast-twitch and slow-twitch muscles. A third type of fast fibre has since been identified and is known as IID or IIX (Pette et al. 1999). In terms of training the fibre types, prolonged aerobic exercise primarily recruits the SO fibres whereas near-maximal efforts (e.g. strength/power training) primarily recruit the FG fibres, resulting in specific adaptations in these specific fibres. In contrast, regular aerobic or anaerobic training can result in adaptation of the FOG fibres to adapt to resemble either the SO or FG fibres, respectively.

For any one motor unit, the characteristic of the muscle fibre type is mirrored by the motor nerve supply (Box 4.1). All muscle fibres that are innervated by the same motor neuron are of the same type; that is, the conduction rate of a motor neuron innervating fast-twitch fibres is faster than that for slow-twitch fibres. The motor neuron determines the characteristic of a muscle fibre and is described as a phasic or tonic motor neurone. Large, phasic high-threshold motor neurons discharge at the high frequency of 30–60/second compared with small, tonic low-threshold motor neurons, with a lower frequency of 10–20/second. The

TABLE 4.3

Characteristics of Skeletal Muscle and Motor Neurones (Newham & Ainscough-Potts 2001)

Characteristic	Type I	Type IIa	Type IIb
Muscle fibre type	Slow oxidative (SO)	Fast oxidative glycolytic (FOG)	Fast glycolytic (FG)
Motor unit type	Slow	Fast fatigue-resistant	Fast fatigable
Motor unit size	Small	Medium	Large
Conduction rate of motor neuron	Slow	Fast	Fast
Twitch tension	Low	Moderate	High
Speed of contraction	Slow	Fast	Fast
Resistance to fatigue	High	High	Low
Mitochondrial enzyme activity	High	Medium	Low
Myoglobin content	High	Medium	Low
Capillary density	High	Medium	Low

BOX 4.1

CHARACTERISTICS OF MOTOR NEURON AND MUSCLE FIBRE TYPE (NEWHAM & AINSCOUGH-POTTS 2001)

Nerve
Large motor neuron
Phasic
High threshold
High frequency

Muscle Fibres
Fast-twitch
Type IIa – fast oxidative glycolytic
Type IIb – fast glycolytic
Large motor unit supplies 300–800 muscle fibres

Nerve
Small motor neuron
Tonic
Low threshold
Low frequency

Muscle Fibres
Slow-twitch
Type I – slow-twitch oxidative
Small motor unit supplies 12–180 muscle fibres

nerve is so influential on muscle fibre type that, if the motor neurons to fast- and slow-twitch fibres are experimentally switched, the muscle fibre types will also switch characteristics (Lomo et al. 1980).

Smaller motor units tend to be composed of slow-twitch muscle fibres and larger motor units composed of fast-twitch fibres. The motor neuron of a slow-twitch motor unit innervates 12–180 muscle fibres compared with 300–800 muscle fibres of a fast-twitch motor unit. The lower number of slow-twitch muscle fibres supplied by a motor neuron enables greater control of muscular action. The fact that any one muscle contains both small and large motor units providing fine control of muscle actions, as well as greater velocity and force of muscle actions, attests to the multiplicity of muscle functions, and it is an oversimplification to define individual muscles as specifically FG or SO twitch, as they will adapt to the environmental-training stresses applied to them.

Nerve Supply of Muscles

Sensory nerve endings in the muscle–tendon units include muscle spindles, Golgi tendon organs and free nerve endings. Large-diameter myelinated group Ia and II fibres supply the muscle spindles, slightly smaller myelinated IIb fibres supply Golgi tendon organs and fine myelinated Aδ (or group III fibres) and unmyelinated C (or group IV) fibres supply the free nerve endings.

Muscle Spindles

Muscle spindles are proprioceptors acting as stretch receptors monitoring the length (or tension) and rate of change in length of muscle. They are sensitive to length changes and also affected by the rate of the length change of the muscle fascicles. The greater the rate of change in length or the greater the magnitude of change in length, the greater the resultant stimulus via the stretch reflex.

Muscle spindles lie within the muscle belly, parallel to extrafusal fibres, and near the musculotendinous junction (Boyd 1976). The muscle spindle consists of intrafusal fibres to distinguish it from the rest of muscle which, in turn, consists of a non-contractile central portion within a capsule with contractile ends. When a muscle is progressively stretched at a constant velocity, the primary endings initially have a burst of activity,

with the rate of activity depending on the velocity of the stretch; increased velocity results in an increased rate of activity (Hunt 1990). Therefore maintaining a low velocity while progressively increasing range of motion during a stretch results in lower stimulation of the muscle spindle and less muscle activation, resulting in a greater range of motion. If the lengthened muscle is then maintained at its new length, there is a reduction in the rate of discharge and the perceived tension in the muscle will reduce. While the lengthened muscle is maintained at its new length the fibres within the muscle spindle exhibit creep, that is, they lengthen (Boyd 1976). The discharge rate from the secondary group II fibres increases with a maintained position, and so they appear to act as position detectors (Hunt 1990). Because the intrafusal fibres lie parallel to the extrafusal fibres, the discharge from the sensory fibres in the muscle spindle diminishes or ceases when the muscle contracts and increases when the muscle is lengthened (Hunt 1990). Stretch of the muscle spindle causes excitation of the alpha motor neurons, leading to contraction of the extrafusal muscle fibres in which the spindle is situated, and inhibition of the antagonistic muscles. This phenomenon is known as the stretch reflex (Fig. 4.10). Muscle spindles protect and limit the muscle from excessive lengthening. Clearly, this is a useful protective mechanism to regulate movement and maintain posture (Hunt 1990).

Where a muscle becomes shortened, treatment may be directed to lengthen it (developmental stretching); slow movements to lengthen a muscle are therefore more effective as they minimize this protective response. In contrast the stimulation of the muscle spindle and the elastic energy from the tendons and fascia aid in the efficiency of movement during activities which utilize the stretch shortening cycle, such as running and jumping.

Summary of the Muscle Spindle. Stimulation of the muscle spindle is highly sensitive to the rate of change in length and therefore when stretching muscles and mobilizing joints movements should be slow to minimize the stimulation of this reflex. In contrast, during jump/plyometric training, the eccentric phase (countermovement) should be rapid to maximize stimulation of the stretch shortening cycle, which results in improved performance in such tasks.

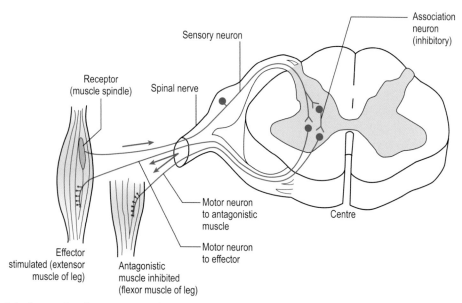

FIG. 4.10 ■ Spindle stretch reflex. Excitation of the muscle spindle causes a reflex contraction of the muscle in which the spindle lies and inhibition of the antagonistic muscle. *(From Crow & Haas 2001, with permission.)*

Golgi Tendon Organs

Golgi tendon organs lie in the musculotendinous junctions, between the fascicles and the collagen strands forming the tendons and aponeurosis; they are rarely found, as their name implies, in the tendon itself (Jami 1992). They are encapsulated corpuscles containing collagen fibres, lying in series with 15–20 muscle fibres and stimulated only by the tension in these muscle fibres in series (Shumway-Cook & Woollacott 1995) (Fig. 4.11). They are proprioceptors, sensitive to changes in tension within the musculotendinous junction and to the rate of change in tension (Houk & Henneman 1967). Golgi tendon organs can be stimulated by passive lengthening of the muscle–tendon unit; however, the threshold for discharge is very high and rarely persists with a maintained muscle stretch (Jami 1992). Each is innervated by a large fast-conducting Ib afferent fibre, with the rate of firing from the Golgi tendon organ proportional to the muscle tension (Crow & Haas 2001). When the muscle fibres contract there is a lengthening of the musculotendinous junction and collagen fibres within the Golgi tendon organ; this compresses the nerve terminals and causes firing of the Ib afferent fibre.

Stimulation of Golgi tendon organs leads to inhibition of the muscle in which they are situated (inhibition of both alpha and gamma motor neurons), a mechanism known as autogenic inhibition, and excitation of the antagonist muscles (Fig. 4.12) (Chalmers 2002, 2004). So, for example, when jumping off an object and landing, the muscles of the lower limbs perform an eccentric action to decelerate the individual; however, if the object was too high and the resultant impact causes excessive force that may damage the musculotendinous junction, the Golgi tendon organs will be stimulated, producing inhibition of the agonist muscles and stimulation of the antagonist. This is a protective mechanism to avoid injury to the musculotendinous junction, even though in the example above the landing would be 'poor'. However, this mechanism is not seen during competitive sport – for example, wrist wrestling can result in ruptured muscles and tendons. In this case the highly motivated athlete disinhibits the process (Brooks & Fahey 1987).

Summary of the Golgi Tendon Organ. Stimulation of the Golgi tendon organ may be advantageous during stretching (contract, relax agonist contract proprioceptive

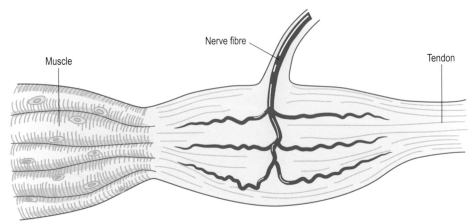

FIG. 4.11 ■ Golgi tendon organ in series with 15–20 muscle fibres. *(From Shumway-Cook & Woollacott 1995, with permission.)*

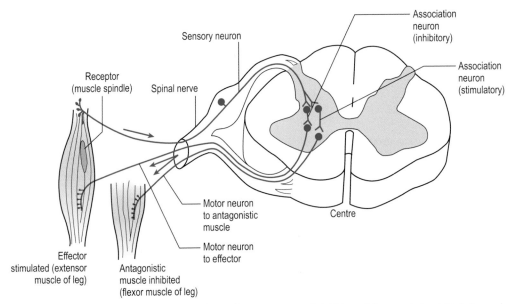

FIG. 4.12 ■ The tendon reflex: stimulation of the Golgi tendon organ causes inhibition of the muscle in which it lies and excitation of the antagonistic muscle. *(From Crow & Haas 2001, with permission.)*

neuromuscular facilitation) as it results in inhibition of the muscle that is being lengthened (Chalmers 2004).

Free Nerve Endings

Free nerve endings lie throughout the muscle, in the connective tissue, between intrafusal and extrafusal fibres, in arterioles and venules, in the capsule of muscle spindles and tendon organs, in tendon tissue at the musculotendinous junction and in fat cells (Reinert & Mense 1992). This is summarized in Box 4.2. Free nerve endings are supplied by myelinated Aδ (group III) and unmyelinated C (group IV) fibres.

Type III afferents act as low-threshold mechanical pressure receptors, contraction-sensitive receptors and nociceptors (Mense & Meyer 1985). Most type IV afferents are mainly nociceptors (to both noxious mechanical and chemical stimulation), with a smaller proportion being low-threshold mechanical pressure receptors, contraction-sensitive receptors and thermo-receptors (Mense & Meyer 1985).

Mechanoreceptors

Mechanoreceptors respond to pressure, active muscle shortening (concentric action) and muscle lengthening (eccentric action). The majority of group III fibres respond to local pressure stimulation (Kaufman et al. 1984a), while very few of the group IV fibres respond to low-threshold innocuous pressure (Franz & Mense 1975).

Group III and IV fibres are activated in a linear fashion to the force of a muscle contraction or the force of a stretch on a muscle (Mense & Stahnke 1983; Mense & Meyer 1985) – the greater the force, the greater the response. Approximately half of the afferents respond to both contraction and lengthening, and half are specific to one or other stimulus (Mense & Meyer 1985).

Afferents responsive to active contraction are often also chemical receptors responsive to bradykinin (Mense & Meyer 1985), a chemical released with inflammation. Group III afferents appear to be stimulated by the mechanical effects of the contraction, whereas group IV receptors seem to be stimulated by the metabolic products produced by muscle actions (Kaufman et al. 1982, 1983).

Chemical Receptors

Some free nerve endings are sensitive to muscle pH, concentrations of extracellular potassium and sodium chloride and changes in oxygen and carbon dioxide. They help to regulate the cardiopulmonary system during exercise or activity (Laughlin & Korthuis 1987). Group IV afferents in muscle are thought to be primarily responsible for producing the reflex changes in cardiorespiratory function with exercise (Kaufman et al. 1982, 1983). Other group IV afferents are activated in the presence of chemicals released with inflammation (Mense 1981; Kaufman et al. 1982). Chemically induced muscle pain in humans is thought to be due to activation of these free nerve endings (Mense 1996).

Thermal Receptors

Some group IV receptors respond to small changes of temperature in muscle (Mense 1996). Others have been identified to have a high threshold for thermal stimulation and are thus thermal nociceptors (Mense & Meyer 1985). A high proportion of thermoreceptors have also been found to be sensitive to noxious mechanical pressure (Mense & Meyer 1985).

Nociceptors

Muscle nociceptors have a high mechanical threshold and some also have a high thermal threshold. The vast majority of group IV afferents in the cat have been found to be high-threshold mechanoreceptors and thus are thought to be nociceptors (Franz & Mense 1975). It is also thought that group III muscle afferents may be capable of acting as nociceptors and thus mediating pain. Bradykinin, a chemical released with inflammation, has been found to sensitize muscle and tendon nociceptors (Mense & Meyer 1985). This sensitization lowers the firing threshold such that an innocuous mechanical stimulus, for example, movement or a light touch, causes excitation, a phenomenon known as allodynia (Raja et al. 1999).

Efferent Nerve Fibres

Generally, the efferent fibres to muscle consist of the large myelinated alpha motor neurones that supply the extrafusal fibres, and the small myelinated gamma (or fusimotor) fibres that supply the intrafusal fibres within the muscle spindle. Type I muscle fibres are innervated by small, low-threshold, slowly conducting motor nerves while type IIb fibres are innervated by large, higher-threshold, fast-conducting motor nerves.

The efferent fibres enter the muscle around the centre of the muscle belly, a region known as the motor point. Motor nerves divide into small branches to supply each muscle fibre; the presynaptic terminal synapses at the neuromuscular junction with the motor end-plate (Fig. 4.13). When an action potential arrives at the presynaptic terminal, a chain of chemical reactions is initiated which causes diffusion of acetylcholine across the synaptic cleft to the postsynaptic membrane. This chemical causes an increase in the permeability of sodium ions which, if sufficient, will initiate an action potential along the muscle fibre.

Each muscle fibre is supplied by a motor neuron. The motor neuron, and the muscle fibres it innervates, is termed a motor unit and is the functional unit of a muscle. Stimulation of the motor neuron initiates and maintains a series of complex events leading to either shortening (concentric contraction) or active lengthening (eccentric contraction) of muscle, and the development of muscle tension. Muscle contraction ceases when the stimulation of the motor nerve stops.

Muscle actions occur via the sliding of myosin and actin filaments so that the length of the sarcomere is shortened (during a concentric muscle action); this is termed the sliding filament theory (Fig. 4.14). Myosin contains proteins that extend towards the actin filaments, in the form of a tail and a head. The head contains a binding site for actin (Fig. 4.15) and forms the cross-bridge between myosin and actin. The reader is directed to a physiology textbook for a more detailed description of the sliding filament theory.

Muscle and Proprioception

Several lines of research support the view that muscle has an important proprioceptive function (Grigg 1994). Isolated movement of a tendon, so as to stretch its muscle, gives a sensation of joint movement (Matthews & Simmonds 1974). In the human hand, it has been found that isolated stimulation of individual spindle afferents is insufficient to cause a perception of joint movement. However, the spatial summation of a number of muscle spindles provides sufficient information for proprioception (Macefield et al. 1990).

In addition, vibration of muscle produces a sensation of joint movement and a sense of joint position (Goodwin et al. 1972). The movement is in the direction that would stretch the muscle being vibrated, so it is the muscle being stretched that provides a sense of joint movement. For example, on elbow extension the elbow flexor muscles will be stretched and give a sense of the extension movement. Because muscle spindles are more sensitive to vibration than Golgi tendon organs, it is thought that the illusion of movement is produced by stimulation of the muscle spindles (Goodwin et al. 1972). Further evidence comes from the fact that, if muscle afferent activity is abolished during joint movement, proprioception is less accurate (Gandevia et al. 1983) and, conversely, when skin and joint receptor activity is abolished, the sense of proprioception remains, albeit poor (Moberg 1983). Additionally, increased tension in a muscle increases the sensitivity of muscle spindles, and increased muscle tension has

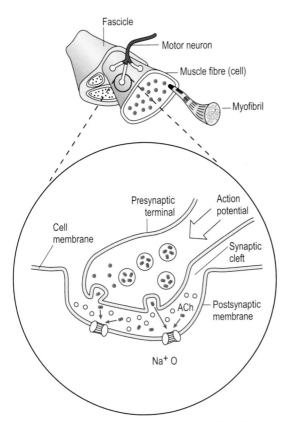

FIG. 4.13 ■ Neuromuscular junction formed by the motor nerve and the motor end-plate. *ACh*, acetylcholine. *(After Herzog 1999, with permission.)*

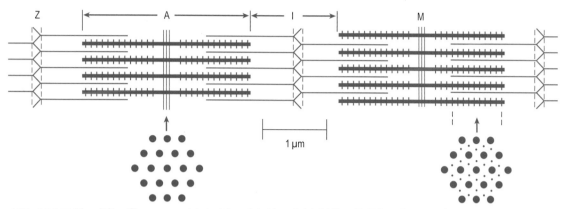

FIG. 4.14 ■ The sliding filament model. A, A band; I, I band; M, M line; Z, Z line. *(From Huxley 2000, with permission.)*

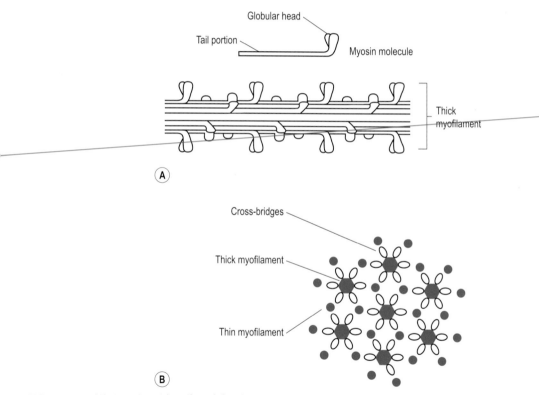

FIG. 4.15 ■ (A) Myosin with tail and head projecting towards the actin filaments. *(From Herzog 1999, with permission.)* (B) Cross-sectional arrangement of actin and myosin. *(After Herzog 1999, with permission.)*

been found to enhance proprioception (Macefield et al. 1990).

The nerve supply to the skin is also relevant as this will be involved in any movement caused by muscle contraction; details of skin sensation can be found under nerve function in Chapter 6.

Muscle Strength

The force of a muscle action depends on the following factors:

1. The type and number of motor units recruited. The recruitment of muscle fibres is directly related

to the size of the motor neuron (Milner-Brown et al. 1973). There is an initial recruitment of small motor neurons and then recruitment of large motor neurons as more force is required (Henneman & Olson 1965; Henneman et al. 1965). This has been referred to as the Henneman size principle, where small motor units (type I) are recruited first and then large motor units (type II). There is a higher predominance of type I muscle fibres in postural muscles, therefore these muscles fire first to provide stability in preparation for movement. The greater the stimulus, the greater the number of muscle fibres stimulated and the greater the strength of the muscle action. The fact that all muscles contain both type I and II muscle fibres enables graded levels of muscle contraction to occur.

2. The initial length of the muscle. The resting length of a muscle fibre affects its strength of contraction. The optimal length is where there is maximum overlap between actin and myosin. Where a muscle fibre is less or more than the optimal length, fewer cross-bridges between actin and myosin are formed and the tension is lessened. This phenomenon produces a length–tension relationship in muscle which can be depicted on a graph (Fig. 4.16). When a single muscle fibre is lengthened there is an uneven lengthening such that the central portion of the muscle fibre lengthens more than the ends of the muscle; so while there is a reduction in the cross-bridges in the central portion there are still cross-bridges at the ends (Huxley 2000).

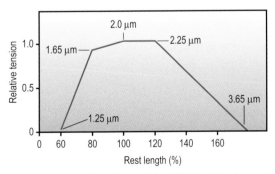

FIG. 4.16 ■ Length–tension relationship in skeletal muscle. *(From Fox 1987, with permission.)*

3. The nature of the neural stimulation of the motor unit. The frequency of the neural stimulation affects the force of the muscular action. A single neural stimulus will result in a muscle twitch. A muscle twitch consists of a brief latent period, then a muscle contraction and then a relaxation period. The total time this takes varies between 10 and 100 ms (Ghez 1991). The force of the action and the total time will depend on the type of muscle fibre, with fast-twitch fibres contracting more quickly, and with more force, than slow-twitch fibres. If a series of neural stimuli are used (1–3 ms apart) (Ghez 1991), the muscle has not had time to relax and so an increase in muscle tension is produced due to the summation of each twitch. If the frequency of the neural stimuli is increased still further, individual contractions are blended together in a single sustained contraction known as fused tetanus (Ghez 1991). This action will continue until the neural stimulus is stopped or the muscle fatigues.

4. Muscle architecture. Architectural properties of skeletal muscle have been shown to affect both force and velocity of muscle actions. A decrease in pennation angle or an increase in fascicle length results in an increase in velocity of contraction due to an increased length of the contractile component (Blazevich 2006; Earp et al. 2010). In contrast, an increase in pennation angle results in an increase in the number of fibers for a given cross-sectional area, which increases force generation capacity (Blazevich 2006; Manal et al. 2006; Earp et al. 2010)

5. The age of the patient. A reduction in isokinetic (Gajdosik et al. 1996) and isometric strength with an increase in age (Grimby 1995; Heyley et al. 1998) have been reported; however this tends to be associated with a decreased level of activity and an associated atrophy (Pedrero-Chamizo et al. 2015). Between the fourth and seventh decades a progressive decline in isokinetic quadriceps strength of approximately 14% per decade appears to be the 'normal' rate of decline (Hughes et al. 2001; Piasecki et al. 2015). However, this decline in force production, which is generally associated with a decrease in cross-sectional area of the muscle, can easily be reduced with increased

activity levels, especially activities requiring high forces to be produced (Mayer et al. 2011; Bouchonville & Villareal 2013).

Muscle strength is proportional to the physiological cross-sectional area of the muscle, reflecting the number of sarcomeres in parallel (Aagaard et al. 2001; Seitz et al. 2016). The cross-sectional area of muscle has been found to reduce with age, although this is generally associated with reduced activity (reduced loading) and is somewhat reversible with appropriate activity (Mayer et al. 2011; Bouchonville & Villareal 2013). The quadriceps femoris cross-sectional area for 20-year-olds compared with 70-year-olds has been found to reduce by 27% men (Trappe et al. 2001) and by 35% in women (Young et al. 1982a).

Muscle Power

Internal muscle power is calculated from the force of contraction and the shortening velocity (force multiplied by velocity), with external power calculated as the force applied to the mass being accelerated, multiplied by the resultant velocity of the object at each specific time point. Muscle power is determined by the number of sarcomeres in series (muscle length), the angle of pennation of the muscle fibres (the more parallel to the direction of force, the greater the fascicle shortening velocity) during a concentric muscle action (de Brito Fontana et al. 2014; Hauraix et al. 2015). For a given muscular force, the fascicle shortening velocity and therefore the external movement velocity are greater in muscles that contain a higher percentage of fast-twitch fibres (Fig. 4.17). For both fast- and slow-twitch muscle fibres, the greatest force occurs at the lowest fascicle shortening velocities, with a progressive decline in force production as fascicle shortening velocity increases (Kojima 1991; Blazevich 2006). Fast-twitch fibres are capable of producing greater force at higher velocities than slow-twitch fibres; hence muscles with predominantly fast-twitch fibres can generate higher forces and greater power than muscles with predominantly slow-twitch fibres. It is worth noting that movement velocity is also related to neuromuscular coordination (Kerr 1998), including the coordination of the relaxation of antagonists. Muscle power reduces with age as a product of muscle atrophy and the aforementioned associated decline in force production capability (Gajdosik et al.

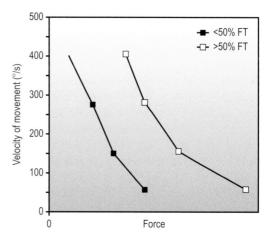

FIG. 4.17 ■ Difference in muscular force and speed of movement between muscles predominantly with fast-twitch (*FT*) and with slow-twitch muscle fibres. *(From Powers & Howley 1997, with permission.)*

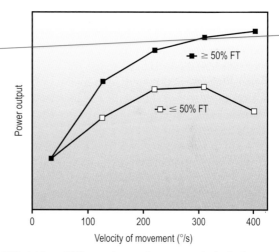

FIG. 4.18 ■ Difference in muscle power and velocity between muscles with predominantly fast-twitch (*FT*) and slow-twitch muscle fibres. *(From Powers & Howley 1997, with permission.)*

1996), although this can easily be reduced with increased activity levels and more specifically resistance training, especially at high intensities (Mayer et al. 2011; Bouchonville & Villareal 2013).

The relationship between muscle power and velocity is depicted in Fig. 4.18. For a given velocity the peak power generated is greater in muscle that contains a high percentage of fast-twitch fibres than in muscle that contains a high percentage of slow-twitch fibres

(Powers & Howley 1997). The peak power generated by any muscle increases with increasing velocity of movement, up to a movement velocity of 200–400°/second, when assessing single joint activities. During multijoint activities the peak power occurs at different loads depending on the type of exercise and the nature of the exercise; for example, peak power during squats occurs at 56% one maximal repetition (1RM), whereas during a squat jump peak power occurs at 0% 1RM back squat (Cormie et al. 2007). This is likely due to the nature of the movement, where the final stages of the squat result in a deceleration phase, whereas acceleration occurs until take-off during jumping activities.

More important than the relationship between power and velocity is the relationship between force and power, as force production directly influences velocity of movement. If force applied to an object increases within the same given time period, acceleration increases (force = mass × acceleration); if acceleration increases, the velocity of movement must also increase. In this case, as both force and velocity have increased, there is a subsequent increase in power (power = force × velocity). Researchers have reported that strength training is more beneficial than power training in individuals who are not already strong, likely due to the increased force increasing both components of the power equations, as described above (Cormie et al. 2010, 2011).

In vitro muscle studies have demonstrated that the type of muscle action affects the force generated by a muscle. The greatest force is produced by an eccentric muscle action, the least force by a concentric muscle action; an isometric muscle action lies somewhere between the two. Increased velocity of an eccentric action increases the force generated, whereas increased velocity of a concentric action reduces the force generated (Fig. 4.19).

Muscle Endurance

Muscle endurance is the ability of a muscle to continue an activity over time. It includes all types of muscle action and so may include repetitive movement, for example, walking, or it may involve holding an isometric muscle action over a period of time, for example, using the rings in gymnastics. Muscle strength is positively associated with the endurance capacity of a muscle. A muscle that is relatively weak, when required to generate force during a functional activity, will do so

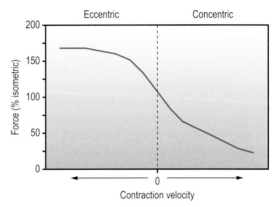

FIG. 4.19 ■ Force–velocity relationship for skeletal muscle. *(From Newham 1993, with permission.)*

at a proportionally greater level of maximum capacity than a muscle that is relatively strong. Other factors affecting muscle endurance include the energy store and blood circulation within the muscle (De Vries & Housh 1994).

There are a variety of ways to measure muscle endurance, and they depend on what specific type of muscle action is being tested. Measuring muscle endurance involves measuring the resultant muscle fatigue, or the number of repetitions performed to failure (when insufficient force can be produced to perform another repetition). Holding an isometric contraction at 60% maximum voluntary contraction (MVC) will increase the pressure within the muscle such that there will be no blood flowing into the muscle. The ability then to continue holding the contraction will depend on accumulation of hydrogen ions and how quickly this inhibits enzyme function within the muscle. A contraction at less than 60% MVC will enable the contraction to be held for longer as blood flow is not completely occluded, and a contraction at more than 60% MVC will result in the contraction being held for less time, due to the reduced blood flow.

Normal control of movement occurs as a result of incoming sensory information of position and movement and is integrated at all levels of the nervous system. Automatic and simple reflex movements occur in the spinal cord. Postural and balance reactions occur at the level of the brainstem and basal ganglia. More complicated movements are initiated and controlled at the motor/sensory cortices, and the cerebellum controls

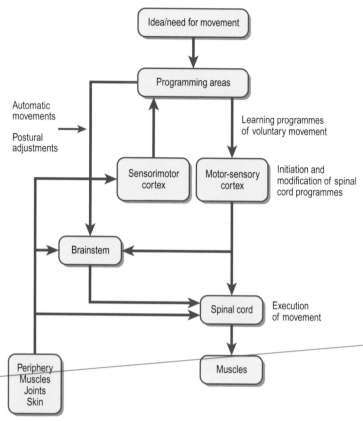

FIG. 4.20 ■ Schematic diagram of the control of movement. *(After Kidd et al. 1992, with permission.)*

and coordinates movement (Crow & Haas 2001) (Fig. 4.20). Motor control depends on 'the spatial and temporal integration of vestibular, visual, and somatosensory information about the motion of the head and body, and the generation of appropriate responses to that motion' (Speers et al. 2002). A discussion of proprioception and motor control is to be found in Chapter 10.

Classification of Muscle Function

Muscle Architecture

Aspects of muscle architecture include the fascicle length, fascicle thickness and pennation angle. Each of these aspects will influence the function of the muscle. Each muscle fibre is capable of shortening to approximately half its total length (Norkin & Levangie 1992). Thus, a longer muscle is able to shorten over a greater distance than a shorter fascicle, resulting in the potential for

higher shortening velocities and therefore higher movement velocities.

The direction of the muscle fibres (pennation angle) differs with each muscle shape and so affects the direction of force during muscle contraction, but this does alter with training, especially in superficial muscles (Blazevich 2006) (Fig. 4.21). A quadrilateral muscle, as the name suggests, is flat and square. The muscle fibres run parallel and extend the length of the muscle. Muscles of this shape, such as pronator quadratus and quadratus lumborum, are well designed to support and stabilize underlying bones and joints.

Strap muscles are long and rectangular in shape, with fibres running the full length of the muscle. They are able to produce movement through a large range, for example sartorius. Rectus abdominis is a strap muscle, but is unusual in that it has three fibrous bands running across it.

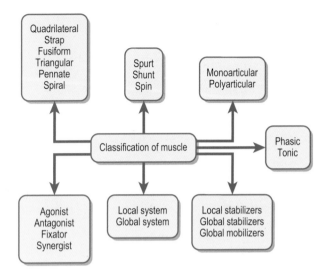

FIG. 4.21 ■ Classification systems for muscle.

Fusiform muscles are in the shape of a spindle with fibres running almost parallel to the line of pull. The two ends of the muscle converge on to a tendon. Biceps brachii consist of two fusiform-shaped muscles, while triceps brachii have three fusiform-shaped muscles.

Triangular muscles have a tendon at one end, and at the other end the muscle attaches to bone via either a flat tendon or an aponeurosis. The shape of the muscle means that some muscle fibres run at quite an oblique angle to the line of pull of the tendon, thus reducing its potential force of contraction. At its flat attachment though, the force of pull is across a broad area. The lower trapezius is an example of a triangular muscle.

Pennate muscles appear like a feather and may be unipennate (fibres attach to only one side of the tendon), bipennate (to both sides of the tendon) or multipennate (a number of bipennate arranged fibres). Examples include flexor pollicis longus (unipennate), rectus femoris (bipennate) and deltoid (multipennate). The oblique direction of muscle fibres to the line of pull means that the force will be relatively less than if they were parallel; only a component of the force (the cosine of the angle) is available to move the bone. Pennate muscles have shorter and more numerous muscle fibres than do fusiform muscles. The greater number of muscle fibres gives pennate muscles, such as deltoid and gluteus maximus, a greater strength than fusiform muscles.

Spiral muscles twist on themselves, and often untwist on muscle contraction, thus producing a rotation force.

Examples include latissimus dorsi twisting 180° through its length to rotate the humerus medially (Lockwood 1998) (Fig. 4.22).

These architectural arrangements provide valuable insight into the function of a muscle and have been shown to have more effect on the force-generating capability of a muscle than its fibre-type composition (Sacks & Roy 1982; Burkholder et al. 1994).

Monoarticular and Polyarticular

Monoarticular muscles cross only one joint whereas polyarticular muscles cross more than one joint. This classification system describes the relationship of muscle to joint, and so provides insight into the movement that will be produced by the muscle. For example, the rectus femoris is a polyarticular muscle crossing the anterior aspect of the hip and knee (biarticular as it crosses two joints) and therefore causing hip flexion and knee extension on concentric contraction. Muscles crossing more than one joint will be longer, and will produce more movement, than a muscle crossing just one joint. This classification system closely relates to the architecture of muscle and, together, they describe anatomical aspects of muscle.

Prime Mover, Antagonist, Fixator and Synergist

This classification system describes the way in which a muscle functions in relation to a specific movement. Any one muscle may act as a prime mover (or agonist),

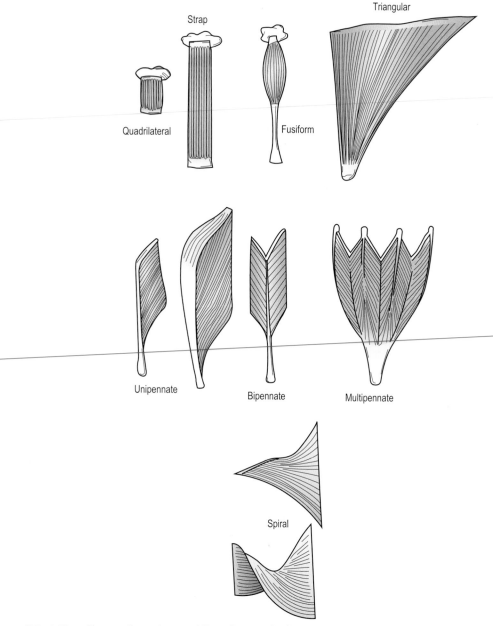

FIG. 4.22 ■ Shapes of muscles: quadrilateral, strap, fusiform, triangular, pennate and spiral. *(From Williams et al. 1995.)*

antagonist, fixator or synergist. The way in which a muscle acts depends on a number of factors which include the start position, the direction and speed of the movement, the phase of the movement and the resistance to movement.

Prime Mover and Antagonist

When a muscle is active in initiating and maintaining a movement it is acting as a prime mover (agonist). A muscle that opposes the prime mover is considered to be the antagonist. For example, during a knee extension exercise the quadriceps are the prime mover (agonist), while the hamstring muscles co-contract to stabilize the knee joint (antagonist); this reverses during the knee flexion exercise.

Co-Contraction of Agonist and Antagonist

It might be assumed that when the prime mover is contracting the antagonist is silent. However, there are numerous examples of co-contraction of agonist and antagonist. During maximal voluntary knee extension, the flexors of the knee are also contracting, albeit to a lesser degree (Baratta et al. 1988). When maintaining trunk extension during a lifting task, there is co-contraction of the trunk flexors and extensors (Granata & Marras 1995), with these muscles performing isometric actions to maintain spinal alignment. With a rapid voluntary movement there is a triphasic pattern of muscle activity, with bursts of activity initially in the agonist, then the antagonist, and then the agonist (Friedli et al. 1984). The effect of co-contraction is to increase stiffness and thus stability of a joint, which is likely to be needed in stressful and complex movements (Fig. 4.23). There is therefore activity of the agonist and antagonist muscles during active movements.

Interestingly, the amount of co-contraction can be altered by activity. Athletes who strongly exercised the quadriceps and not the hamstrings had reduced co-contraction of the hamstrings on active knee extension compared with those who exercised both groups of muscles (Baratta et al. 1988). The amount of co-contraction is related to motor control; co-contraction is greater when motor skill is poor and reduces when motor skill is improved (Osu et al. 2002).

Increased levels of co-contraction of the hamstrings and quadriceps during gait appear to be related to increased severity of knee osteoarthritis (Mills et al. 2013) and decreasing levels of co-contraction reduce knee osteoarthritis symptoms (Al-Khaifat et al. 2016). Co-contraction of the latissimus dorsi muscle during tackling tasks appears to stabilize the shoulder in the presence of superior labrum, anterior and posterior (SLAP) lesions (Horsley et al. 2010).

The amount of co-contraction increases with age: elderly women compared with young women were found to have over 100% greater activity of hamstring muscles just before and during a step-down movement (Hortobagyi & DeVita 2000) and both men and women

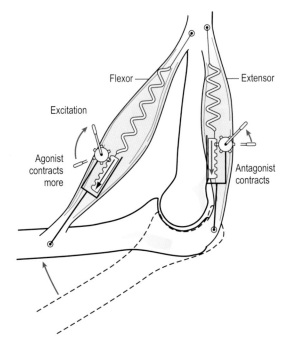

FIG. 4.23 ■ Co-contraction of elbow flexors and extensors to increase joint stiffness and stability. *(From Ghez 1991, with permission.)*

were found to have greater co-contraction of biceps femoris during a maximum isometric contraction and 1RM of quadriceps femoris muscle (Tracy & Enoka 2002). This increased co-contraction functions to increase joint stiffness and is thought to compensate for the neuromotor impairments (atrophy/sarcopenia, reduced strength and proprioception) associated with the elderly (Hortobagyi & DeVita 2000).

Fixators

As the name implies, this is when muscles contract to fix a bone. Muscles on either side of a joint sometimes contract together to create a fixed base on which another muscle can contract. For example, the muscles acting around the wrist contract together to fix the wrist when a strong fist is made.

Synergists

When a muscle acts over two or more joints, but the required movement is only over one joint, other muscles contract to eliminate the movement. When a muscle acts in this way it is said to act as a synergist (derived from *syn*, together, and *ergon*, work). Contraction of the finger flexors would produce flexion at both the wrist and fingers. The wrist extensors contract to eliminate wrist flexion during a power grip and thus act as a synergist. Similarly, during elbow flexion with a pronated forearm, the contraction of biceps brachii will produce both elbow flexion and supination. To maintain the pronated forearm, the pronator quadratus and pronator teres contract and thus act as synergists. In the same way, when muscles around the shoulder contract to produce movement at the glenohumeral joint, muscles around the cervical spine, thoracic spine and scapula must contract to prevent unwanted movement and are therefore acting as synergists.

Any clinician attempting to analyse muscle activity during movement will immediately appreciate the difficulty in doing this. Visual and palpatory cues are simply inadequate to sense whether a particular muscle is active and in what way it is active.

Because almost all muscles contain type I and type II muscle fibres, it can be presumed that the characteristics of whole muscles reflect both characteristics, although the proportion of each fibre type varies across muscles, depending on their roles, and also alter due to activity/training. That is, all muscles can contract slowly and gently for a long period of time, exhibiting endurance, and all muscles can contract quickly and forcefully, exhibiting strength and power; the actual amount will depend on factors such as ratio of fast- and slow-twitch fibres, cross-sectional area of the muscle, leverage and architecture. It seems reasonable to suggest that all muscles will have a role in posture and balance, and all muscles will have a role in movement. The central nervous system (CNS) will activate type I fibres in all types of muscle in order to provide the necessary posture and balance and will activate the type II fibres in all types of muscle in order to provide strength and power. The relative amounts of activation, and in which muscles, will depend on the specific position and the movement that is being carried out.

SKELETAL MUSCLE DYSFUNCTION

Just as the function of muscles depends on the function of joints and nerves, so dysfunction of muscles can lead to dysfunction of joints and nerves. They are dependent on each other in both normal and abnormal conditions (Fig. 4.24).

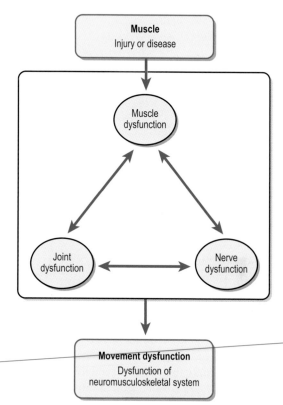

FIG. 4.24 ■ Dysfunction of muscle can produce joint and/or nerve dysfunction, and can lead to movement dysfunction.

Dysfunctions in muscles and joints often occur together. For example, abnormality of the eccentric muscle force of the quadriceps muscle may be a contributing factor in anterior knee pain (Bennett & Stauber 1986) and lateral epicondylitis is associated with tears of the lateral collateral ligament of the elbow (Bredella et al. 1999). This evidence highlights the close relationship of muscle and joint dysfunction.

There is overwhelming evidence that weakness of a muscle occurs with joint pathology and dysfunction. This has been demonstrated in the knee in the presence of a variety of pathologies: rheumatoid arthritis and osteoarthritis (Hurley & Newham 1993), ligamentous knee injuries (DeVita et al. 1997; Urbach & Awiszus 2002) and following meniscectomy (Hurley et al. 1994; Suter et al. 1998a); and in the glenohumeral joint in the presence of anterior dislocation (Keating & Crossan 1992). The inhibition of muscle is thought to be due to inhibitory input (Suter & Herzog 2000; Torry et al.

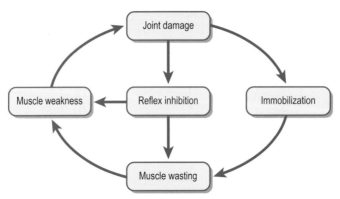

FIG. 4.25 ■ Effect of joint damage and/or immobilization on muscle and nerve tissues. *(From Stokes, M., Young, A. 1984 Clinical Science 67: 7–14. © The Biochemical Society and the Medical Research Society (http://www.clinsci.org), with permission.)*

2000) or abnormal input from joint afferents (Hurley et al. 1991; Hurley & Newham 1993). Thus, joint pathology leads to altered neural activity, which alters muscle activity. A muscle that is inhibited will, over time, atrophy and weaken and this may make the joint vulnerable to further injury (Stokes & Young 1984). For example, it is thought that weakness of the posterior rotator cuff muscles may make the glenohumeral joint vulnerable to recurrent anterior dislocation (Keating & Crossan 1992) (Fig. 4.25).

Muscle activity around a joint is altered in the presence of ligament insufficiency and joint instability. During throwing, electromyogram (EMG) activity of the elbow muscles is altered with ligament insufficiency of the elbow (Glousman et al. 1992). Similarly, during throwing, the EMG activity around the shoulder region is altered with shoulder instability (Glousman et al. 1988). In the lower limb, the EMG activity of quadriceps and hamstring muscle groups is altered with ACL deficiency during knee movement and during gait and functional activities (Frank et al. 2016). Fig. 4.26 identifies a proposed cycle of events of progressive knee instability following an initial ligament injury (Kennedy et al. 1982).

Muscle activity is directly affected by joint nociceptor activity. Pain around the knee causes a nociceptive flexor withdrawal response: hip and knee flexion and ankle dorsiflexion. There is increased alpha motor neuron excitability of the muscles to produce this movement and reciprocal inhibition of the knee extensors. For example, pressure or tension on a partially ruptured medial collateral ligament results in an increased activity

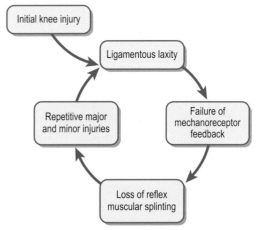

FIG. 4.26 ■ A proposed cycle of progressive knee instability following an initial ligament injury. *(From Kennedy et al. 1982, with permission.)*

of sartorius and semimembranosus (knee flexors) with inhibition of the vastus medialis (extensor) resulting in reduced external force during knee extension.

Nociceptor activity is thought to influence muscle activity via the alpha motor neuron (Wyke & Polacek 1975). Nociceptor activity is thought to have a greater inhibitory effect upon the low-threshold motor units supplying type I muscle fibres than on the high-threshold motor units supplying type II fibres (Gydikov 1976). If this is true, it might be speculated that a muscle containing a relatively higher proportion of type I fibres, such as soleus and tibialis anterior, may be more affected by nociceptor activity than a muscle that has a more equal proportion of type I and II fibres.

The functions of a muscle are essentially to produce and allow movement to occur. That is, it will contract with strength, power and endurance, it will lengthen and shorten with movement and, under the control of the CNS (motor control), it will produce coordinated movement. The signs and symptoms of muscle dysfunction are related to these functions, that is, there may be one or more of the following: reduced muscle strength (which is accompanied by a reduction in both muscle power and muscle endurance), reduced muscle power, reduced muscle endurance, altered motor control, reduced muscle length or production of symptoms. Box 4.3 highlights these characteristics of muscle function and dysfunction.

Reduced Muscle Strength

Reduced muscle strength can occur as a result of disuse such as immobility (Berg et al. 1997), immobilization (Vaughan 1989; Labarque et al. 2002), trauma (DeVita et al. 1997; Urbach & Awiszus 2002), weightlessness (Fitts et al. 2000, 2001) and pathology (Zhao et al. 2000; Yoshihara et al. 2001). As will be seen later, a reduction in muscle strength will result in a reduction in muscle power (if force generation decreases, so does acceleration and therefore velocity of movement; as power = force × velocity, it is clear that a reduction in force directly impacts muscle power) and a reduction in endurance.

A body of knowledge is emerging on the effects of space flight on the musculoskeletal system. While the reader is unlikely to be managing patients recovering from the effects of space flight, the effects on muscle are of interest in furthering our understanding of the plastic nature of the muscle. Space flight causes a reduction in muscle strength and power (Fitts et al. 2000, 2001), associated with progressive atrophy over

the first 110 days (Antonutto et al. 1999; Fitts et al. 2000). Such observations may have implications for muscle atrophy during bed rest and immobilization.

Muscle atrophy has been found to occur with pathology. For example, in patients who underwent surgery for a chronic lumbar disc herniation there was atrophy of the multifidus and longissimus muscles (Sirca & Kostevc 1985). In another similar study a biopsy of multifidus at L4–L5 and L5–S1 levels also revealed muscle atrophy on the side of herniation, with smaller type I and type II fibres (Zhao et al. 2000). Patients with an L4–L5 disc herniation and L5 nerve root compression (identified at surgery) were found to have atrophy of multifidus with a 6.4% reduction in cross-section area of type I fibres and a 9.8% reduction in type II fibres at the level of the herniation; interestingly, no atrophy was found at the L4 level (Yoshihara et al. 2001).

It should be remembered that there are normal age-related changes in muscle strength (Piasecki et al. 2015). Between the fourth and seventh decades there is a 14% reduction in isokinetic quadriceps strength per decade (Hughes et al. 2001). However, such decreases are associated with a reduction in activity and the decline in strength can be slowed with appropriate and progressive training. In fact, in weak individuals strength will noticeably increase with appropriate training.

Immobilization

Immobilization affects the contractile portion of muscle, the musculotendinous junction and the tendon. The reduced strength resulting from immobilization is thought to be due to muscle atrophy and reduced neural input to the muscle (Young et al. 1982b; Berg et al. 1997), although architectural changes are also likely to occur in trained individuals. The effects of immobilization on muscle depend on the length of time, the position of the muscle when immobilized and the predominant muscle fibre type within the muscle.

Time of Immobilization. If a muscle does not contract at all muscle strength will decrease by approximately 5% per day, but one contraction at 50% of MVC is considered sufficient to prevent this reduction (Muller 1970). Normally, some muscle actions may occur while a muscle is immobilized, giving a more realistic estimate of 2–3% reduction in muscle strength per day (Appell

1990); bed rest is estimated to cause a 1–1.5% reduction per day (Muller 1970).

Position of the Muscle. The effects of immobilization on muscle depend on the position in which the muscle is held, whether it is in a shortened or lengthened position. The effects of immobilization in a shortened position are summarized in Box 4.4. The decrease in the number of sarcomeres and increase in length of each sarcomere ensure that the muscle is able to contract maximally in the shortened immobilized position. The connective tissue loss, due to immobilization, occurs at a lower rate than the loss of contractile tissue, resulting in a relative increase in connective tissue; this can occur as early as 2 days after immobilization (Williams & Goldspink 1984). In addition, the connective tissue remodels during immobilization to produce a thicker perimysium and endomysium. These changes produce an increased stiffness to passive lengthening, which is thought to occur to prevent the muscle from being overstretched (Goldspink & Williams 1979). Tendon stiffness appears to decrease due to immobilization at a similar rate in both young and old men (Couppe et al. 2012). Interestingly, collagen turnover after an acute bout of exercise is not affected by a period of immobilization (Moerch et al. 2013).

The increase in connective tissue associated with immobilization in a shortened position can be prevented by 15 minutes of passive stretch on alternate days. This intermittent stretching regime, however, does not influence the reduction in muscle fibre length and subsequent reduction in range of movement (Williams 1988).

When the immobilization ceases the muscle will be weak and shortened and will have an increased resistance to passive lengthening, therefore restoration of muscle length, active and passive range of motion and strength is essential. A 2-week period of immobilization of the knee, close to full extension (shortened position for knee extensors and relative lengthened position for knee flexors) resulted in a 27% reduction in knee extensor torque and an 11% reduction in knee flexor torque (Labarque et al. 2002). The reduction in knee extensor torque agrees with the estimate of 2–3% reduction per day in muscle strength (Appell 1990).

The effects of immobilization of muscle in a lengthened position are summarized in Box 4.5. There is an increase in the number of sarcomeres that lie in series, thus lengthening the muscle (Goldspink 1976; Williams & Goldspink 1978); however, the length of the sarcomeres is reduced (Williams & Goldspink 1978, 1984). Functionally the muscle has a greater capacity to generate

---

BOX 4.4
EFFECTS OF IMMOBILIZATION ON MUSCLE IN A SHORTENED POSITION

Decrease in muscle weight and fibre size	Williams & Goldspink 1978 Witzmann 1988
Decrease in the number of sarcomeres	Goldspink 1976 Tabary et al. 1972 Williams & Goldspink 1973 Williams & Goldspink 1978
Increase in the sarcomere length	Williams & Goldspink 1978, 1984
Increase in amount of perimysium	Williams & Goldspink 1984
Increase in ratio of collagen concentration	Goldspink & Williams 1979 Williams & Goldspink 1984
Increase in ratio of connective tissue to muscle fibre tissue	Goldspink & Williams 1979 Williams & Goldspink 1984
Reduction in the cross-sectional area of the intrafusal fibres of the muscle spindle	Jozsa et al. 1988
Increase in the thickness of the capsule surrounding the muscle spindle	Jozsa et al. 1988

BOX 4.5
EFFECTS OF IMMOBILIZATION ON MUSCLE IN A LENGTHENED POSITION

Increase in the number of sarcomeres in series	Goldspink 1976 Tabary et al. 1972 Williams & Goldspink 1973, 1976, 1978
Decrease in the length of sarcomeres	Tabary et al. 1972 Williams & Goldspink 1978, 1984
Muscle hypertrophy that may be followed by atrophy	Williams & Goldspink 1984

tension at longer lengths, but this will be offset by the resultant atrophy from immobilization.

Predominant Type of Muscle Fibre Within the Muscle

There is some suggestion that the effect of immobilization on a muscle is affected by its proportion of type I and type II muscle fibres. The effect of immobilization in near-resting length of a guinea pig soleus (predominantly type I muscle fibres) has been compared with immobilization of gastrocnemius (predominantly type II muscle fibres) (Maier et al. 1976). In both muscles type I fibre atrophied to a greater extent than type II fibres, and interestingly the capacity of gastrocnemius to create tension was reduced; however, there was no change in soleus (Maier et al. 1976). In contrast, another study found that type II fibres atrophied more than type I fibres with a 30% reduction in cross-sectional area of type II fibres and a 25% reduction in type I fibres following 5–6 weeks of elbow immobilization (MacDougall et al. 1980).

Effect of Immobilization on the Musculotendinous Junction and the Tendon

Immobilization has widespread effects on the musculotendinous junction and the tendon (Box 4.6). As tendons adapt in response to the load that is applied to them via muscular actions, reduction in loading of the tendon or musculotendinous junction results in a decrease in strength and stiffness of the tendon. At the musculotendinous junction, 3 weeks of immobilization of the rat gastrocnemius–soleus–tendon unit in a shortened position resulted in over 40% reduction in the contact area between the muscle and the tendon (Kannus et al. 1992). Other changes included an increase in scar tissue in the area, reduced glycosaminoglycans and an increase in weaker type III collagen fibres (Kannus et al. 1992).

Collectively, these changes will reduce the tensile strength of the musculotendinous junction. An experimental muscle strain and 2 days of immobilization have been shown to result in a reduction in tensile strength and stiffness at the musculotendinous junction (Almekinders & Gilbert 1986). In addition, a 30% reduction in blood vessels in the musculotendinous junction has been observed following immobilization (Kvist et al. 1995), along with a reduced energy supply, oxygen consumption and enzyme activity within the

---

BOX 4.6

EFFECTS OF IMMOBILIZATION ON THE MUSCULOTENDINOUS JUNCTION AND TENDON

MUSCULOTENDINOUS JUNCTION

Reduction in the contact area between muscle and tendon	Kannus et al. 1992
Increase in scar tissue	Kannus et al. 1992
Reduced glycosaminoglycans	Kannus et al. 1992
Increase in the weaker type III collagen fibres	Kannus et al. 1992
Reduced tensile strength	Almekinders & Gilbert 1986 Kannus et al. 1992
Reduced stiffness	Almekinders & Gilbert 1986
Reduction in blood vessels	Kvist et al. 1995
Increase in the thickness of the capsule of the Golgi tendon organ	Jozsa et al. 1988

TENDON

Reduced collagen fibres	Nakagawa et al. 1989
Reduced energy supply, oxygen consumption and enzyme activity	Jozsa & Kannus 1997

---

tendon following a period of immobilization (Jozsa & Kannus 1997).

The effect of remobilization of tendon following a period of immobilization is still largely unclear. The 30% loss of vascularity at the musculotendinous junction can be restored following remobilization (Kvist et al. 1995). There is acceleration of collagen synthesis and enzyme activity; however, the collagen content and orientation of remobilized tendon may continue to be inferior despite remobilization (Jozsa & Kannus 1997).

Measurement of Muscle Strength

Quadriceps muscle wasting has been measured clinically by using a tape measure around the circumference of the thigh; however, there are clear difficulties with this measure as it includes the subcutaneous fat and hamstring muscle group, which can conceal the quadriceps muscle wasting (Young et al. 1982b). The measurement underestimates the extent of the quadriceps muscle atrophy (Young et al. 1982b, 1983; Arangio et al. 1997) and is of questionable value in the clinical environment

(Arangio et al. 1997). If used to identify thigh muscle atrophy this may be more useful. More importantly, such measures provide very little regarding muscle strength with a decrease in circumference only indicating muscle atrophy and therefore a likely decrease in strength. A more objective measure of atrophy is muscle cross-sectional area, which can be measured by ultrasound, computed axial tomography and magnetic resonance imaging. The physiological cross-sectional area, however, underestimates muscle strength; Young et al. (1983) found a 15% increase in isometric strength of the quadriceps following a training period, but only a 6% increase in physiological cross-sectional area. Therefore such measurements should not be used as a proxy for strength assessments.

Muscle strength is often clinically assessed using manual muscle testing with a subjective scale from 0 (no contraction) to 5 ('normal' strength); this also leads to the question, 'What is normal?' The value of this is severely limited as the accuracy and sensitivity are very poor; for example, in one study a muscle which was only 8% of 'normal' strength was rated as grade 4, clearly underestimating true muscle strength (Agre & Rodriquez 1989).

Force can be measured using devices such as the hand-held dynamometer for isometric strength and the large isotonic or isokinetic dynamometers for larger muscle groups (Watkins et al. 1984). In both situations only single joint actions and therefore individual groups of muscles are assessed; although this can be useful, it is limited by the fact that force assessed during such tasks does not reflect functional performance in the normal population or athletes (Augustsson et al. 1998; Blackburn & Morrissey 1998; Ostenberg et al. 1998). Where isometric strength is measured muscle length will affect the resultant force and therefore the joint angle used during assessment must be consistent to ensure comparable measures. In addition the motivation and subsequent effort by an individual will affect the force measurement.

Muscle strength testing is further complicated by the fact that asymptomatic subjects have been found to vary the maximal voluntary contraction over different days of testing (Allen et al. 1995; Suter & Herzog 1997), although the reliability of multijoint assessments, such as the isometric midthigh pull, has been shown to be highly reliable between sessions, with smallest detectable differences of >1.3% and 10.3%, for peak force and rate of force development, demonstrating meaningful differences between sessions (Comfort et al. 2015). Peak force and rate of force development during the isometric midthigh pull have also been shown to be related to performance in athletic tasks (Winchester et al. 2010; Spiteri et al. 2014; Thomas et al. 2015).

Other useful methods of assessing strength include repetition maximum testing, with a high reliability of 1RM testing reported in recreationally training individuals (Comfort & McMahon 2015), adolescents (Faigenbaum et al. 2012) and older females (Amarante do Nascimento et al. 2013), with similarly high reliability using 8RM (Taylor & Fletcher 2012). For individuals not used to strength training or the specific exercises, a period of familiarization is recommended (Taylor & Fletcher 2012; Amarante do Nascimento et al. 2013). Assessing strength, a repetition maximum test may be easier for most individuals when using resistance machines and those not familiar with such practices; higher repetitions (e.g. 6–12RM) are potentially safer and more useful: for example, performance in a 6RM can be used directly to prescribe strength training loads for the exercise assessed. It is also possible to predict 1RM performance from maximal performance during higher repetitions in some exercises (Julio et al. 2012).

Reduced Muscle Power

Muscle power is a function of force and velocity and if either is reduced there will be a subsequent reduction in power. Where there is a reduction in muscle strength, there will be, by definition, a reduction in power. Force applied to a mass determines its acceleration (force = mass × acceleration) and therefore its resultant velocity. It has already been identified that immobilization in a shortened position causes a reduction in strength and a reduction in length; both of these changes will cause a reduction in muscle power, as fascicle length also determines fascicle shortening velocity and therefore movement velocity and power (Blazevich 2006; Earp et al. 2010).

The velocity of a contraction is determined, in part, by the proportion of fibre types within the muscle – the greater the proportion of type II fibres, the greater the power. Any reduction in type II fibres within a muscle would potentially reduce its power. Additionally the pennation angle and fascicle length are associated with power output, and have been shown to change adversely in response to detraining, sarcopenia, injury and immobilization (Narici et al. 2016).

No difference in atrophy of type I and type II fibres in vastus lateralis was found in healthy volunteers confined to 6 weeks' bed rest (Berg et al. 1997). Any reduction in muscle power would not be as a result of a reduction in type II fibres; however, all subjects had an 18% reduction in cross-sectional area of the muscle and this would reduce muscle strength, and hence power.

A number of studies have investigated the effect of knee immobilization on the proportion of type I and type II fibres in vastus lateralis (MacDougall et al. 1980; Hortobagyi et al. 2000). Three weeks of knee immobilization resulted in a 13% reduction in type I fibres and a 10% reduction in type II fibres (Hortobagyi et al. 2000). Following a lower-limb fracture and knee immobilization for up to 7 weeks there was a 46% reduction in type I fibres and a 37% reduction in type II fibres (Sargeant et al. 1977). Following knee surgery and 5 weeks of knee immobilization there was a reduction only in the cross-sectional area of type I fibres with no alteration in type II fibres (Haggmark et al. 1981). These studies suggest that knee immobilization causes a greater atrophy of type I fibres than of type II fibres in vastus lateralis, but more importantly, both force and power decrease.

The effect of immobilization on the atrophy of type I and type II fibres has also been investigated in triceps muscle. Researchers have investigated type I and II atrophy following elbow immobilization and found greater reduction in type II fibres (MacDougall et al. 1980). Following 6 weeks of elbow immobilization there was a 38% reduction in cross-sectional area of type II fibres and a 31% reduction in type I fibres (MacDougall et al. 1980). In a similar study, 5–6 weeks of elbow immobilization resulted in a 33% reduction in type II fibres and a 25% reduction in type I fibres (MacDougall et al. 1980). In the triceps muscles it appears that immobilization causes greater atrophy in type II fibres than in type I fibres; irrespective of this both force and therefore power decrease.

Reduced Muscle Endurance

Reduced muscle endurance may be manifested by a reduced ability to repeat a muscle action, or a reduced ability to hold an isometric action over a period of time. In order to avoid testing muscle strength it is suggested that the resistance is sufficiently low (usually 60–70% 1RM) to allow 8–15 repetitions.

Altered Motor Control

Aspects of altered motor control include:

- muscle inhibition
- timing of onset
- increased muscle activation
- altered activation of agonist and antagonist.

Muscle Inhibition

Muscle inhibition may be identified by the clinician by visual and/or palpatory cues. While these methods are clearly practical in the clinical setting and require no special equipment, they may have questionable reliability. Some muscles are superficial and may be relatively easy to identify – for example, sternocleidomastoid; the vast majority of muscles overlap with other muscles or lie deep underneath a whole muscle, so that identification of decreased activity in these muscles is extremely difficult, if not impossible. This has led to the development of instrumentation to help the clinician identify muscle inhibition; it includes ultrasound imaging (Hides et al. 1995) and EMG biofeedback (Richardson et al. 1999). In research, voluntary muscle activity can be measured using the interpolated twitch technique (ITT) and involuntary muscle activity by a reduction in the Hoffman (H)-reflex.

The ITT involves applying a single electrical twitch to a nerve during a maximal isometric contraction and indicates the motor unit activity (Hales & Gandevia 1988; Gandevia et al. 1998), although a high-frequency train of stimuli is considered to be a more sensitive measure than the single twitch (Kent-Braun & Le Blanc 1996). A dynamometer measures muscle torque during the active contraction, and if there is full motor unit activity then the addition of nerve stimulation will not produce any increase in torque. Any increase in torque (referred to as 'interpolated twitch torque': Suter & Herzog 2000) indicates muscle inhibition due to incomplete activation.

In asymptomatic subjects, the ITT will produce, on average, a 4% increase in isometric quadriceps muscle torque at 90° flexion (Suter et al. 1996). It should be noted that the extent of muscle inhibition measured by the ITT is dependent on the joint angle; at 60°, knee flexion muscle inhibition is three times greater than with the knee in extension (Suter & Herzog 1997).

Involuntary muscle activity is measured by a reduction in the H-reflex, indicating an inhibition of the alpha motor neuron pool. The H-reflex is a small muscle contraction (via alpha motor neurons) in response to low-intensity stimulation of a mixed nerve (via stimulation of group Ia fibres from muscle spindles). This reflex inhibition continues to be present during active contraction of the muscle (Iles et al. 1990).

Both acute and chronic joint pathology, effusion, pain and immobilization have been found to lead to inhibition of the overlying muscle, a response sometimes referred to as arthrogenous muscle inhibition (Stokes & Young 1984). All of the research studies identified in Box 4.7 have been carried out on the knee, apart from those on rheumatoid arthritis of the elbow joint. The muscle inhibition of an active voluntary contraction seems to be related to the extent of the joint damage: the greater the injury, the greater the inhibition of muscle (Urbach & Awiszus 2002).

The presence of pain can cause muscle inhibition (Arvidsson et al. 1986; Rutherford et al. 1986), although the mechanism is not fully understood. It has been suggested that muscle inhibition can be due to inhibitory input (Suter & Herzog 2000; Torry et al. 2000) or abnormal input (Hurley & Newham 1993) from joint afferents, which reduces the motor drive to muscles acting over the joint.

The presence of effusion can cause muscle inhibition (Fahrer et al. 1988; Torry et al. 2000), although one study found no effect on quadriceps strength or power (McNair et al. 1994). Knee joint effusion and muscle inhibition however do have a marked effect on gait (Torry et al. 2000). This inhibition is thought to be due to increased intraarticular pressure causing an increase in tension in the joint capsule that stimulates mechanoreceptors in the intracapsular receptors and causes a reflex inhibition of the alpha motor neuron pool (Torry et al. 2000).

In experimentally produced effusion there is a linear relationship between the volume of the effusion and the reduction in the H-reflex amplitude; that is, the greater the effusion the greater the muscle inhibition (Iles et al. 1990). In chronic effusions, associated with arthritis, the degree of effusion is not related to the

BOX 4.7
POSSIBLE CAUSES OF ARTHROGENIC MUSCLE INHIBITION

Causes	References
Rheumatoid arthritis of the knee	deAndrade et al. 1965
Rheumatoid arthritis of the elbow	Hurley et al. 1991
Osteoarthritis (knee joint) with no pain or effusion	deAndrade et al. 1965 Hurley & Newham 1993
Articular cartilage	Suter et al. 1998a
Degeneration of the patellar or tibial plateau	Hurley & Newham 1993
Subperiosteal tumour of the femur	Stener 1969
Anterior knee pain	Suter et al. 1998a, b
Muscle pain	Rutherford et al. 1986
Ligamentous knee injuries without pain or effusion	DeVita et al. 1997 Hurley et al. 1992 Newham et al. 1989 Hurley et al. 1994 Snyder-Mackler et al. 1994 Urbach & Awiszus 2002
Postmeniscectomy (knee joint)	Hurley et al. 1994 Shakespeare et al. 1985 Stokes & Young 1984 Suter et al. 1998a
Presence of pain	Arvidsson et al. 1986 Rutherford et al. 1986
Effusion of the knee joint	deAndrade et al. 1965 Fahrer et al. 1988 Kennedy et al. 1982 Jones et al. 1987 Iles et al. 1990 Spencer et al. 1984 Stratford 1981 L. Wood et al. 1988
Anterior cruciate ligament Deficiency of the knee joint	Newham et al. 1989 Hurley et al. 1994 Snyder-Mackler et al. 1994 Suter et al. 1998a, b
Immobilization	Vaughan 1989

amount of inhibition (Jones et al. 1987). With experimentally induced knee joint effusion, aspiration reduces the muscle inhibition (Spencer et al. 1984), whereas in chronic or recurrent knee joint effusions muscle inhibition remains the same post aspiration (Jones et al. 1987). The amount of inhibition of the muscle is related to the angle of the joint, with greater inhibition occurring with the knee in extension than in flexion (Stokes & Young 1984; Jones et al. 1987). This is thought to be due to the difference in intraarticular pressure, which is greater in full extension than in a few degrees of flexion (Levick 1983).

Interestingly, a number of studies have found that muscle inhibition is not just restricted to the local muscles but also occurs in the contralateral limb (Suter et al. 1998a, b; Urbach & Awiszus 2002). The clinician needs to be aware of this when comparing muscle function on the side of injury with the unaffected side as the degree of inhibition may be underestimated. The reason for the change on the unaffected side is unclear: it has been suggested to be due to altered movement patterns (Berchuck et al. 1990; Frank et al. 1994). Another explanation may be the connection of nerve pathways in the spinal cord.

Timing of Onset

The timing of onset of muscle activation during movement and functional activities has been identified in patients. Patients with chronic low-back pain have exhibited delayed activation of transversus abdominis muscle when asked to perform rapid arm movements (Hodges & Richardson 1996). A delayed activation was also found in the internal oblique, external oblique and rectus abdominis muscles during rapid shoulder flexion (Hodges & Richardson 1996), though the true biological significance of these differences has been challenged recently even by the authors of these papers. It should be noted that there are normal age-related changes in the activation of muscles. For example, with age there is increased coactivation of quadriceps and hamstring muscle groups during a step-down movement (Hortobagyi & DeVita 2000). In addition, older subjects have been found to have a delay in muscle activation in the lower limb when stepping to regain balance during a fall (Thelen et al. 2000).

Increased Muscle Activation

Increased muscle activation is brought about by an increase in the activation of the alpha motor neuron pool supplying the muscle. The alpha motor neuron pool can be activated by the CNS, as part of motor control, or by peripheral input from muscle spindles, skin, joint, nerve and muscle afferents, including nociceptors. The underlying causes are therefore wide-ranging, and could include the perception of pain, as well as joint, nerve or muscle dysfunction.

Baseball players with known elbow medial collateral ligament insufficiency have been found to have increased EMG activity of extensor carpi radialis longus and brevis and reduced EMG activity of triceps, flexor carpi radialis and pronator teres compared with a control group (Glousman et al. 1992). Flexor carpi radialis and pronator teres might have been expected to demonstrate increased activity to compensate for the ligamentous insufficiency, but this was not the case. Additionally, baseball players with known anterior shoulder instability have been found to have reduced EMG activity of pectoralis major, subscapularis, latissimus dorsi and serratus anterior and increased activity of biceps and supraspinatus compared with a control group (Glousman et al. 1988). The authors postulate that the reduced muscle activity exacerbates the anterior shoulder instability while the increased activity of biceps and supraspinatus compensates for the anterior instability. Similarly, in rugby players with SLAP lesions in the shoulder, Horsley et al. (2010) found increased latissimus dorsi muscle activity, which appeared to be compensating for poor activity elsewhere in an attempt to stabilize the shoulder.

Altered Activation of Agonist and Antagonist

This alteration in the relative activation of agonist and antagonist can result from the above consequences of increased or decreased muscle activation. In addition to these dysfunctions, there is evidence of a specific alteration in the agonist and antagonist activation patterns. Pain around the knee causes a nociceptive flexor withdrawal response: hip and knee flexion and ankle dorsiflexion. To produce this movement there is increased alpha motor neuron excitability of the hip and knee flexors and ankle dorsiflexors (Stener & Petersen 1963) and reciprocal inhibition of the knee extensors (Young et al. 1987).

Patients with chronic ACL deficiency (16 months–21 years) have been found to have less quadriceps and gastrocnemius activity and greater hamstring activity during the stance phase, and increased hamstring activity during the swing phase of gait (Branch et al. 1989). However, in another study of patients with chronic ACL deficiency (2–3 years), horizontal walking failed to show any difference in EMG activity of quadriceps and hamstrings but on walking uphill the hamstring muscle was activated much earlier than in control subjects (Kalund et al. 1990). Patients with an ACL-deficient knee following 6 months' rehabilitation continued to exhibit increased EMG activity of vastus lateralis, biceps femoris and tibialis anterior muscles during functional movements, compared with a control group (Ciccotti et al. 1994). This indicates a change in recruitment strategy of the muscles around the knee and possible subsequent muscle atrophy from disuse.

A number of studies have demonstrated that chronic ACL deficiency and reconstruction cause an alteration of motor control around the knee (Ciccotti et al. 1994; Beard et al. 1996; DeVita et al. 1997), with patients demonstrating what has been call a quadriceps avoidance strategy. Patients who have had an ACL reconstruction were found to have an altered gait pattern such that, compared with control subjects and the uninjured limb, the knee was in more flexion at heel contact and midstance, and a greater range of extensor torque was present during the stance phase (DeVita et al. 1997). Patients with chronic ACL deficiency, longer than 6 months without repair, were found to walk with the knee in more flexion at heel contact and midstance and this correlated with an increased duration of hamstring activity (Beard et al. 1996), though later studies dispute these findings (Lepley et al. 2016). During running, landing and cutting, decreased knee flexion and knee extensor movements are often reported (Trigsted et al. 2015).

Altered Muscle Length

The most obvious reduction in muscle length is seen following immobilization of a joint, when the muscle is held in a shortened position. In this situation the muscle will be shortened and will have an increased resistance to passive lengthening (Goldspink 1976; Goldspink & Williams 1979). When muscle is immobilized in a lengthened position it increases the number of sarcomeres and thus becomes longer; there is no change in resistance to passive lengthening, though this might have consequences for the length–tension relationship of the muscle. Muscle length can be approximated by lengthening muscle fully and measuring the range of motion based on the final joint angle using a goniometer; when compared to a previous measurement

changes in musculotenidinous length can be inferred. To measure muscle length (fascicle length) diagnostic ultrasound is required. The passive resistance of muscle to lengthening is more difficult to measure, if not impossible to distinguish between when there is passive or active resistance to elongation; this can only truly be tested with the patient under anaesthetic.

Production of Symptoms

Symptoms from muscle dysfunction are commonly a pain or an ache. Symptoms may be felt when the muscle is at rest, when it is lengthened or when it contracts. Muscle can be a primary source of pain with both free nerve endings activated by noxious thermal, mechanical and chemical stimuli (Mense 1996). The last two, noxious mechanical and chemical forms of irritation, are the probable causes in patients with muscle pain seen in the musculoskeletal field. The pain from muscle can therefore be classified as mechanical or chemical nociceptive pain (Gifford 1998).

Mechanical pain occurs when certain movements stress injured tissue, increasing the mechanical deformation and activation of nociceptors; other movements may reduce the stress on injured tissue, reducing the mechanical deformation and activation of nociceptors. Thus, with mechanical pain, there are particular movements which aggravate and ease the pain, sometimes referred to as 'on/off' pain. The magnitude of the mechanical deformation may be directly related to the magnitude of nociceptor activity (Garell et al. 1996).

Ischaemic nociceptive pain in muscle is not yet fully understood (Mense 1996). It may be related to chemical irritation, build-up of potassium ions or lack of oxidation of metabolic products. Experimentally induced ischaemia of muscle activated only 10% of muscle nociceptors. However, when a muscle contracts under ischaemic conditions there is much stronger activation of group IV nociceptors (Mense & Stahnke 1983; Kaufman et al. 1984b). With muscle hypoxia there is an increase in group III and IV mechanoreceptor and nociceptor afferent activity (Kieschke et al. 1988). The underlying mechanism of ischaemic contraction causing nociceptor activity appears to be related to chemical sensitization of muscle nociceptors (Mense 1996).

Clinical features of ischaemic pain are thought to be symptoms produced after prolonged or unusual activities, rapid ease of symptoms after a change in posture, symptoms towards the end of the day or after the accumulation of activity, a poor response to anti-inflammatory medication and sometimes absence of trauma (Butler 2000).

The sympathetic nervous system can cause pain. Increased concentrations of adrenaline (epinephrine) in muscle cause an increased discharge frequency of muscle nociceptors, and this response is enhanced with the addition of noxious mechanical stimulation (Kieschke et al. 1988). In the presence of tissue injury or inflammation, sympathetic nervous system activity can maintain the perception of pain or enhance nociception in inflamed tissue (Raja et al. 1999). Sympathetically maintained pain can occur with complex regional pain syndromes and may play a part in chronic arthritis and soft-tissue trauma (Raja et al. 1999). Thus, it appears that the sympathetic nervous system can cause muscle pain.

Constant experimentally induced muscle pain in humans has been found to cause an increase in the stretch reflex of the relaxed muscle, suggesting that muscle pain increases the sensitivity of the muscle spindle to stretch (Matre et al. 1998). In the same study, muscle pain did not alter the H-reflex, suggesting that muscle pain does not directly alter the sensitivity of alpha motor neuron activity, although it may have an indirect effect by causing a reduction in descending inhibition on the alpha motor neuron activity and thus cause an increase in the stretch reflex. Inducing muscle pain also increases the stretch reflex of the antagonist muscle group; pain in tibialis anterior increases the stretch reflex of soleus (Matre et al. 1998).

Referral of Pain From Muscle

In the upper and lower limbs, muscle pain is often felt over the joint that the muscle moves, provided that the joint has the same segmental innervation as the muscle. Some generalizations can be made about the pattern of pain referral from muscle. The segmental distribution of muscle is given in Fig. 4.27. The chart of pain referral for various muscles is shown in Fig. 4.28. There are differences in the quality of pain from muscle, from tendon and from fascia. Fascia and tendon tended to produce sharp localized pain, while muscle tended to produce some localized pain and a diffuse referred pain with tenderness of structures deep to the skin.

The limb muscles are generally innervated by more than one spinal segment; for example, infraspinatus is supplied by C5 and C6 and this produces a more widespread area of referral than the dermatome areas for skin. Pain from muscle appears to be referred to regions corresponding to the spinal segments from which it obtains its motor supply; this is clearer in the upper limb than in the lower limb.

Pain from muscle may be poorly localized to muscle. Pain from the lumbar erector spine muscle produces pain similar to that caused by injection of the gluteal fascia. Some muscles, such as rectus abdominis and muscles in the hand, are much more sensitive and produce more severe pain than biceps brachii and glutei muscles. Metabolic muscle disease, in contrast, typically causes pain that the patient is able to locate as 'in the muscle'; it is not vague and does not refer (Petty 2003).

The mechanism of referred pain is thought to be due to the convergence of afferents in the periphery and in the dorsal horn (Torebjork et al. 1984). This is depicted in Fig. 4.29. In the periphery, proximal to the spinal cord, sensory neurons from skin and muscle converge (Wells et al. 1994). In the dorsal horn, there is convergence of skin afferents and group III and IV muscle afferents on to wide dynamic range cells (Foreman et al. 1979). In both cases, activation of nociceptors from the muscle, for example, is perceived by the brain to come from the skin; the brain thus misinterprets the information.

Tendon Injury and Repair

The elastic properties (compliance vs. stiffness) of tendons are associated with the force production characteristics of the muscle they attach to (Muraoka et al. 2005), as they adapt in response to the stress and strain which the muscles impart on them.

Tendons can tear in the middle region, by avulsion of bone, and more rarely at the insertion site (Woo et al. 1988). Repetitive strain of a tendon can produce micro- and macrotrauma of the tendon. The amount of strain needed to cause micro- and macrotrauma is given in Fig. 4.30. Repetitive strain may alter the collagenous structure of tendon, with resultant inflammation, oedema and pain (Jozsa & Kannus 1997). Overuse injury occurs where this repetitive strain, causing tissue damage, is greater than the natural repair and

Text continued on p. 110

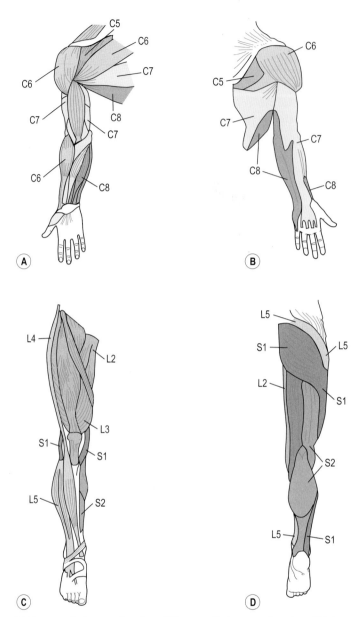

FIG. 4.27 ■ Myotomes of (A) upper limb, anterior view; (B) upper limb, posterior view; (C) lower limb, anterior view; and (D) lower limb, posterior view. *(Reproduced with permission from Kellgren 1939. © The Biochemical Society and the Medical Research Society.)*

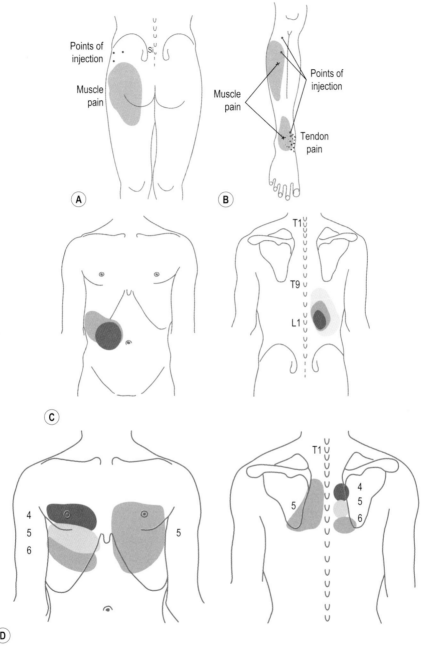

FIG. 4.28 ■ Referred pain from muscle. (A) Gluteus medius. (B) Tibialis anterior; stippling is tendon pain. (C) Horizontal hatching from multifidus, vertical hatching from intercostals and stippling from rectus abdominis. (D) From fourth, fifth and sixth intercostal muscles.   *Continued*

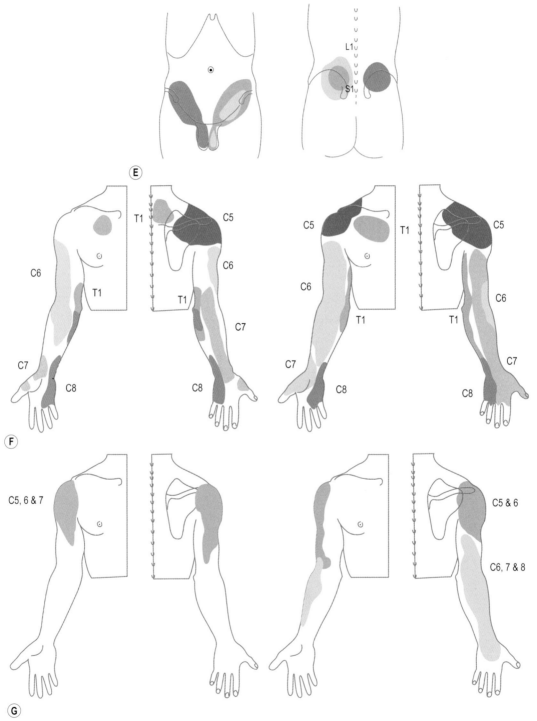

FIG. 4.28, cont'd ■ (E) Vertical hatching from testis, horizontal hatching from abdominal obliques and stippling from multifidus. (F) Crosses from rhomboids, oblique hatching from flexor carpi radialis, stippling from abductor pollicis longus, vertical hatching from third dorsal interosseous, horizontal hatching from first intercostal space. (G) Vertical hatching from serratus anterior, oblique hatching from infraspinatus and stippling from latissimus dorsi.

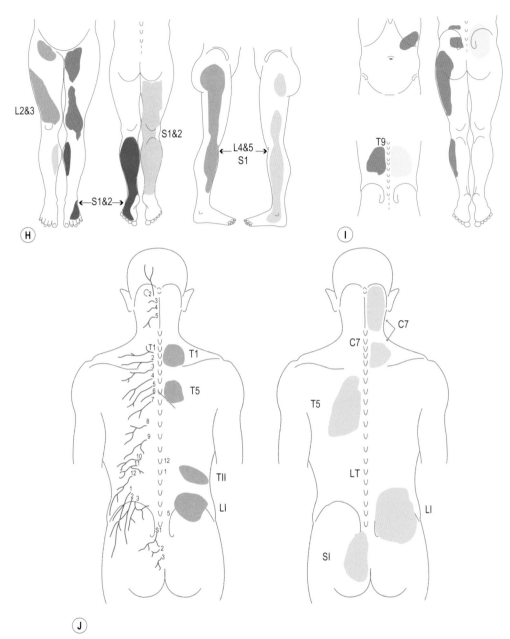

FIG. 4.28, cont'd ■ (H) Left leg with oblique hatching from adductor longus, right leg with oblique hatching from sartorius, vertical hatching from gastrocnemius, horizontal hatching from first interosseous, crosses from tensor fasciae latae and stippling from peroneus longus. (I) Vertical hatching from erector spinae and horizontal hatching from multifidus stimulated opposite T9 and L5. (J) Left figure represents anterior aspect of erector spinae and right figure posterior aspect of erector spinae at the spinal level indicated. *(From Kellgren 1938. © The Biochemical Society and the Medical Research Society, with permission.)*

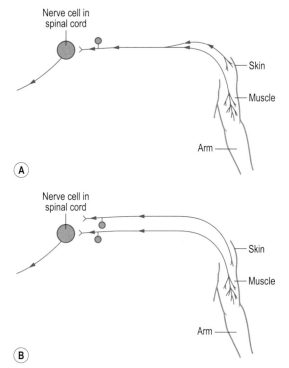

FIG. 4.29 ■ Referred pain due to convergence of afferents (A) in the periphery and (B) in the spinal cord. *(After Wells et al. 1994, with permission.)*

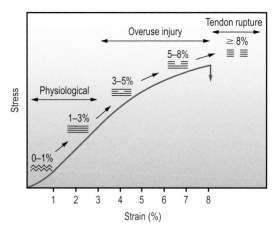

FIG. 4.30 ■ Stress–strain curve of tendon depicting the amount of stress involved in microtrauma (3–8%) and macrotrauma (<8%). *(From Jozsa & Kannus 1997.)*

healing process and this may lead, with further strain, to partial or complete rupture of the tendon (Archambault et al. 1995; Jozsa & Kannus 1997). Evidence suggests that very little inflammation exists within the tendon (Rees et al. 2006; Woodley et al. 2007). Often, these overuse injuries are seen in the upper extremity in occupations that require repetitive movement of the hands and forearms, and in the lower extremities (usually Achilles and patellar tendons) in sports-related injuries.

The aetiology of sports-related lower-limb tendon injuries is thought to include vascularity of the tendon, malalignments, leg length discrepancy, age and weight (Jozsa & Kannus 1997), as well as extrinsic factors such as type of sport, training errors, environmental conditions, equipment and ineffective rules (Jozsa & Kannus 1997). Interestingly, a recent review and metaanalysis concluded that strength training appears to be the most effective method of preventing sports-related injuries to the muscle and tendon (Lauersen et al. 2014).

Vascularity is thought to be an important aetiological factor because tendon injuries often occur where there is a relatively poor blood supply (Archambault et al. 1995). For example, the tendocalcaneus tendon has an avascular area 2–6 cm proximal to its distal attachment (Carr & Norris 1989), and it is in this region where the most severe tendon degeneration and spontaneous ruptures occur (Jozsa & Kannus 1997). The posterior tibial tendon has an area of poor vascularity posterior and distal to the medial malleolus, and it is in this region that it frequently ruptures (Frey et al. 1990). The supraspinatus tendon has poor vascularity where it inserts on to the humerus (Chansky & Iannotti 1991), and, again, it is in this region where the tendon ruptures (Jozsa & Kannus 1997). Age-related degenerative changes within the tendon can cause narrowing or obliteration of blood vessels, further reducing the vascularity of the tendon (Kannus & Jozsa 1991).

In work-related upper-limb tendon injuries the strain placed on tendons may not be excessive, but the repetitive nature of the task may be sufficient to cause change in the tissue. It is proposed that, initially, in the first 5 days, there is ischaemia, metabolic disturbance and cell membrane damage leading to inflammation (Jozsa & Kannus 1997). The increase in tissue pressure further impairs the circulation and enhances the ischaemic changes. In the proliferation phase (5–21 days) there is fibrin clotting and proliferation of fibroblasts, synovial cells and capillaries. This is followed by the maturation phase (<21 days) in which adhesions and thickening of the tenosynovium and paratenon occur (Jozsa & Kannus 1997).

Spontaneous tendon rupture is associated with degenerative changes (Jozsa et al. 1989b). The diameter of collagen fibres decreases in degenerative tendon, suggesting an increase in weaker type III collagen fibres (Jozsa et al. 1989a). Degenerative changes were found in 97% of ruptured tendons, which included the Achilles tendon, biceps brachii and extensor pollicis longus from nearly 900, compared with 35% in a control group (Kannus & Jozsa 1991).

Tendon Repair

Healing of tendon is similar to that of other soft tissues and consists of three phases: lag or inflammation phase (1–7 days), regeneration or proliferation phase (7–21 days) and remodelling or maturation phase (21 days to 1 year) (Jozsa & Kannus 1997). Initially type III collagen is laid down; this is replaced by type I collagen tissue during the late proliferation stage and maturation phase (Coombs et al. 1980).

Muscle Injury and Repair

Muscle strain injury can occur predominantly with eccentric exercise, producing delayed muscle soreness. Pain, weakness and muscle stiffness are felt after unaccustomed eccentric exercise. There is disruption of the Z band, predominantly of type II fibres, with repair largely completed by 6 days (Jones et al. 1986). The reason for the delayed-onset muscle soreness (DOMS) following eccentric action may be due to the fact that eccentric action produces greater force than other types of muscle action. It is important to note that DOMS reduces within a few training sessions, after the individual becomes familiar with a new mode of exercise, and should not be considered to be a 'real' injury. The myotendinous region is the weakest part of the tendon–muscle unit and is the region most susceptible to strain injuries (Garrett 1990; Tidball 1991).

Muscle Repair

Repair of muscle injury follows the typical healing process of all soft tissues: the lag phase, regeneration and remodelling. There is initially the development of a necrotic zone at the site of damage and the adjacent uninjured myofibrils retract and begin the repair process, with activation of satellite cells (McComas 1996). The satellite cells migrate into the necrotic area and differentiate into myotubes, which begin to bridge the gap between the retracted uninjured myofibrils.

REFERENCES

Aagaard, P., Andersen, J.L., Dyhre-Poulsen, P., et al., 2001. A mechanism for increased contractile strength of human pennate muscle in response to strength training: changes in muscle architecture. J. Physiol. 534, 613–623.

Agre, J.C., Rodriquez, A.A., 1989. Validity of manual muscle testing in post-polio subjects with good or normal strength. Arch. Phys. Med. Rehabil. 70 (Suppl.), A17–A18.

Al-Khaifat, L., Herrington, L., Hammond, A., et al., 2016. The effectiveness of an exercise programme on knee loading, muscle co-contraction, and pain in patients with medial knee osteoarthritis. Knee 23, 63–69.

Allen, G.M., Gandevia, S.C., McKenzie, D.K., 1995. Reliability of measurements of muscle strength and voluntary activation using twitch interpolation. Muscle Nerve 18, 593–600.

Almekinders, L.C., Gilbert, J.A., 1986. Healing of experimental muscle strains and the effects of nonsteroidal antiinflammatory medication. Am. J. Sports Med. 14, 303–308.

Alter, M.J., 1996. Science of flexibility, second ed. Human Kinetics, Champaign, IL.

Amarante do Nascimento, M., Januario, R.S., Gerage, A.M., et al., 2013. Familiarization and reliability of one repetition maximum strength testing in older women. J. Strength Cond. Res. 27, 1636–1642.

Antonutto, G., Capelli, C., Girardis, M., et al., 1999. Effects of microgravity on maximal power of lower limbs during very short efforts in humans. J. Appl. Physiol. 86, 85–92.

Appell, H.J., 1990. Muscular atrophy following immobilisation, a review. Sports Med. 10, 42–58.

Arangio, G.A., Chen, C., Kalady, M., et al., 1997. Thigh muscle size and strength after anterior cruciate ligament reconstruction and rehabilitation. J. Orthop. Sports Phys. Ther. 26, 238–243.

Archambault, J.M., Wiley, J.P., Bray, R.C., 1995. Exercise loading of tendons and the development of overuse injuries, a review of current literature. Sports Med. 20, 77–89.

Arvidsson, I., Eriksson, E., Knutsson, E., et al., 1986. Reduction of pain inhibition on voluntary muscle activation by epidural analgesia. Orthopaedics 9, 1415–1419.

Augustsson, J., Esko, A., Thomee, R., et al., 1998. Weight training of the thigh muscles using closed vs open kinetic chain exercises: a comparison of performance enhancement. J. Orthop. Sports Phys. Ther. 27, 3–8.

Baratta, R., Solomonow, M., Zhou, B.H., et al., 1988. Muscular coactivation. The role of the antagonist musculature in maintaining knee stability. Am. J. Sports Med. 16, 113–122.

Beard, D.J., Soundarapandian, R.S., O'Connor, J.J., et al., 1996. Gait and electromyographic analysis of anterior cruciate ligament deficient subjects. Gait Posture 4, 83–88.

Bennett, J.G., Stauber, W.T., 1986. Evaluation and treatment of anterior knee pain using eccentric exercise. Med. Sci. Sports Exerc. 18, 526–530.

Berchuck, M., Andriacchi, T.P., Bach, B.R., et al., 1990. Gait adaptations by patients who have a deficient anterior cruciate ligament. J. Bone Joint Surg. Am. 72A, 871–877.

Berg, H.E., Larsson, L., Tesch, P.A., 1997. Lower limb skeletal muscle function after 6 weeks of bed rest. J. Appl. Physiol. 82, 182–188.

Blackburn, J.R., Morrissey, M.C., 1998. The relationship between open and closed kinetic chain strength of the lower limb and jumping performance. J. Orthop. Sports Phys. Ther. 27, 430–435.

Blazevich, A.J., 2006. Effects of physical training and detraining, immobilisation, growth and aging on human fascicle geometry. Sports Med. 36, 1003–1017.

Bogduk, N., MacIntosh, J.E., 1984. The applied anatomy of the thoracolumbar fascia. Spine 9, 164–170.

Bouchonville, M.F., Villareal, D.T., 2013. Sarcopenic obesity – how do we treat it? Curr. Opin. Endocrinol. Diabetes Obes. 20, 412–419.

Boyd, I.A., 1976. The mechanical properties of dynamic nuclear bag fibres, static nuclear bag fibres and nuclear chain fibres in isolated cat muscle spindles. Prog. Brain Res. 44, 33–50.

Branch, T.P., Hunter, R., Donath, M., 1989. Dynamic EMG analysis of anterior cruciate deficient legs with and without bracing during cutting. Am. J. Sports Med. 17, 35–41.

Bredella, M.A., Tirman, P.F.J., Fritz, R.C., et al., 1999. MR imaging findings of lateral ulnar collateral ligament abnormalities in patients with lateral epicondylitis. AJR Am. J. Roentgenol. 173, 1379–1382.

Brooks, G.A., Fahey, T.D., 1987. Fundamentals of human performance. Macmillan, New York.

Brumitt, J., Cuddeford, T., 2015. Current concepts of muscle and tendon adaptation to strength and conditioning. Int. J. Sports Phys. Ther. 10, 748–759.

Burkholder, T.J., Fingado, B., Baron, S., et al., 1994. Relationship between muscle fiber types and sizes and muscle architectural properties in the mouse hindlimb. J. Morphol. 221, 177–190.

Butler, D.S., 2000. The sensitive nervous system. Noigroup, Adelaide.

Carr, A.J., Norris, S.H., 1989. The blood supply of the calcaneal tendon. J. Bone Joint Surg. Am. 71B, 100–101.

Chalmers, G., 2002. Do Golgi tendon organs really inhibit muscle activity at high force levels to save muscles from injury, and adapt with strength training? Sports Biomech. 1, 239.

Chalmers, G., 2004. Re-examination of the possible role of Golgi tendon organ and muscle spindle reflexes in proprioceptive neuromuscular facilitation. Sports Biomech. 3, 159–183.

Chansky, H.A., Iannotti, J.P., 1991. The vascularity of the rotator cuff. Clin. Sports Med. 10, 807–822.

Ciccotti, M.G., Kerlan, R.K., Perry, J., et al., 1994. An electromyographic analysis of the knee during functional activities. II. The anterior cruciate ligament-deficient and -reconstructed profiles. Am. J. Sports Med. 22, 651–658.

Comfort, P., McMahon, J.J., 2015. Reliability of maximal back squat and power clean performances in inexperienced athletes. J. Strength Cond. Res. 29, 3089–3096.

Comfort, P., Jones, P.A., McMahon, J.J., et al., 2015. Effect of knee and trunk angle on kinetic variables during the isometric midthigh pull: test–retest reliability. Int. J. Sports Physiol. Perform. 10, 58–63.

Coombs, R.R.H., Klenerman, L., Narcisi, P., et al., 1980. Collagen typing in Achilles tendon rupture. J. Bone Joint Surg. Am. 62B, 258.

Cormie, P., McBride, J.M., McCaulley, G.O., 2007. Validation of power measurement techniques in dynamic lower body resistance exercises. J. Appl. Biomech. 23, 103–118.

Cormie, P., McGuigan, M.R., Newton, R.U., 2010. Influence of strength on magnitude and mechanisms of adaptation to power training. Med. Sci. Sports Exerc. 42, 1566–1581.

Cormie, P., McGuigan, M.R., Newton, R.U., 2011. Developing maximal neuromuscular power: part 2 – training considerations for improving maximal power production. Sports Med. 41, 125–146.

Couppe, C., Suetta, C., Kongsgaard, M., et al., 2012. The effects of immobilization on the mechanical properties of the patellar tendon in younger and older men. Clin. Biomech. (Bristol, Avon) 27, 949–954.

Crow, J.L., Haas, B.M., 2001. The neural control of human movement. In: Trew, M., Everett, T. (Eds.), Human movement, an introductory text, fourth ed. Churchill Livingstone, Edinburgh.

deAndrade, J.R., Grant, C., DixonSt, A.J., 1965. Joint distension and reflex muscle inhibition in the knee. J. Bone Joint Surg. Am. 47A, 313–322.

de Brito Fontana, H., Roesler, H., Herzog, W., 2014. In vivo vastus lateralis force–velocity relationship at the fascicle and muscle tendon unit level. J. Electromyogr. Kinesiol. 24, 934–940.

DeVita, P., Hortobagyi, T., Barrier, J., et al., 1997. Gait adaptations before and after anterior cruciate ligament reconstruction surgery. Med. Sci. Sports Exerc. 29, 853–859.

De Vries, H.A., Housh, T.J., 1994. Physiology of exercise for physical education, athletics and sports science, fifth ed. Brown & Benchmark, Madison, WI.

Earp, J.E., Kraemer, W.J., Newton, R.U., et al., 2010. Lower-body muscle structure and its role in jump performance during squat, countermovement, and depth drop jumps. J. Strength Cond. Res. 24, 722–729.

Fahrer, H., Rentsch, H.U., Gerber, N.J., et al., 1988. Knee effusion and reflex inhibition of the quadriceps – a bar to effective retraining. J. Bone Joint Surg. Am. 70B, 635–638.

Faigenbaum, A.D., McFarland, J.E., Herman, R.E., et al., 2012. Reliability of the one-repetition-maximum power clean test in adolescent athletes. J. Strength Cond. Res. 26, 432–437.

Fitts, R.H., Riley, D.R., Widrick, J.J., 2000. Microgravity and skeletal muscle. J. Appl. Physiol. 89, 823–839.

Fitts, R.H., Riley, D.R., Widrick, J.J., 2001. Functional and structural adaptations of skeletal muscle to microgravity. J. Expe. Biol. 204, 3201–3208.

Foreman, R.D., Schmidt, R.F., Willis, W.D., 1979. Effects of mechanical and chemical stimulation of fine muscle afferents upon primate spinothalamic tract cells. J. Physiol. 286, 215–231.

Fox, S.I., 1987. Human Physiology, second ed. Times Mirror Higher Education Group, Inc.

Frank, C.B., Loitz, B., Bray, R., et al., 1994. Abnormality of the contralateral ligament after injuries of the medial collateral ligament – an experimental study in rabbits. J. Bone Joint Surg. Am. 76A, 403–412.

Frank, R.M., Lundberg, H., Wimmer, M.A., et al., 2016. Hamstring activity in the ACL injured patient: injury implications and comparison with quadriceps activity. Arthroscopy 32, 1651–1659.

Franz, M., Mense, S., 1975. Muscle receptors with group IV afferent fibres responding to application of bradykinin. Brain Res. 92, 369–383.

Frey, C., Shereff, M., Greenidge, N., 1990. Vascularity of the posterior tibial tendon. J. Bone Joint Surg. Am. 72A, 884–888.

Friedli, W.G., Hallett, M., Simon, S.R., 1984. Postural adjustments associated with rapid voluntary arm movements. 1. Electromyographic data. J. Neurol. Neurosurg. Psychiatry 47, 611–622.

Fung, Y.C., 1993. Biomechanics, biomechanical properties of living tissues, second ed. Springer-Verlag, New York.

Gajdosik, R.L., Linden, D.W.V., Williams, A.K., 1996. Influence of age on concentric isokinetic torque and passive extensibility variables of the calf muscles of women. Eur. J. Appl. Physiol. 74, 279–286.

Gandevia, S.C., Hall, L.A., McCloskey, D.I., et al., 1983. Proprioceptive sensation at the terminal joint of the middle finger. J. Physiol. 335, 507–517.

Gandevia, S.C., Herbert, R.D., Leeper, J.B., 1998. Voluntary activation of human elbow flexor muscles during maximal concentric contractions. J. Physiol. 512, 595–602.

Garell, P.C., McGillis, S.L.B., Greenspan, J.D., 1996. Mechanical response properties of nociceptors innervating feline hairy skin. J. Neurophysiol. 75 (3), 1177–1189.

Garrett, W.E., 1990. Muscle strain injuries: clinical and basic aspects. Med. Sci. Sports Exerc. 22, 436–443.

Ghez, C., 1991. Muscles: effectors of the motor systems. In: Kandel, E.R., Schwartz, J.H., Jessell, T.M. (Eds.), Principles of neural science, third ed. Elsevier, New York, pp. 548–563.

Gifford, L., 1998. Pain. In: Pitt-Brooke, J., Reid, H., Lockwood, J., et al. (Eds.), Rehabilitation of movement, theoretical basis of clinical practice. W.B. Saunders, London, pp. 196–232.

Glousman, R., Jobe, F., Tibone, J., et al., 1988. Dynamic electromyographic analysis of the throwing shoulder with glenohumeral instability. J. Bone Joint Surg. Am. 70A, 220–226.

Glousman, R.E., Barron, J., Jobe, F.W., et al., 1992. An electromyographic analysis of the elbow in normal and injured pitchers with medial collateral ligament insufficiency. Am. J. Sports Med. 20, 311–317.

Goldspink, G., 1976. The adaptation of muscle to a new functional length. In: Anderson, D.J., Matthews, B. (Eds.), Mastication. Wright, Bristol, pp. 90–99.

Goldspink, G., Williams, P.E., 1979. The nature of the increased passive resistance in muscle following immobilization of the mouse soleus muscle. J. Physiol. 289, 55. (Proceedings of the Physiological Society December 15/16th 1978).

Goodwin, G.M., McCloskey, D.I., Matthews, P.B.C., 1972. The contribution of muscle afferents to kinaesthesia shown by vibration induced illusions of movement and by the effects of paralysing joint afferents. Brain 95, 705–748.

Granata, K.P., Marras, W.S., 1995. The influence of trunk muscle coactivity on dynamic spinal loads. Spine 20, 913–919.

Grigg, P., 1994. Peripheral neural mechanisms in proprioception. J. Sport Rehabil. 3, 2–17.

Grimby, G., 1995. Muscle performance and structure in the elderly as studied cross-sectionally and longitudinally. J. Gerontol. 50A, 17–22 (special issue).

Gydikov, A.A., 1976. Pattern of discharge of different types of alpha motoneurones and motor units during voluntary and reflex activities under normal physiological conditions. In: Komi, P.V. (Ed.), Biomechanics. V-A University Park, Baltimore, MD, pp. 45–57.

Haggmark, T., Jansson, E., Eriksson, E., 1981. Fibre type area and metabolic potential of the thigh muscle in man after knee surgery and immobilization. Int. J. Sports Med. 2, 12–17.

Hales, J.P., Gandevia, S.C., 1988. Assessment of maximal voluntary contraction with twitch interpolation: an instrument to measure twitch responses. J. Neurosci. Methods 25, 97–102.

Hauraix, H., Nordez, A., Guilhem, G., Rabita, G., Dorel, S., 2015. In vivo maximal fascicle-shortening velocity during plantar flexion in humans. J. Appl. Physiol. 119 (11), 1262–1271.

Henneman, E., Olson, C.B., 1965. Relations between structure and function in the design of skeletal muscles. J. Neurophysiol. 28, 581–598.

Henneman, E., Somjen, G., Carpenter, D.O., 1965. Functional significance of cell size in spinal motoneurons. J. Neurophysiol. 28, 560–580.

Herzog, W., Gal, J., 1999. Tendon. In: Nigg, B.M., Herzog, W. (Eds.), Biomechanics of the musculo-skeletal system, second ed. John Wiley, Chichester, pp. 127–147.

Herzog, W., Gal, J., 2007. Tendon. In: Nigg, B.M., Herzog, W. (Eds.), Biomechanics of the musculo-skeletal system, third ed. John Wiley, Chichester, pp. 127–147.

Hess, G.P., Cappiello, W.L., Poole, R.M., et al., 1989. Prevention and treatment of overuse tendon injuries. Sports Med. 8, 371–384.

Heyley, M.V., Rees, J., Newham, D.J., 1998. Quadriceps function, proprioceptive acuity and functional performance in healthy young, middle-aged and elderly subjects. Age. Ageing 27, 55–62.

Hides, J., Richardson, C., Jull, G., et al., 1995. Ultrasound imaging in rehabilitation. Aust. J. Physiother. 41, 187–193.

Hirsch, C., 1974. Tensile properties during tendon healing. A comparative study of intact and sutured rabbit peroneus brevis tendons. Acta Orthop. Scand. 153 (Suppl.), 11.

Hodges, P.W., Richardson, C.A., 1996. Inefficient muscular stabilization of the lumbar spine associated with low back pain. A motor control evaluation of transversus abdominis. Spine 21, 2640–2650.

Horowits, R., Maruyama, K., Podolsky, R.J., 1989. Elastic behavior of connectin filaments during thick filament movement in activated skeletal muscle. J. Cell Biol. 109, 2169–2176.

Horsley, I., Herrington, L.C., Rolf, C., 2010. Does SLAP lesion affect muscle recruitment as measured by EMG activity during a rugby tackle? Sports Med. Arthrosc. Rehabil. Ther. Technol. 5, 67–71.

Hortobagyi, T., DeVita, P., 2000. Muscle pre- and coactivity during downward stepping are associated with leg stiffness in aging. J. Electromyogr. Kinesiol. 10, 117–126.

Hortobagyi, T., Dempsey, L., Fraser, D., et al., 2000. Changes in muscle strength, muscle fibre size and myofibrillar gene expression after immobilization and retraining in humans. J. Physiol. 524, 293–304.

Houk, J., Henneman, E., 1967. Responses of Golgi tendon organs to active contractions of the soleus muscle of the cat. J. Neurophysiol. 30, 466–481.

Hughes, V.A., Frontera, W.R., Wood, M., et al., 2001. Longitudinal muscle strength changes in older adults: influence of muscle mass, physical activity, and health. J. Gerontol. 56A, B209B217.

Hunt, C.C., 1990. Mammalian muscle spindle: peripheral mechanisms. Physiol. Rev. 70, 643–663.

Hurley, M.V., Newham, D.J., 1993. The influence of arthrogenous muscle inhibition on quadriceps rehabilitation of patients with early, unilateral osteoarthritic knees. Br. J. Rheumatol. 32, 127–131.

Hurley, M.V., O'Flanagan, S.J., Newham, D.J., 1991. Isokinetic and isometric muscle strength and inhibition after elbow arthroplasty. J. Orthop. Rheumatol. 4, 83–95.

Hurley, M.V., Jones, D.W., Wilson, D., et al., 1992. Rehabilitation of quadriceps inhibited due to isolated rupture of the anterior cruciate ligament. J. Orthop. Rheumatol. 5, 145–154.

Hurley, M.V., Jones, D.W., Newham, D.J., 1994. Arthrogenic quadriceps inhibition and rehabilitation of patients with extensive traumatic knee injuries. Clin. Sci. 86, 305–310.

Huxley, A.F., 2000. Cross-bridge action: present views, prospects, and unknowns. In: Herzog, W. (Ed.), Skeletal muscle mechanics: from mechanisms to function. John Wiley, Chichester, pp. 7–31.

Iles, J.F., Stokes, M., Young, A., 1990. Reflex actions of knee joint afferents during contraction of the human quadriceps. Clin. Physiol. 10, 489–500.

Jami, L., 1992. Golgi tendon organs in mammalian skeletal muscle: functional properties and central actions. Physiol. Rev. 72, 623–666.

Jones, D.A., Newham, D.J., Round, J.M., et al., 1986. Experimental human muscle damage: morphological changes in relation to other indices of damage. J. Physiol. 375, 435–448.

Jones, D.W., Jones, D.A., Newham, D.J., 1987. Chronic knee effusion and aspiration: the effect on quadriceps inhibition. Br. J. Rheumatol. 26, 370–374.

Jozsa, L., Kannus, P., 1997. Human tendons: anatomy, physiology and pathology. Human Kinetics, Champaign, IL.

Jozsa, L., Kvist, M., Kannus, P., et al., 1988. The effect of tenotomy and immobilization on muscle spindles and tendon organs of the rat calf muscles. Acta Neuropathol. 76, 465–470.

Jozsa, L., Lehto, M., Kvist, M., et al., 1989a. Alterations in dry mass content of collagen fibers in degenerative tendinopathy and tendon-rupture. Matrix 9, 140–146.

Jozsa, L., Kvist, M., Balint, B.J., et al., 1989b. The role of recreational sport activity in Achilles tendon rupture, a clinical, pathoanatomical, and sociological study of 292 cases. Am. J. Sports Med. 17, 338–343.

Julio, U.F., Panissa, V.L.G., Franchini, E., 2012. Prediction of one repetition maximum from the maximum number of repetitions with submaximal loads in recreationally strength-trained men. Sci. Sports 27, e69–e76.

Kalund, S., Sinkjaer, T., Arendt-Nielsen, L., et al., 1990. Altered timing of hamstring muscle action in anterior cruciate ligament deficient patients. Am. J. Sports Med. 18, 245–248.

Kannus, P., Jozsa, L., 1991. Histopathological changes preceding spontaneous rupture of a tendon. J. Bone Joint Surg. Am. 73A, 1507–1525.

Kannus, P., Jozsa, L., Kvist, M., et al., 1992. The effect of immobilization on myotendinous junction: an ultrastructural, histochemical and immunohistochemical study. Acta Physiol. Scand. 144, 387–394.

Kaufman, M.P., Iwamoto, G.A., Longhurst, J.C., et al., 1982. Effects of capsaicin and bradykinin on afferent fibers with endings in skeletal muscle. Circ. Res. 50, 133–139.

Kaufman, M.P., Longhurst, J.C., Rybicki, K.J., et al., 1983. Effects of static muscular contraction on impulse activity of groups III and IV afferents in cats. J. Appl. Physiol. 55, 105–112.

Kaufman, M.P., Waldrop, T.G., Rybicki, K.J., et al., 1984a. Effects of static and rhythmic twitch contractions on the discharge of group III and IV muscle afferents. Cardiovasc. Res. 18, 663–668.

Kaufman, M.P., Rybicki, K.J., Waldrop, T.G., et al., 1984b. Effect of ischaemia on responses of group III and IV afferents to contraction. J. Appl. Physiol. 57, 644–650.

Keating, J.F., Crossan, J.F., 1992. Evaluation of rotator cuff function following anterior dislocation of the shoulder. J. Orthop. Rheumatol. 5, 135–140.

Kellgren, J.H., 1938. Observations on referred pain arising from muscle. Clin. Sci. 3, 175–190.

Kellgren, J.H., 1939. On the distribution of pain arising from deep somatic structures with charts of segmental pain areas. Clin. Sci. 4, 35–46.

Kennedy, J.C., Alexander, I.J., Hayes, K.C., 1982. Nerve supply of the human knee and its functional importance. Am. J. Sports Med. 10, 329–335.

Kent-Braun, J.A., Le Blanc, R., 1996. Quantification of central activation failure during maximal voluntary contractions in humans. Muscle Nerve 19, 861–869.

Kerr, K., 1998. Exercise in rehabilitation. In: Pitt-Brooke, J., Reid, H., Lockwood, J. (Eds.), Rehabilitation of movement, theoretical basis of clinical practice. W.B. Saunders, London, pp. 423–457.

Kidd, G., Lawes, N., Musa, I., 1992. Understanding neuromuscular plasticity: a basis for clinical rehabilitation. Edward Arnold, London.

Kieschke, J., Mense, S., Prabhakar, N.R., 1988. Influence of adrenaline and hypoxia on rat muscle receptors in vitro. In: Hamann, W., Iggo, A. (Eds.), Progress in brain research 74. Elsevier, Amsterdam, pp. 91–97.

Kojima, T., 1991. Force–velocity relationship of human elbow flexors in voluntary isotonic contraction under heavy loads. Int. J. Sports Med. 12, 208–213.

Kolz, C.W., Suter, T., Henninger, H.B., 2015. Regional mechanical properties of the long head of the biceps tendon. Clin. Biomech. (Bristol, Avon) 30, 940–945.

Kvist, M., Jozsa, L., Kannus, P., et al., 1991. Morphology and histochemistry of the myotendineal junction of the rat calf muscles. Histochemical, immunohistochemical and electron-microscopic study. Acta Anat. (Basel) 141, 199–205.

Kvist, M., Hurme, T., Kannus, P., et al., 1995. Vascular density at the myotendinous junction of the rat gastrocnemius muscle after immobilization and remobilization. Am. J. Sports Med. 23, 359–364.

Labarque, V.L., EijndeOp't, B., Van Leemputte, M., 2002. Effect of immobilization and retraining on torque–velocity relationship of human knee flexor and extensor muscles. Eur. J. Appl. Physiol. 86, 251–257.

Lauersen, J.B., Bertelsen, D.M., Andersen, L.B., 2014. The effectiveness of exercise interventions to prevent sports injuries: a systematic review and meta-analysis of randomised controlled trials. Br. J. Sports Med. 48, 871–877.

Laughlin, M.H., Korthuis, R.J., 1987. Control of muscle blood flow during sustained physiological exercise. Can. J. Sport Sci. 12 (Suppl.), 77S–83S.

Lepley, A., Gribble, P., Thomas, A., et al., 2016. Longitudinal evaluation of stair walking in patients with ACL injury. Med. Sci. Sports Exerc. 48, 7–15.

Levick, J.R., 1983. Joint pressure–volume studies: their importance, design and interpretation. J. Rheumatol. 10, 353–357.

Lockwood, J., 1998. Musculoskeletal requirements for normal movement. In: Pitt-Brooke, J., Reid, H., Lockwood, J. (Eds.), Rehabilitation of movement, theoretical basis of clinical practice. W.B. Saunders, London.

Lomo, T., Westgaard, R.H., Engebretsen, L., 1980. Different stimulation patterns affect contractile properties of denervated rat soleus muscles. In: Pette, D. (Ed.), Plasticity of muscle. Walter de Gruyter, Berlin.

Louie, J.K., Mote, C.D., 1987. Contribution of the musculature to rotatory laxity and torsional stiffness at the knee. J. Biomech. 20, 281–300.

MacDougall, J.D., Elder, G.C.B., Sale, D.G., et al., 1980. Effects of strength training and immobilisation on human muscle fibres. Eur. J. Appl. Physiol. Occup. Physiol. 43, 25–34.

Macefield, G., Gandevia, S.C., Burke, D., 1990. Perceptual responses to microstimulation of single afferents innervating joints, muscles and skin of the human hand. J. Physiol. 429, 113–129.

Maier, A., Crockett, J.L., Simpson, D.R., et al., 1976. Properties of immobilized guinea pig hindlimb muscles. Am. J. Physiol. 231, 1520–1526.

Manal, K., Roberts, D.P., Buchanan, T.S., 2006. Optimal pennation angle of the primary ankle plantar and dorsiflexors: variations with sex, contraction intensity, and limb. J. Appl. Biomech. 22, 255–263.

Matthews, P.B.C., Simmonds, A., 1974. Sensations of finger movement elicited by pulling upon flexor tendons in man. J. Physiol. 239, 27P–28P.

Matre, D.A., Sinkjaer, T., Svensson, P., et al., 1998. Experimental muscle pain increases the human stretch reflex. Pain 75, 331–339.

Mayer, F., Scharhag-Rosenberger, F., Carlsohn, A., et al., 2011. The intensity and effects of strength training in the elderly. Dtsch. Arztebl. Int. 108, 359–364.

McBryde, A.M., Anderson, R.B., 1988. Sesamoid foot problems in the athlete. Clin. Sports Med. 7, 51–60.

McComas, A.J., 1996. Skeletal muscle: form and function. Human Kinetics, Champaign, IL.

McGill, S.M., Norman, R.W., 1986. Partitioning of the L4–L5 dynamic moment into disc, ligamentous, and muscular components during lifting. Spine 11, 666–678.

McNair, P.J., Marshall, R.N., Maguire, K., 1994. Knee effusion and quadriceps muscle strength. Clin. Biomech. (Bristol, Avon) 9, 331–334.

Mense, S., 1981. Sensitization of group IV muscle receptors to bradykinin by 5-hyroxytryptamine and prostaglandin E^2. Brain Res. 225, 95–105.

Mense, S., 1996. Group III and IV receptors in skeletal muscle: are they specific or polymodal? In: Kumazawa, T., Kruger, L., Mizumura, K. (Eds.), Progress in brain research, vol. 113. Elsevier Science, Amsterdam, pp. 83–100.

Mense, S., Meyer, H., 1985. Different types of slowly conducting afferent units in cat skeletal muscle and tendon. J. Physiol. 363, 403–417.

Mense, S., Stahnke, M., 1983. Responses in muscle afferent fibres of slow conduction velocity to contractions and ischaemia in the cat. J. Physiol. 342, 383–397.

Mills, K., Hunt, M., Leigh, R., et al., 2013. A systematic review and meta-analysis of lower limb neuromuscular alterations associated with knee osteoarthritis during level walking. Clin. Biomech. (Bristol, Avon) 28, 713–724.

Milner-Brown, H.S., Stein, R.B., Yemm, R., 1973. The orderly recruitment of human motor units during voluntary isometric contractions. J. Physiol. 230, 359–370.

Moberg, E., 1983. The role of cutaneous afferents in position sense, kinaesthesia, and motor function of the hand. Brain 106, 1–19.

Moerch, L., Pingel, J., Boesen, M., et al., 2013. The effect of acute exercise on collagen turnover in human tendons: influence of prior immobilization period. Eur. J. Appl. Physiol. 113, 449–455.

Muller, E.A., 1970. Influence of training and of inactivity on muscle strength. Arch. Phys. Med. Rehabil. 51, 449–462.

Muraoka, T., Muramatsu, T., Fukunaga, T., et al., 2005. Elastic properties of human Achilles tendon are correlated to muscle strength. J. Appl. Physiol. 99, 665–669.

Nakagawa, Y., Totsuka, M., Sato, T., et al., 1989. Effect of disuse on the ultrastructure of the Achilles tendon in rats. Eur. J. Appl. Physiol. 59, 239–242.

Narici, M., Franchi, M., Maganaris, C., 2016. Muscle structural assembly and functional consequences. J. Exp. Biol. 219, 276–284.

Newham, D.J., 1993. Eccentric muscle activity in theory and practice. In: Harms-Ringdahl, K. (Ed.), Muscle strength. Churchill Livingstone, Edinburgh, p. 63.

Newham, D.J., Ainscough-Potts, A.-M., 2001. Musculoskeletal basis for movement. In: Trew, M., Everett, T. (Eds.), Human movement, fourth ed. Churchill Livingstone, Edinburgh, pp. 105–128.

Newham, D.J., Hurley, M.V., Jones, D.W., 1989. Ligamentous knee injuries and muscle inhibition. J. Orthop. Rheumatol. 2, 163–173.

Nordin, M., Frankel, V.H., 1989. Basic biomechanics of the musculoskeletal system, second ed. Lea & Febiger, Philadelphia.

Norkin, C.C., Levangie, P.K., 1992. Joint structure and function, a comprehensive analysis, second ed. F.A. Davis, Philadelphia, pp. 101–115.

Ostenberg, A., Roos, E., Ekdahl, C., et al., 1998. Isokinetic knee extensor strength and functional performance in healthy female soccer players. Scand. J. Med. Sci. Sports 8, 275–284.

Osu, R., Franklin, D.W., Kato, H., et al., 2002. Short- and long-term changes in joint co-contraction associated with motor learning as revealed from surface EMG. J. Neurophysiol. 88, 991–1004.

Panjabi, M.M., 1992. The stabilizing system of the spine. Part 1. Function, dysfunction, adaptation, and enhancement. J. Spinal Disord. 5, 383–389.

Panjabi, M.M., White, A.A., 2001. Biomechanics in the musculoskeletal system. Churchill Livingstone, New York.

Panjabi, M., Abumi, K., Duranceau, J., et al., 1989. Spinal stability and intersegmental muscle forces: a biomechanical model. Spine 14, 194–200.

Pearson, S.J., Hussain, S.R., 2014. Region-specific tendon properties and patellar tendinopathy: a wider understanding. Sports Med. 44, 1101–1112.

Pedrero-Chamizo, R., Gomez-Cabello, A., Melendez, A., et al., 2015. Higher levels of physical fitness are associated with a reduced risk of suffering sarcopenic obesity and better perceived health among the elderly: the EXERNET multi-center study. J. Nutr. Health. Aging 19, 211–217.

Pette, D., Staron, R.S., 1990. Cellular and molecular diversities of mammalian skeletal muscle fibres. Rev. Physiol. Biochem. Pharmacol. 116, 1–76.

Pette, D., Peuker, H., Staron, R.S., 1999. The impact of biochemical methods for single muscle fibre analysis. Acta Physiol. Scand. 166, 261–277.

Petty, R., 2003. Evaluating muscle symptoms. J. Neurol. Neurosurg. Psychiatry 74 (Suppl. 11), ii38ii42.

Piasecki, M., Ireland, A., Jones, D.A., et al., 2015. Age-dependent motor unit remodelling in human limb muscles. Biogerontology 1–12.

Powers, S.K., Howley, E.T., 1997. Exercise physiology: theory and application to fitness and performance, third ed. Brown & Benchmark Publishers.

Raja, S.N., Meyer, R.A., Ringkamp, M., et al., 1999. Peripheral neural mechanisms of nociception. In: Wall, P.D., Melzack, R. (Eds.), Textbook of pain, fourth ed. Churchill Livingstone, Edinburgh.

Rees, J.D., Wilson, A.M., Wolman, R.L., 2006. Current concepts in the management of tendon disorders. Rheumatology 45, 508–521.

Reinert, A., Mense, S., 1992. Free nerve endings in the skeletal muscle of the rat exhibiting immunoreactivity to substance P and calcitonin gene-related peptide. Pflugers Arch. 420 (Suppl. 1), R54.

Renstrom, P., Arms, S.W., Stanwyck, T.S., 1986. Strain within the anterior cruciate ligament during hamstring and quadriceps activity. Am. J. Sports Med. 14, 83–87.

Richardson, C., Jull, G., Hodges, P., et al., 1999. Therapeutic exercise for spinal segmental stabilization in low back pain, scientific basis and clinical approach. Churchill Livingstone, Edinburgh.

Rutherford, O.M., Jones, D.A., Newham, D.J., 1986. Clinical and experimental application of the percutaneous twitch superimposition technique for the study of human muscle activation. J. Neurol. Neurosurg. Psychiatry 49, 1288–1291.

Sacks, R.D., Roy, R.R., 1982. Architecture of the hind limb muscles of cats: functional significance. J. Morphol. 173, 185–195.

Sargeant, A.J., Davies, C.T.M., Edwards, R.H.T., et al., 1977. Functional and structural changes after disuse of human muscle. Clin. Sci. Mol. Med. 52, 337–342.

Scott, W., Stevens, J., Binder-Macleod, S.A., 2001. Human skeletal muscle fiber type classifications. Phys. Ther. 81, 1810–1816.

Seitz, L.B., Trajano, G.S., Haff, G.G., et al., 2016. Relationships between maximal strength, muscle size, and myosin heavy chain isoform composition and postactivation potentiation. Appl. Physiol. Nutr. Metab. 41, 491–497.

Shakespeare, D.T., Stokes, M., Sherman, K.P., et al., 1985. Reflex inhibition of the quadriceps after meniscectomy: lack of association with pain. Clinical Physiology 5, 137–144.

Shumway-Cook, A., Woollacott, M.H., 1995. Motor control, theory and practical applications. Williams & Wilkins, Baltimore.

Sirca, A., Kostevc, V., 1985. The fibre type composition of thoracic and lumbar paravertebral muscles in man. J. Anat. 141, 131–137.

Snyder-Mackler, L., De Luca, P.F., Williams, P.R., et al., 1994. Reflex inhibition of the quadriceps femoris muscle after injury or reconstruction of the anterior cruciate ligament. J. Bone Joint Surg. Am. 76-A, 555–560.

Solomonow, M., Guzzi, A., Baratta, R., et al., 1986. EMG-force model of the elbows antagonistic muscle pair: the effect of joint position, gravity and recruitment. Am. J. Phys. Med. 65, 223–244.

Solomonow, M., Baratta, R., Zhou, B.-H., et al., 1987. The synergistic action of the anterior cruciate ligament and thigh muscles in maintaining joint stability. Am. J. Sports Med. 15, 207–213.

Speers, R.A., Kuo, A.D., Horak, F.B., 2002. Contributions of altered sensation and feedback responses to changes in coordination of postural control due to aging. Gait Posture 16, 20–30.

Spencer, J.D., Hayes, K.C., Alexander, I.J., 1984. Knee joint effusion and quadriceps reflex inhibition in man. Arch. Phys. Med. Rehabil. 65, 171–177.

Spiteri, T., Nimphius, S., Hart, N.H., et al., 2014. Contribution of strength characteristics to change of direction and agility performance in female basketball athletes. J. Strength Cond. Res. 28, 2415–2423.

Staron, R.S., 1997. Human skeletal muscle fiber types: delineation, development, and distribution. Can. J. Appl. Physiol. 22, 307–327.

Stener, B., 1969. Reflex inhibition of the quadriceps elicited from a subperiosteal tumour of the femur. Acta Orthop. Scand. 40, 86–91.

Stener, B., Petersen, I., 1963. Excitatory and inhibitory reflex motor effects from the partially ruptured medial collateral ligament of the knee joint. Acta Orthop. Scand. 33, 359.

Stokes, M., Young, A., 1984. The contribution of reflex inhibition to arthrogenous muscle weakness. Clin. Sci. 67, 7–14.

Stratford, P., 1981. Electromyography of the quadriceps femoris muscles in subjects with normal knees and acutely effused knees. Phys. Ther. 62, 279–283.

Suter, E., Herzog, W., 1997. Extent of muscle inhibition as a function of knee angle. J. Electromyogr. Kinesiol. 7, 123–130.

Suter, E., Herzog, W., 2000. Muscle inhibition and functional deficiencies associated with knee pathologies. In: Herzog, W. (Ed.), Skeletal muscle mechanics, from mechanisms to function. Wiley, Chichester, p. 365.

Suter, E., Herzog, W., Huber, A., 1996. Extent of motor unit activation in the quadriceps muscles of healthy subjects. Muscle Nerve 19, 1046–1048.

Suter, E., Herzog, W., Bray, R.C., 1998a. Quadriceps inhibition following arthroscopy in patients with anterior knee pain. Clin. Biomech. (Bristol, Avon) 13, 314–319.

Suter, E., Herzog, W., De Souza, K.D., et al., 1998b. Inhibition of the quadriceps muscles in patients with anterior knee pain. J. Appl. Biomech. 14, 360–373.

Tabary, J.C., Tabary, C., Tardieu, C., et al., 1972. Physiological and structural changes in the cat's soleus muscle due to immobilization at different lengths by plaster casts. J. Physiol. 224, 231–244.

Taylor, J.D., Fletcher, J.P., 2012. Reliability of the 8-repetition maximum test in men and women. J. Sci. Med. Sport 15, 69–73.

Taylor, D.C., Dalton, J.D., Seaber, A.V., et al., 1990. Viscoelastic properties of muscle–tendon units, the biomechanical effects of stretching. Am. J. Sports Med. 18, 300–309.

Thelen, D.G., Muriuki, M., James, J., et al., 2000. Muscle activities used by young and old adults when stepping to regain balance during a forward fall. J. Electromyogr. Kinesiol. 10, 93–101.

Thomas, C., Jones, P.A., Rothwell, J., et al., 2015. An investigation into the relationship between maximum isometric strength and vertical jump performance. J. Strength Cond. Res. 29, 2176–2185.

Threlkeld, A.J., 1992. The effects of manual therapy on connective tissue. Phys. Ther. 72, 893–902.

Tidball, J.G., 1991. Myotendinous junction injury in relation to junction structure and molecular composition. Exerc. Sport Sci. Rev. 19, 419–445.

Torebjork, H.E., Ochoa, J.L., Schady, W., 1984. Referred pain from intraneural stimulation of muscle fascicles in the median nerve. Pain 18, 145–156.

Torry, M.R., Decker, M.J., Viola, R.W., et al., 2000. Intra-articular knee joint effusion induces quadriceps avoidance gait patterns. Clin. Biomech. (Bristol, Avon) 15, 147–159.

Tracy, B.L., Enoka, R.M., 2002. Older adults are less steady during submaximal isometric contractions with the knee extensor muscles. J. Appl. Physiol. 92, 1004–1012.

Trappe, T.A., Lindquist, D.M., Carrithers, J.A., 2001. Muscle-specific atrophy of the quadriceps femoris with aging. J. Appl. Physiol. 90, 2070–2074.

Trigsted, S.M., Post, E.G., Bell, D.R., 2015. Landing mechanics during single hop for distance in females following anterior cruciate ligament reconstruction compared to healthy controls. Knee Surg. Sports Traumatol. Arthrosc. 1–8.

Urbach, D., Awiszus, F., 2002. Impaired ability of voluntary quadriceps activation bilaterally interferes with function testing after knee injuries. A twitch interpolation study. Int. J. Sports Med. 23, 231–236.

Vaughan, V.G., 1989. Effects of upper limb immobilization on isometric muscle strength, movement time, and triphasic electromyographic characteristics. Phys. Ther. 69, 36–46.

Wainwright, S.A., Biggs, W.D., Currey, J.D., et al., 1982. Mechanical design in organisms. Princeton UniversityPress, Princeton, NJ.

Watkins, M.P., Harris, B.A., Kozlowski, B.A., 1984. Isokinetic testing in patients with hemiparesis. A pilot study. Phys. Ther. 64, 184–189.

Wells, P.E., Frampton, V., Bowsher, D., 1994. Pain management by physiotherapy, second ed. Butterworth-Heinemann, Oxford.

Wilke, H.-J., Wolf, S., Claes, L.E., et al., 1995. Stability increase of the lumbar spine with different muscle groups: a biomechanical in vitro study. Spine 20, 192–198.

Williams, P.E., 1988. Effect of intermittent stretch on immobilised muscle. Ann. Rheum. Dis. 47, 1014–1016.

Williams, P.E., Goldspink, G., 1973. The effect of immobilization on the longitudinal growth of striated muscle fibres. J. Anat. 116, 45–55.

Williams, P.E., Goldspink, G., 1976. The effect of denervation and dystrophy on the adaptation of sarcomere number to the functional length of the muscle in young and adult mice. J. Anat. 122, 455–465.

Williams, P.E., Goldspink, G., 1978. Changes in sarcomere length and physiological properties in immobilized muscle. J. Anat. 127, 459–468.

Williams, P.E., Goldspink, G., 1984. Connective tissue changes in immobilized muscle. J. Anat. 138, 343–350.

Williams, P.L., Bannister, L.H., Berry, M.M., et al., 1995. Gray's anatomy, thirty-eighth ed. Churchill Livingstone, New York.

Winchester, J., McGuigan, M.R., Nelson, A.G., et al., 2010. The relationship between isometric and dynamic strength in college aged males. J. Strength Cond. Res. 24, 1.

Witzmann, F.A., 1988. Soleus muscle atrophy in rats induced by cast immobilization: lack of effect by anabolic steroids. Arch. Phys. Med. Rehabil. 69, 81–85.

Woo, S., Maynard, J., Butler, D., et al., 1988. Ligament, tendon, and joint capsule insertions to bone. In: Woo, S.L.-Y., Buckwalter, J. (Eds.), Injury and repair of the musculoskeletal soft tissues. American Academy of Orthopaedic Surgeons, Park Ridge, IL, pp. 133–166.

Wood, L., Ferrell, W.R., Baxendale, R.H., 1988. Pressures in normal and acutely distended human knee joints and effects on quadriceps maximal voluntary contractions. Q. J. Exp. Physiol. 73, 305–314.

Wood, T.O., Cooke, P.H., Goodship, A.E., 1988. The effect of exercise and anabolic steroids on the mechanical properties and crimp morphology of the rat tendon. Am. J. Sports Med. 16, 153–158.

Woodley, B.L., Newsham-West, R.J., Baxter, D., et al., 2007. Chronic tendinopathy: effectiveness of eccentric exercise. Br. J. Sports Med. 41, 188–198.

Wyke, B.D., Polacek, P., 1975. Articular neurology: the present position. J. Bone Joint Surg. Am. 57B, 401.

Yoshihara, K., Shirai, Y., Nakayama, Y., et al., 2001. Histochemical changes in the multifidus muscle in patients with lumbar intervertebral disc herniation. Spine 26, 622–626.

Young, A., Stokes, M., Crowe, M., 1982a. The relationship between quadriceps size and strength in elderly women. Clin. Sci. 63, 35P–36P.

Young, A., Hughes, I., Round, J.M., et al., 1982b. The effect of knee injury on the number of muscle fibres in the human quadriceps femoris. Clin. Sci. 62, 227–234.

Young, A., Stokes, M., Round, J.M., et al., 1983. The effect of high-resistance training on the strength and cross-sectional area of the human quadriceps. Eur. J. Clin. Invest. 13, 411–417.

Young, A., Stokes, M., Iles, J.F., 1987. Effects of joint pathology on muscle. Clin. Orthop. Relat. Res. 219, 21–27.

Zhang, L.Q., Nuber, G., Butler, J., et al., 1998. In vivo human knee joint dynamic properties as functions of muscle contraction and joint position. J. Biomech. 31, 71–76.

Zhao, W.P., Kawaguchi, Y., Matsui, H., et al., 2000. Histochemistry and morphology of the multifidus muscle in lumbar disc herniation comparative study between diseased and normal sides. Spine 25, 2191–2199.

5

PRINCIPLES OF MUSCLE AND TENDON TREATMENT

PAUL COMFORT ■ LEE HERRINGTON

CHAPTER CONTENTS

I t is not possible to treat muscle tissue in isolation; any management approaches applied to muscle will always to a greater or lesser extent affect tendons, joints and/or nerve tissue. In this text a 'muscle treatment' is defined as a 'treatment to effect a change in muscle'; that is, the intention of the clinician is to produce a change in muscle and therefore it is described as a muscle treatment. Similarly, where a technique is used to effect a change in a joint, it will be referred to as a 'joint treatment', and where a technique is used to effect a change in nerve, it will be referred to as a 'nerve treatment'. Thus, treatments are classified according to which tissue the clinician is predominantly attempting to affect.

This relationship of treatment of muscle, joint and nerve is depicted in Fig. 5.1.

There are a variety of muscle treatments, categorized in this text from the dysfunctions identified in the previous chapter, namely, reduced muscular strength, power and endurance, altered motor control, reduced length and production of symptoms (Table 5.1). From this, a classification of muscle treatment can be identified: to increase muscle strength, power and endurance, alter motor control (increase muscle activation, reduce muscle activation, change timing of onset, alter activation of agonist and antagonist), increase muscle length and reduce muscle-related symptoms.

TABLE 5.1
Muscle Dysfunction, Aims of Muscle Treatment and Treatment Techniques

Muscle Dysfunction	Aims of Muscle Treatment	Treatment Techniques
Reduced strength, power and endurance	Increase strength, power and endurance	Training regimes using free weights, springs, pulleys, TheraBand, dynamometers, PNF
Altered motor control	Increase muscle activation	Active assisted movements, rapid stretch mechanical vibration, PNF, touch, use of overflow, ice and taping
Muscle inhibition delayed timing of onset	Increase time of onset	Challenge posture and balance using, for example, SitFit, gym ball
Increased muscle activation	Reduce muscle activation	Made aware of the unwanted muscle activity using a mirror, verbal feedback, touch, electromyogram feedback. Positioning, PNF, trigger points, deep inhibitory massage and taping
Reduced length	Increase length	Stretching: ballistic or static, passively by clinician or actively by patient PNF
Symptom production	Reduce symptoms	Soft-tissue mobilization: massage, connective tissue massage, specific soft-tissue mobilizations, trigger points, frictions Joint mobilizations Taping Electrotherapy

PNF, proprioceptive neuromuscular facilitation.

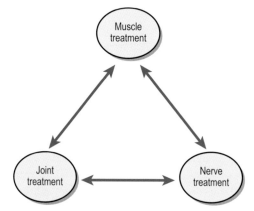

FIG. 5.1 ■ Relationship of treatment techniques of muscle, joint and nerve. Treatment of muscle will also affect joints and nerves.

PRINCIPLES OF INCREASING MUSCLE STRENGTH, POWER AND ENDURANCE

There are a variety of exercise regimes used to increase muscle strength, power and endurance and the reader is referred to the numerous exercise physiology and strength and conditioning textbooks for further details on these.

BOX 5.1
PRINCIPLES OF INCREASING MUSCLE STRENGTH, POWER AND ENDURANCE

Overload	Learning
Specificity	Reversibility
Individuality	Diminishing returns
Motivation	

This text reviews the principles involved in increasing muscle strength, power and endurance. The principles are overload, specificity, individuality, motivation, learning, reversibility and diminishing returns (Box 5.1).

Overload

For any of the systems within the body to adapt the stimuli must be sufficient to create overload; that is, expose the tissue to a load greater than it is currently experiencing. To improve the strength, power or endurance of a muscle it must be progressively and appropriately overloaded (Bruton 2002). To create overload when strengthening a muscle, the resistance (load) must be greater than the muscles are accustomed to during everyday activities, and as the muscle gains strength the resistance must be progressively increased. Overload in this case can be achieved initially through a slight increase in repetitions (2–6) or sets (3–6), but once the maximum number of repetitions is achieved at a given resistance, the resistance (external load) must be increased. To increase repetitions further would alter the focus from muscular strength to endurance. When increasing muscle endurance, there must be a progressive increase in volume of exercise, again via an increase in repetitions (10–15) of sets (3–4), although as with strength, if the maximum number of repetitions can be achieved with a given resistance the resistance must be increased. It is this progressive nature which ensures that overload continues across the rehabilitation/training session.

Specificity

This relates to the specific adaptation of muscle to the imposed demands (DiNubile 1991). The effect on muscle is specific to the nature of the exercise:

1. High resistance and low repetition (usually 2–6 repetitions) will result in an increase in muscle strength (Staron et al. 1994; Hakkinen et al. 1998). It is worth noting that increasing strength also increases muscular endurance, as the relative effort required to move a submaximal load multiple times decreases with an increase in strength, meaning additional repetitions can be performed. Training to the point of momentary muscle failure (no further repetitions can be performed within the set) is not necessary (Izquierdo et al. 2006), as long as exercise is performed in sufficient load (usually ≥80% 1RM).
2. Low resistance (60–75% one-repetition maximum [1RM]) and high repetition (10–15 repetitions) will result in an increase in muscle endurance; only small increases in strength associated with the hypertrophic response to muscular endurance training will result in an increased cross-sectional area of a muscle. Training to momentary muscle failure appears advantageous (Izquierdo et al. 2006).
3. Low resistances (≤40% 1RM) moved at a high velocity will increase muscle power, that is, an increase in fascicle shortening velocity. Power can also be increased with higher loads (≥60% 1RM) as long as the intention is to move quickly, even

if the level of resistance results in a relatively low movement velocity (Behm & Sale 1993). In addition increasing strength increases power output as a result of increased force production and therefore greater acceleration (Cormie et al. 2011; Haff & Nimphius 2012).

The implication of specificity is that the prescribed exercise does not need to mirror the movement pattern of the functional activity it aims to improve, i.e. it does not need to look like the movement in terms of its kinematics. The activity needs to target the appropriate musculature and the loading and/or velocity of movement need to be specific to the aim, e.g. strength for the quadriceps should be high resistance and low repetition, but the exercise could be a squat or lunge variation or a simple knee extension exercise, although the transfer from knee extension to sit to stand will be less effective than from a squat or lunge variation (Augustsson et al. 1998; Blackburn & Morrissey 1998).

Individuality

Individuals will respond differently to the same exercise; this response is determined by genetics, cellular growth rates, metabolism and neural and endocrine regulation. For example, over the age of 60 years the number of fast-twitch fibres diminishes; therefore, an exercise given to an 80-year-old and a 26-year-old will have different effects. With differences in strength levels between middle-aged and older men partly explained by the decrease in anabolic hormones associated with ageing (Izquierdo et al. 2001), although these decreases in strength are somewhat reversible with appropriate strength training (Suetta et al. 2004). Training status, based on strength levels, also determines the response to subsequent training, with individuals who are already strong progressing at a slower rate (Cormie et al. 2010) due to the law of diminishing returns.

Motivation

Only those motivated enough will make the physical and mental effort of following a training programme. The clinician can help to motivate the patient by the use of voice, explanation and enthusiasm. During prolonged and frequent periods of rehabilitation variety is also required. Improving compliance can also be aided by educating the patient as to the relevance and importance of the exercise programme and also by clear goal setting.

Learning

The clinician educates the patient about the required exercise so that it is carried out effectively. Where the movement is unfamiliar, motor learning will have to occur.

Diminishing Returns

An exercise regime will produce a greater improvement in people in poor physical condition than in those already in a good physical condition. However, even in athletic populations many individuals may not have reached such high levels of development, especially in terms of strength, where diminishing returns have only been reported once the athlete can squat to 90° internal knee angle with an external load of >2 × body mass (Cormie et al. 2010), for example.

Endurance training gains take longer to have an effect but are longer-lasting, whereas power can be achieved more quickly but tends to diminish faster.

Reversibility

This rather disappointing principle states that, when training stops, any strength or endurance gains will be progressively lost (Bruton 2002), as can be clearly observed when a limb is immobilized.

Increasing Muscle Strength

The above principles need to be applied when attempting to increase muscle strength. The resistance to a muscle contraction needed to strengthen a muscle can be provided by: gravity, the clinician, the patient, free weights, pulleys, springs, elastic resistance bands and isokinetic dynamometers. Interestingly, an isotonic exercise programme using free weights has been found to be as effective in strengthening the quadricep femoris muscle as the more expensive dynamometer machine (DeLateur et al. 1972). One benefit of free weights is the versatility and greater transference of the adaptive responses to activities of daily living and athletic tasks.

Recommended strengthening regimes for sedentary adults have been advocated by the American College of Sports Medicine (ACSM); but it is important to be aware that these are recommendations for strengthening (resulting in an increase in muscular endurance, muscle

mass and some increase in strength), not strength training, where the primary focus is increasing muscular strength. Such programmes recommend three sets of 8–10 repetitions at least twice a week using the major muscle groups, using a 10RM load. A 10RM would be the maximum amount of weight that could be lifted 10 times before fatigue or loss of technique occurs. This type of training has been used extensively for over 60 years, since it was first formally introduced by DeLorme in 1948 (Todd et al. 2012).

The daily adjustable progressive resistance exercise (DAPRE) system was introduced nearly 30 years ago as a simple tool to take the guesswork out of prescribing training loads and 1RM numbers. Although there have been many advances in periodization models for athletes, the DAPRE method has stood the test of time as an effective method to strengthen novice weight trainers and in rehabilitation (Knight 1985). Table 5.2 explains the basic principles of application.

The optimum frequency of exercise has also been investigated by a number of studies, with varying results. An optimum frequency for strengthening the muscles has been found to be three times a week (Leggett et al. 1991; Pollock et al. 1993; DeMichele et al. 1997). A reasonable guideline for frequency would be a minimum of twice per week (Feigenbaum & Pollock 1999), although if motor learning is the goal and the intensity of the exercise is low, more frequent performance of the task will result in greater improvements in motor control.

TABLE 5.2		
Progressive Resistance Exercise (PRE) Programme[a]		
Number of Repetitions	**Adjustment for Set 3**	**Adjustment for Next Day**
0–2	Decrease by 2.5–5 kg; repeat set	Decrease by 2.5–5 kg
3–4	Decrease by 2.5–5 kg	Keep weight the same
5–7	Keep weight the same	Increase by 2.5–5 kg
8–12	Increase by 2.5–5 kg	Increase by 2.5–7.5 kg
13+	Increase by 2.5–7.5 kg	Increase by 7.5–10 kg

[a]Adjustment of the weight for the exercise programme using the daily adjustable progressive resistive exercise (DAPRE) technique. The number of repetitions during set number 2 is used to adjust weight for set number 3. The number of repetitions during set number 4 is used to adjust the weight for the next session.

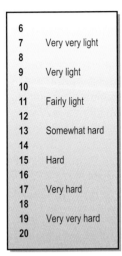

6	
7	Very very light
8	
9	Very light
10	
11	Fairly light
12	
13	Somewhat hard
14	
15	Hard
16	
17	Very hard
18	
19	Very very hard
20	

FIG. 5.2 ■ Fifteen-point scale for ratings of perceived exertion – the RPE scale. *(From Borg 1982, with permission.)*

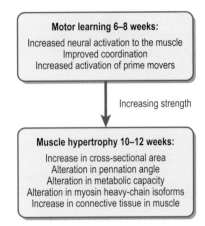

FIG. 5.3 ■ The underlying effects of strengthening muscle.

A strengthening regime would normally start slowly with a low intensity of exercise (American College of Sports Medicine 2013; Feigenbaum & Pollock 1999). Initially, loads that permit three sets of 10 repetitions, without reaching momentary muscle failure, should be used. Once three sets of 12 repetitions can be performed (with a rating of perceived exertion [RPE] of 12–14 RPE [Borg 1982]), a 5% increase in load can be added to the next training session (Fig. 5.2). Exercising near to maximal effort, that is, to 19–20 RPE, produces the greatest gains in strength (American College of Sports Medicine 2013), with progression of weight every 1–2 weeks. However, such intensities tend to result in additional delayed-onset muscle soreness (DOMS), which can discourage unaccustomed individuals from further participation.

It is recommended that, for the elderly and those with clinically significant chronic conditions, the intensity be reduced to one set of 10–15RM, increasing the weight every 2–4 weeks (Feigenbaum & Pollock 1999; Nelson et al. 2007). Using 1RM to assess strength in those with musculoskeletal injuries and chronic diseases can increase injury risk, so a 10RM is a more appropriate estimation. While muscle strength is less in the older person, the potential to strengthen muscle with a training programme is much the same as with a young person (Grimby 1995).

In conformity with the principle of specificity, the type of muscle contraction used in an exercise regime affects the change in muscle strength. Eccentric muscle actions appear to be more effective and efficient in increasing muscle strength. Eccentric exercises have been found to cause a greater increase in eccentric, isometric and concentric muscle strength than either concentric exercises or a mixed exercise regime (Hortobagyi et al. 2000). Eccentric exercise performed three times a week for 12 weeks has been found to increase eccentric strength three and a half times more than concentric exercises (Hortobagyi et al. 1996). However, such exercise is associated with pronounced DOMS, due to the associated muscle damage, in those unaccustomed to eccentric muscle loading.

Underlying Effect of Strengthening a Muscle

A low number of repetitions against a high resistance will strengthen muscle (Staron et al. 1994; Hakkinen et al. 1998). The underlying effects are, first, neural adaptations, including increased recruitment and synchronization of motor units along with reduced activation of antagonists, as part of improved motor learning, and, second, a change in muscle tissue, including hypertrophy, although this is preceded by architectural adaptations (alterations in fascicle length, pennation angle) (Seynnes et al. 2007) (Fig. 5.3). The stimulus for a strength change is the force of muscle action determined by the load applied, and this is reflected in the nature of the adaptations.

Motor Learning

The first stage, which lasts for 6–8 weeks, is where motor learning occurs; performance improves but strength remains the same.

The changes include:

- increased neural activation to the muscle (Sale et al. 1983; Komi 1986) which parallels the increase in muscle strength
- increased activation of prime movers (Sale 1988)
- improved coordination (Sale 1988)
- decreased activation of antagonists.

These neural changes alone can produce an increase in force production (Enoka 1988). During an 8-week training programme neural changes were responsible for almost all the strength gains in older subjects (~70 years), while in younger subjects (~22 years), neural changes were responsible for most of the increased strength in the first 4 weeks, with muscle hypertrophy after 4–6 weeks (Moritani & DeVries 1979). These differences are likely to be related to activity levels and initial muscle strength.

In symptomatic individuals changes in neural activation may be responsible for improved strength and endurance beyond the suggested 6–8 weeks (Kaser et al. 2001; Mannion et al. 2001). Patients with chronic low-back pain followed a 3-month back exercise programme (Mannion et al. 2001), and, although activation, strength and endurance improved, this was not accompanied by any change in the size of the muscle fibres or proportion of muscle fibre type (Kaser et al. 2001). It is likely that in such cases neural activation was initially impaired due to neural inhibition of the muscle.

Muscle Hypertrophy

After the initial neurological adaptations subsequent increases in strength are attributable to muscle architectural adaptations and increases in cross-sectional area (hypertrophy). The changes are:

1. An increase in the cross-sectional area of the muscle (Housh et al. 1992; Narici et al. 1996) and muscle fibres (Melissa et al. 1997; Andersen & Aagaard 2000) visible after a few weeks of training. The increase in cross-sectional area of the muscle is due to hypertrophy of muscle fibres (see below) and an increase in the connective tissue in muscle.

In addition, where the strength training involves a group of muscles, the increase in cross-sectional area is not equal in each muscle (Housh et al. 1992; Narici et al. 1996). For example, with quadriceps strength training, using the knee extension, greatest hypertrophy was seen in rectus femoris and least hypertrophy in vastus intermedius (Narici et al. 1996). In contrast, the rectus femoris was the only muscle to show no adaptation after 8 weeks of heavy squat or squat jump training (Earp et al. 2015). Such findings demonstrating differential adaptations to specific exercises highlight the importance of appropriate selection of exercises.

2. Alteration in muscle fibre types. Some studies have found no change in proportion of type I or type II fibres (Terrados et al. 1990; Labarque et al. 2002), whereas other studies have found an increase in the proportion of type IIa fibres and a decrease in type IIb fibres following strength training (Hortobagyi et al. 1996; Andersen & Aagaard 2000).

3. An alteration in pennation angles (Kawakami et al. 1993, 1995).

4. An alteration in metabolic capacity of muscle has been demonstrated; this effect appears to be genetically determined (Simoneau et al. 1986).

5. An alteration in myosin heavy-chain (MHC) isoforms (Gea 1997; Andersen & Aagaard 2000). The myosin head, which binds with actin during a muscle contraction, contains the MHC isoforms (Scott et al. 2001).

6. An increase in the connective tissue found in muscle structures proportional to muscle hypertrophy.

Increasing Muscle Power

Muscle power is a function of muscle force and velocity; improvement in either or both of these aspects will result in an increase in muscle power. Additionally, repeated practice of the movement, or a component of the movement, at speed, is thought to produce an improvement in muscle power likely due to increased efficiency of movement and decreased antagonist activation (deVries & Housh 1994).

Force production (strength) is the key determinant of power, with an increase in force production resulting in an increased ability to accelerate an object ($F = M \times A$). If acceleration of an object increases from an increase in force production there is a resultant increase in velocity of movement, therefore increasing both force and velocity results in a greater improvement in power ($P = F \times V$).

It has been suggested that movement should be carried out as fast as possible against a resistance of 30% maximal isometric force, although exercises performed with low loads resulted in improvement in power at low loads, whereas exercises using moderate or heavy loads increased power across all loads (Kaneko et al. 1983; Toji & Kaneko 2004). In line with the principle of specificity, the load and resultant velocity result in the greatest increases in power at those loads and velocities; however, the heavy load training results in greater improvements in power across a range of loads (Kaneko et al. 1983; Toji et al. 1997; Toji & Kaneko 2004; Harris et al. 2008). The key factor in power development appears to be the ability to produce force rapidly, which is best training with a focus on strength development rather than power, unless the individual is already strong (Cormie et al. 2010).

Increasing Muscle Endurance

Muscle endurance refers to the ability of a muscle to produce a specific force repetitively or to sustain an isometric action for a period of time (Bruton 2002). To increase muscle endurance a muscle must contract at 50–70% of its maximum force, for 8–20 repetitions, for 3–4 sets at each session. It is worth noting that such intensity and repetition ranges help to increase work capacity of the muscles, but due to the high volume of exercise associated with such training, this is most likely to result in a hypertrophic response. In addition, for individuals who are weak, initially increasing strength increases endurance of the muscles purely by ensuring that activities of daily living are no longer near maximal intensity.

Underlying Effects of Increasing Muscle Endurance

A high number of repetitions of muscle actions against a moderate resistance will increase muscle endurance by effecting a change in the muscle (increased cross-sectional area, increased glycolytic enzymes and increased glycogen storage). The stimulus is the

---

BOX 5.2
UNDERLYING EFFECT OF INCREASING MUSCLE ENDURANCE

Increase in number of I and IIa fibres, and a decrease in type IIb fibres
Increase in cross-sectional area of type I fibres
Increase in number of capillaries
Increase in myoglobin content
Increase in oxidative power and enzyme activity of mitochondria
Increase in oxidative enzymes
Increased store of muscle glycogen and fat
Increased activity of enzymes
Higher threshold level of lactate
Altered myosin heavy-chain isoforms

---

metabolic demand and tensile stress on the muscle and this is reflected in the nature of the changes (Box 5.2) and includes:

- an increase in the number of type I and IIa fibres and a decrease in type IIb fibres (Ingjer 1979; Demirel et al. 1999)
- an increase in the cross-sectional area of type I and IIb fibres (Ingjer 1979)
- an increase in the number of capillaries surrounding each muscle fibre (Ingjer 1979)
- an increase in blood flow in muscle (Vanderhoof et al. 1961; Rohter et al. 1963)
- an increase in myoglobin content (Holloszy 1976).

Aerobic Endurance

Where endurance training incorporates general cardiorespiratory exercises, such as walking, running, swimming and cycling, the ACSM provides guidance for healthy adults recommending moderate exercise intensity sufficient to raise the heart rate to 60–90% of maximum, and it should be carried out for 30 minutes five times a week, or 20 minutes of vigorous intensity (80–90% maximum heart rate) three times per week (Haskell et al. 2007). For the older adult and those with clinically significant chronic conditions the recommendations are similar except the heart rate should be raised to 50–85%, where 5–6 is moderate (50%) and 7–8 (80%) is vigorous intensity on a 10-point scale.

Clinical Implications of Strength, Power and Endurance Training

Exercise prescription is a core skill of therapists that combines management of disorders of movement, knowledge of exercise regimens and clinical reasoning skills to ensure that the exercises prescribed are appropriate for the individual (Taylor et al. 2007). For example, there is strong evidence that strengthening and aerobic exercises reduce pain and improve activity levels in people with osteoarthritis of the knee (Brosseau et al. 2004). A patient with osteoarthritis of the knee is likely to have weak quadriceps and pain, and may be unable to perform a functional activity such as sit to stand, stair climbing and walking for more than 10 minutes. Therefore a training programme needs to reflect each of these elements. It requires strength training to enable the patient to carry out sit to stand, improvements in muscular endurance to climb stairs and cardiovascular endurance to enable the patient to walk for extended periods of time. Consideration needs to be taken for the load, repetition, rest period and order of exercise. As with any exercise regimen the most complex and fatiguing tasks should be performed at the start of the session, with adequate rest between sets (usually 2–3 minutes) to ensure that the subsequent set does not commence when the muscles are still fatigued.

Altering Motor Control

Signs of altered motor control have been considered in the previous chapter, such as muscle inhibition, delayed timing of onset, increased muscle activation and altered relative activation of agonist and antagonist. The aim of treatment, in this case, would therefore be to increase muscle activation, increase the speed of onset of muscle contraction, reduce muscle activation or alter relative activation of agonist and antagonist. The common theme for each of these aims is to alter the pattern of muscle activation, which is to alter motor control. Aspects of motor learning will be covered in Chapter 10.

To Increase Muscle Activation

Methods for increasing muscle activation, that is, for facilitating muscle contraction, include active assisted movements, rapid stretch mechanical vibration, proprioceptive neuromuscular facilitation (PNF), touch,

---

BOX 5.3
TREATMENT TO INCREASE MUSCLE ACTIVATION

Active assisted movements
Rapid stretch
Proprioceptive neuromuscular facilitation
Touch
Use of overflow
Mechanical vibration
Ice
Taping

---

use of overflow, ice and taping (Box 5.3). Electrical stimulation of muscle is also available and has been shown to be very successful, especially in combination with a volitional muscle contraction being undertaken at the same time. With the muscle contracting and in a lengthened position, a rapid stretch is applied to the muscle; this stimulates the muscle spindles to facilitate extrafusal muscle contraction. Vibration similarly stimulates the muscle spindles, such as using vibration platforms. PNF may also prove helpful in facilitating muscle contraction. Touch can be used to facilitate muscle contraction; stimulation of the skin has been shown to enhance alpha and gamma motor neuron activity in the underlying muscles and cause inhibition of more distal muscles (Eldred & Hagbarth 1954). Taping is thought to increase activation of the underlying muscle (Gilleard et al. 1998; Cowan et al. 2002).

Inhibition of an active voluntary contraction was eliminated with a fast-velocity isotonic contraction (Newham et al. 1989). This can be explained by the relationship of force and speed, where increased speed of concentric contraction reduces the force generated (Hill 1938).

Increase Speed of Onset

Using the principles of motor learning, it would seem reasonable to suggest that, to increase the speed of onset of muscle action, treatment needs to use normal functional activities that will produce a need for the muscle to contract. With delayed activation of transversus abdominis in patients with low-back pain (Hodges & Richardson 1996), treatment would include functional postures and movements that challenge postural stability and this would need to be continued repetitively over a period of time. In patients with anterior knee pain, a combination of specific muscle exercise with biofeedback, muscle stretches, taping and patellofemoral accessory movements has been shown, over a 6-week period, to increase the timing of muscle onset of vastus medialis, when going up and down stairs (Gilleard et al. 1998; Cowan et al. 2002). The mechanism by which the tape increased the onset of vastus medialis is unclear. Cutaneous stimulation has been shown to alter the recruitment threshold and recruitment order of motor units (Garnett & Stephens 1981; Jenner & Stephens 1982).

To Reduce Muscle Activation

This may be needed where the clinician feels there is overactivity of muscles. For example, in the early stages of motor learning there is co-contraction of the agonist and antagonist when carrying out a movement (Moore & Marteniuk 1986). Similarly, there may be unwanted muscle activity as a patient attempts to produce a specific muscle contraction, for example, flexion of the lumbar spine, while trying to isolate contraction of the transversus abdominis and lumbar multifidus. The patient may have overactivity of muscles because of pain, which may be sufficient to produce muscle spasm. In all of these examples, the clinician may need to reduce the muscle activity. To do this the patient may need to be made aware of the unwanted muscle activity using a mirror, verbal feedback, touch or EMG feedback. Other methods for reducing muscle activation include positioning, PNF, massage, relaxation techniques and taping (Box 5.4). It has been speculated that tape to the posterior thigh inhibits overactive hamstring muscles (McConnell 2002) and some other studies would

---

BOX 5.4
TREATMENT TO REDUCE MUSCLE ACTIVITY

Mirror
Verbal feedback
Touch
Electromyogram feedback
Positioning
Proprioceptive neuromuscular facilitation
Trigger points
Deep inhibitory massage
Taping

---

support this (Tobin & Robinson 2000). Tape over the lower fibres of trapezius of asymptomatic subjects was found to inhibit the muscle by as much as 22% when measured using the Hoffman reflex (Alexander et al. 2003). The underlying mechanism is not known; it has been postulated that it could be due to an alteration in muscle length and/or stimulation of cutaneous afferents, leading to inhibition of the underlying muscle and/or decrease in descending drive of the motor neuron pool (Alexander et al. 2003).

Altering Muscle Length

Treatment may aim to decrease or increase length. The reason a muscle may be considered long, and why treatment should be aimed at reducing its length, is likely to be associated with reduced muscle tone. Where the clinician identifies reduced tone, treatment would be directed at increasing the strength of the muscle, which has been discussed above.

Increasing Muscle Length

When considering muscle stretching, it can be helpful to categorize muscle into the active contractile unit and the non-contractile connective tissue, within the muscle belly and tendon. Treatment can be classified according to which effect the clinician is attempting to have on the muscle. Increasing the length of a muscle can be achieved by passively lengthening the connective tissue such that there is a permanent increase in length, or by attempting to produce physiological relaxation of the active contractile unit of the muscle belly using, for example, PNF (autogenic or reciprocal inhibitory techniques). Clearly, the contractile and non-contractile elements are inseparable and what is not being stated here is that treatment to lengthen the connective tissue affects the connective tissue alone and has no effect on the contractile unit, or vice versa. The classification of treatment is used simply to aid communication between clinicians and is not attempting to describe the effect of the treatment. Muscle can be stretched passively with the aim of treatment to produce a permanent lengthening of the muscle and tendon.

Passive Muscle Stretching by the Clinician

An effective passive stretch is produced when a force moves the proximal and distal muscle attachments further apart; often, this involves fixing the proximal attachment while passively moving the distal attachment away. Positioning can often be used to help fix the proximal attachment; for example, supine with one leg flexed on to the chest helps to fix the pelvis as the other hip is moved into extension to lengthen the iliopsoas muscle.

Direction of Movement. There is no single direction of movement that will stretch all parts of a muscle because the muscle line of action often lies across multiple planes; the clinician needs to explore fully and treat all aspects of muscle length by combining movements (Hunter 1998). The muscle attachments, direction of its fibres, position of the muscle and the relationship of the muscle to other structures enable the clinician to decide how to combine movements for any particular muscle. For example, to lengthen biceps femoris fully, a combination of hip flexion, medial rotation and adduction with knee extension and medial tibial rotation needs to be used. Similarly, to lengthen extensor carpi radialis brevis fully, elbow extension with forearm pronation, wrist flexion, ulnar deviation and individual finger flexion need to be combined (Hunter 1998).

Magnitude of Force. When a muscle is stretched the force is distributed throughout the connective tissue framework of the muscle (Hill 1950). Whenever a permanent lengthening is achieved, there is initially some degree of mechanical weakening. Interestingly, the amount of weakening depends on the way the muscle has been lengthened, as well as how much it has been lengthened. A small force for a long duration will induce less weakening than a large force for a short duration (Sapega et al. 1981; Taylor et al. 1990).

Speed of Movement. The speed of the movement can be described as slow or fast, and the rhythm should be smooth. The connective tissue in muscle is viscoelastic and is therefore sensitive to the speed of the applied force. A force applied quickly will produce less movement, provoking a greater stiffness; that is, the gradient of the resistance curve will increase; a force applied more slowly, on the other hand, will cause more movement as the stiffness is relatively less. If the intention of treatment is to maximize the range of movement by lengthening connective tissue then a slow speed would seem preferable.

In addition, as the muscle spindles detect both the magnitude and rate of change in length, rapidly moving the limb into a position where the muscle is stretched results in early stimulation of this sensory receptor. Such stimulation results in reflection stimulation of the muscle, creating a shortening rather than a lengthening of the muscle fascicles and therefore a less effective stretch.

Duration. In terms of treatment dose, time relates to the duration of the stretch, the number of times this is repeated and the frequency of the appointments. Hamstring muscle length has been found to be as effectively lengthened with daily static stretches using a 30-second stretch as with three repetitions of 1-minute stretches (Bandy et al. 1997). Reassessment after each repetition enables the clinician to determine the effect of treatment on the patient's signs and symptoms. Depending on this change (better, same or worse), the clinician may alter the time and number of repetitions within a treatment session. A permanent (plastic) lengthening of the connective tissue of muscle and tendon with minimal structural weakness is enhanced by a long-duration stretch (Sapega et al. 1981).

Temperature. Temperature influences the mechanical behaviour of connective tissue under tensile load. As temperature rises to about 40–45°C, stiffness decreases and extensibility increases (Rigby 1964; Lehmann et al. 1970). At about 40°C a change in the microstructure of collagen occurs, which significantly enhances the extensibility and potential for a permanent (plastic) change in length (Rigby 1964). The viscoelastic properties can be increased by as much as 170% when muscle temperature is raised to 43°C and a higher temperature will induce less weakening than a lower temperature (Sapega et al. 1981). Once the heat is removed, it has been found that maintaining the tension as the tissue cools enhances the plastic deformation (Lehmann et al. 1970; Sapega et al. 1981). Increasing the temperature of a tissue depends on its depth; it will obviously be easier to heat more superficial muscles.

The ability of short-wave diathermy, hot-water baths and ultrasound to increase muscle and tendon temperature has been investigated. Twenty minutes of short-wave diathermy has been shown to raise muscle temperature by as much as 4°C (Millard 1961). If normal muscle temperature is assumed to be the same as normal body temperature, 37°C, then this would raise the temperature of muscle to 41°C, sufficient to enhance the effect of stretching. Twenty minutes of immersion in a water bath at 42.5°C has been found to increase forearm muscle temperature to 39°C (Barcroft & Edholm 1943), which may be sufficient to enhance the effect of a stretch. Ultrasound at a frequency of 1 megacycle with a 12.5 cm² head at an intensity of 1 W/cm² for 7 minutes caused the muscle temperature (3.5 cm below the surface of the skin) to rise to 40°C (Lehmann et al. 1966). This research suggests that heating muscle and tendon with short-wave diathermy, hot water or ultrasound will enhance the effect of muscle stretching.

Symptom Response. The clinician decides which symptom, and to what extent, is to be provoked during treatment. Choices include:

- no provocation
- provocation to the point of onset or increase in resting symptoms
- partial reproduction
- total reproduction.

The decision as to what extent symptoms are provoked during treatment depends on the severity and irritability of the symptom(s) and the nature of the condition. If the symptoms are severe, that is, the patient is unable to tolerate the symptom being produced, the clinician would choose not to provoke the symptoms. The clinician may also choose not to provoke symptoms if they are irritable, that is, once symptoms are provoked they take some time to ease. If, however, the symptoms are not severe and not irritable then the clinician is able to reproduce the patient's symptoms during treatment, and the extent to which symptoms are reproduced will depend on the tolerance of the patient. The nature of

the condition may limit the extent to which symptoms are produced, such as a recent traumatic injury. Treatment is progressed or regressed by altering appropriate aspects of the treatment dose: patient position, movement, direction of force, magnitude of force, amplitude of oscillation, speed, rhythm, time or symptom response. Table 5.3 suggests the ways in which each aspect of the treatment dose can be progressed and regressed.

Table 5.4 provides an example of how a treatment dose for lengthening the upper fibres of trapezius may be progressed and regressed. An increase in time from 30 seconds to 1 minute provides a progression of the treatment dose, and a reduction in the amount of symptoms accounts for the regression. Other aspects of treatment dose which are closely linked are the length of time for each repetition and the number of repetitions; these, together, provide a dose of time and so each can be altered at the same time.

TABLE 5.3		
Progression and Regression of Treatment Dose		
Treatment Dose	**Progression**	**Regression**
Position	Muscle towards end of available range	Muscle towards beginning of available range
Direction of force	More provocative	Less provocative
Magnitude of force	Increased	Decreased
Amplitude of oscillation	Decreased	Increased
Rhythm	Staccato	Smoother
Time	Longer	Shorter
Speed	Slower or faster	Slower
Symptom response	Allowing more symptoms to be provoked	Allowing fewer symptoms to be provoked

TABLE 5.4		
Example of How a Treatment Dose for Increasing the Passive Length of the Upper Fibres of Trapezius Can Be Progressed and Regressed		
Regression	**Dose**	**Progression**
In full cervical flexion and 1/2 range contralateral flexion, static hold for 30 seconds to partial reproduction of patient's neck pain	In full cervical flexion and 1/2 range contralateral flexion, static hold for 30 seconds to full reproduction of patient's neck pain	In full cervical flexion and 1/2 range contralateral flexion, static hold for 1 minute to full reproduction of patient's neck pain

TABLE 5.5

Treatment Dose for Passive Stretching by the Clinician and Active Stretching by the Patient

Factors	Passive Stretching by the Clinician	Active Stretching by the Patient
Patient's position	E.g. supine	E.g. sitting, standing with heel of foot on a stool with knee extended
Direction of movement	E.g. hip flexion	E.g. active knee extension
Magnitude of force applied	Related to therapist's perception of resistance: grades I–V	Related to patient's perception of stretch
Amplitude of oscillation	Static or small or large	Static or small or large
Speed	Slow or fast	Slow or fast (if fast, may be referred to as ballistic)
Rhythm	Smooth or staccato	Smooth or staccato
Time	Of repetitions and number of repetitions	Of repetitions and number of repetitions
Temperature	Room temperature or heat with short-wave diathermy	Room temperature
Symptom response	Short of symptom production	Short of symptom production
	Point of onset or increase in resting symptom	Point of onset or increase in resting symptom
	Partial reproduction of symptom	Partial reproduction of symptom
	Full reproduction of symptom	Full reproduction of symptom

Passive Muscle Stretching by the Patient

The patient can actively stretch a muscle. The factors defining the treatment dose are exactly the same as passive muscle stretching carried out by the clinician (Table 5.5). The only difference is that, with passive stretching by the patient, the patient is in total control of the stretching movement and relies on his or her own perception of stretch and symptom production to determine the way the stretch is carried out. The patient needs to be fully informed as to how to carry out the stretch, that is, how forceful to be and to what extent to reproduce the symptoms. The clinician in this case takes on a more educational and advisory role.

In sports medicine, two types of stretching are advocated: ballistic and static stretching. Ballistic stretching involves the person performing bouncing, rhythmic end-range movements. While such stretching may be beneficial during a warm-up in preparation for participation in sport, due to the rate of lengthening the muscle spindle is stimulated, resulting in a less effective stretch. Static stretching involves a simple hold at the end of range. Controversy exists over the effectiveness of each type of stretching in producing an increase in muscle length. One study found that both methods were ineffective; only hold–relax produced an increase in muscle length (Sady et al. 1982).

Summary of Increasing Muscle Length

The important factors that affect a permanent increase in length of muscle following a passive stretch include the magnitude of force, time of force application and temperature of the muscle (Sapega et al. 1981). From research to date, it appears that a permanent (plastic) lengthening of the connective tissue of muscle and tendon with minimal structural weakness will be enhanced by a relatively low force for a long-duration stretch (Sapega et al. 1981) at high temperatures (Talishev & Fedina 1976; Sapega et al. 1981).

Increasing Length via the Contractile Unit of Muscle

The aim of this type of treatment is to cause a relaxation of the contractile unit of muscle in order to increase muscle length. Muscle energy techniques and positional release techniques can also be used to cause muscle relaxation (Chaitow 2013, 2015). PNF is advocated to achieve this muscle relaxation. These are rotational movement patterns through full range of movement, hold–relax, contract–relax and agonist–contract.

Hold–Relax. The muscle is positioned in its stretched position, either actively or passively. A strong isometric contraction of the muscle is achieved by the clinician providing manual resistance. The muscle contraction needs to be carefully controlled by the clinician. This is achieved by saying to the patient, 'don't let me move you' or 'hold' and by slowly and smoothly increasing the manual resistance to maximum contraction. Following contraction the patient is asked to relax, the clinician gradually reduces the resistance and time is allowed for muscle relaxation to occur. The clinician then moves further into range to increase the length of the muscle. The procedure of contraction followed by relaxation is then repeated until no further increase in muscle length can be achieved.

Contract–Relax. This is the same as hold–relax except that, following the isometric contraction, the patient actively contracts to lengthen the antagonistic muscle further, rather than the clinician passively lengthening the muscle. For example, to lengthen quadriceps the patient isometrically contracts the quadriceps at, for example, 60° flexion for 3–6 seconds. The patient is then asked to relax and actively to contract the hamstrings in an attempt to increase knee flexion and stretch the quadriceps muscle group. As in hold–relax, the procedure is repeated in the new range of movement and repeated until no further increase in muscle length is achieved.

Agonist–Contract. The muscle is put in a position of stretch and a contraction of the agonist attempts to increase movement and thus increase stretch of the muscle. The clinician facilitates this movement by carefully applying a passive force. For example, to lengthen quadriceps the knee is positioned in 60° flexion. The patient actively contracts the hamstrings in an attempt to increase knee flexion and stretch the quadriceps muscle group. The clinician applies a force to the lower leg to enhance this movement.

Reducing Symptoms

A useful premise for the clinician is to consider that the symptom is whatever patients say it is, existing whenever they say it is. This was originally used for pain, but can be widened to any symptom the patient feels.

The assumption in this text is that the cause of the muscle pain is some sort of injury to the muscle and/or tendon. In this situation, the pain will be a result of mechanical and/or chemical irritation of the muscle

nociceptors. The subjective information from the patient, particularly the behaviour of symptoms and mechanism of injury, may enable the clinician to identify whether it is the contractile unit of muscle and/or connective tissue of muscle that is involved in the pain. For example, an overstretch injury may affect the connective tissue of muscle and require treatment to increase the muscle length and, by so doing, reduce pain.

Various palpatory techniques can be used to reduce symptoms emanating from muscle, including specific soft-tissue mobilization massage, connective tissue massage trigger points and frictions. Joint mobilizations, taping and electrotherapy can also be used. Specific soft-tissue mobilization has been described above. The reader is referred to reviews by Watson (2000) and Hainan et al. (2016).

Massage can be applied to muscle to reduce pain, using stroking, effleurage, kneading, picking up, wringing and skin rolling. Additional effects are thought to include an increase in the flow of the circulation, muscle relaxation, lengthening of tissues and increased tissue drainage and pain relief (Waters-Banker et al. 2014).

Connective tissue massage involves applying specific strokes to the skin and subcutaneous tissues from the lumbar spine to the upper limbs or from the lumbar spine to the lower limbs. It has been suggested that it affects the autonomic nervous system and, via this system, increases circulation which may aid healing and ease pain (Waters-Banker et al. 2014).

A trigger point is defined as a focus of hyperirritability of a muscle and is thought to contribute to muscle tightness. On palpation of the muscle, an area of local tightness with tenderness, possible muscle twitch and referral of pain in a typical pattern is found. Having identified this, treatment involves applying manual pressure over the area. The underlying cause of the phenomenon of trigger points has been proposed as secondary hyperalgesia originating from peripheral nerves (Quintner & Cohen 1994).

Frictions are small-amplitude deep pressures applied to tissue such as muscle and tendon. The clinician's finger or thumb moves with the patient's skin across the tissue. The tissue is often positioned such that it is in a lengthened position. It has been proposed that frictions cause hyperaemia, break down adhesions and stimulate mechanoreceptors (Cyriax 1984). In an experimental study on New Zealand white rabbits, 10 minutes of frictions caused mechanical trauma to muscle tissue, which, after 6 days, had largely healed (Gregory et al. 2003). Whether this traumatic effect may be therapeutic in the presence of a muscle injury remains unknown, but it certainly highlights the mechanical effects of force on muscle.

Joint mobilizations may be used to reduce pain and change muscle. For example, anterior knee pain often involves the dysfunction of the quadriceps muscle group and the patellofemoral joint. Treatment to the muscle will affect the joint, and, similarly, treatment to the joint will affect the muscle. Accessory movements applied to the patellofemoral joint, with or without concentric, eccentric or isometric quadriceps contraction, may be useful. Similarly, with lateral elbow pain there may be dysfunction of the extensor muscles of the forearm as well as a radiohumeral joint dysfunction. Again, accessory movements may be applied to the joint with or without concentric, eccentric or isometric contraction of the wrist and finger extensor muscles. For example, a lateral glide combined with the patient performing an isometric grip with the hand has been found in a randomized double-blind placebo-controlled study to increase by approximately 10% the pressure pain threshold and increase by almost 60% the painfree grip strength (Vicenzino et al. 2001). In another study, spinal accessory movements have been found to reduce pain and improve muscle activation in the cervical spine (Sterling et al. 2001). Further information on accessory movements combined with active muscle contractions can be found elsewhere (Mulligan 1995; Vicenzino 2003). The mechanism by which joint accessory movements reduce pain and cause a change in muscle activity is discussed in Chapter 7.

Tape may be used to relieve muscle pain. A useful principle is to apply the tape in such a way that it replicates the direction of the pain-relieving force applied by the clinician during treatment. For details of methods of taping the reader is referred to other texts (Vicenzino 2003; Macdonald 2004).

The mechanism by which pain is relieved with each of these manual techniques is still unclear. Large-diameter type III afferents are distributed throughout muscle tissue and are stimulated by pressure, mechanical force caused by lengthening muscle or by muscle contraction (Mense & Meyer 1985). It is possible that the manual techniques described above may stimulate

the type III afferents and cause a reflex inhibition of the type IV muscle nociceptors according to the pain gate theory (Melzack & Wall 1965). Clearly, large-diameter afferents in the skin and joint may also contribute to this pain inhibition. The pain may also be reduced via a descending inhibitory system explained below and expanded upon rather more in Chapter 7 on nerve treatment.

Descending Inhibition of Pain

The periaqueductal grey (PAG) area has been found to be important in the control of nociception. PAG projects to the dorsal horn and has a descending control of nociception (Fig. 5.4). It also projects upwards to the medial thalamus and orbital frontal cortex, and so may have an ascending control of nociception (Heinricher & Fields 2013). The PAG has two distinct regions, the dorsolateral PAG (dPAG) and the ventrolateral PAG (vPAG).

dPAG

The dPAG runs to the dorsolateral pons and ventrolateral medulla, which is involved in autonomic control (Heinricher & Fields 2013). In the rat, stimulation of the dPAG causes analgesia, increased blood pressure, increased heart rate, vasodilation of the hindlimb muscles, increased rate and depth of respiration and coordinated hindlimb, jaw and tail movements, suggesting increased activity of the sympathetic nervous system, and alpha motor neurons (Lovick 2007). The neurotransmitter from dPAG is noradrenaline (norepinephrine), and the analgesic effect appears to mediate morphine analgesia of mechanical nociceptor stimuli (Kuraishi et al. 1983). At the spinal cord level, dPAG causes inhibition of substance P from peripheral noxious mechanical stimulation (Kuraishi 1990).

vPAG

The vPAG runs mainly to the nucleus raphe magnus. In the rat, stimulation of vPAG causes analgesia with decreased blood pressure, decreased heart rate, vasodilation of the hindlimb muscles and reduced hindlimb, jaw and tail movements, suggesting inhibition of the sympathetic nervous system and inhibition of alpha motor neurons (Lovick 2007). The neurotransmitter used in vPAG is serotonin, and the analgesic effect appears to mediate morphine analgesia of thermal

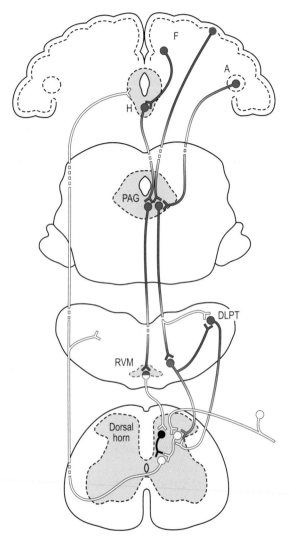

FIG. 5.4 ■ Pain-modulating pathway. Periaqueductal grey (*PAG*) receives input from the frontal lobe (*F*), the amygdala (*A*) and the hypothalamus (*H*). Afferents from PAG travel to the rostral ventromedial medulla (*RVM*) and the dorsolateral pontomesencephalic tegmentum (*DLPT*) and on to the dorsal horn. The RVM has bidirectional control of nociceptive transmission. There are inhibitory (filled) and excitatory (unfilled) interneurons. *(From Fields & Basbaum 1999, with permission.)*

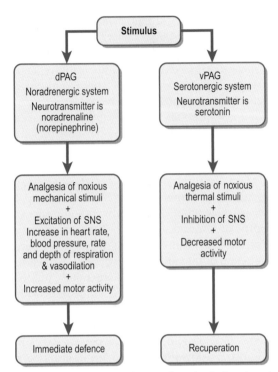

FIG. 5.5 ■ Descending inhibition of mechanical nociception from the dorsolateral periqueductal grey (*dPAG*: noradrenergic system) and thermal nociception from the ventrolateral periaqueductal grey (*vPAG*: serotonergic system). *SNS*, sympathetic nervous system.

nociceptive stimuli (Kuraishi et al. 1983). At the dorsal horn vPAG inhibits the release of somatostatin, produced by peripheral noxious thermal stimulation (Kuraishi 1990). These mechanisms have been linked to the behaviour of an animal under threat, which initially acts with a defensive flight-or-fight response, followed by recuperation (Fanselow 2007; Lovick 2007); this is summarized in Fig. 5.5.

Noxious stimuli can cause activation of the descending control system (Yaksh & Elde 1981; Heinricher & Fields 2013), which may reduce nociceptive transmission. Noxious stimulation has been found to cause release of enkephalins at the supraspinal and spinal levels (Yaksh & Elde 1981). It has also been found that stimulation of the spinothalamic tract, transmitting nociceptive information from one foot, can be inhibited by noxious input from the contralateral foot, hand, face or trunk (Gerhart et al. 1981). It has been suggested that this may explain the relief of pain with acupuncture, and pain behaviours such as 'biting your lip' (Melzack 1975). Painful treatment of muscle may also activate the descending control system.

Addressing the Biopsychosocial Aspects of Symptoms

Injury, or the perception of injury, produces anxiety and fear (Craig 1999). Who has ever injured themselves, however minimally, and not experienced an emotional reaction? We all will have a cognitive and emotional response to injury, because injury interrupts our lives. It seems reasonable to suggest, therefore, that all patients with neuromusculoskeletal dysfunction will have thoughts and feelings about their problem, and it would be an oversight on the part of the clinician not to enquire about these. This enquiry involves the clinician understanding the patient's thoughts and feelings. This is no easy task, and to do it well requires a high level of skill in active listening. Active listening involves putting our own thoughts, beliefs and feelings to one side and choosing, instead, to hear what the patient has to say. It involves trying to understand patients and their world, through their eyes, and avoiding the all-too-easy error of reinterpreting through our eyes. It requires the clinician to listen with compassion and patience and without judgement. It involves the clinician using words carefully and meaningfully and using open-ended questions to search for information, until understanding is reached. It involves sensitive verbal and non-verbal communication, encouraging safe and open communication.

Following the enquiry of patients as to their thoughts and feelings, two further steps are recommended: education and exposure (Vlaeyen & Crombez 1999). Education involves the clinician carefully facilitating the patient's understanding of his or her problem. How this is carried out with patients will vary according to a number of factors, including their prior knowledge, thoughts and beliefs, and how they feel about the problem. All the listening skills discussed above will be essential in this process. The ability of the clinician to be honest is important. The clinician needs to explain the problem to the patient in a careful way. There is a world of difference between, 'The pain in your back is from the disc' and 'I think the pain in your back could be coming from the disc'. The former explanation suggests that you know that the pain is coming from the disc, and yet there is overwhelming evidence that you cannot make such claims; it has been estimated that a definite diagnosis of pathology can be made in

about only 15% of cases (Waddell 2004). Furthermore, there is a long-term problem with being so confident as the patient may, in the future, have a recurrence of the same pain and may see another clinician who may say, 'The pain in your back is from your sacroiliac joint'. The patient is aware that this is a repeat episode and now, quite rightly, begins to have doubts about the ability of these two clinicians. This will be a familiar story to experienced clinicians, who will have come across patients who may have received three, four or even more confident 'diagnoses' of the same problem, and who come to you depressed, cynical and disillusioned with the medical profession.

The final aspect is exposure, which involves careful and graded exposure to the movements or postures that provoke pain (Vlaeyen & Crombez 1999). While this is designed for chronic pain patients who learn to avoid movements and posture through fear (Waddell & Main 2004), it may also be an important part of the treatment of acute tissue damage. Using movements and postures in a careful, controlled and graded way may help to avoid long-term movement dysfunctions; the principles of graded exposure and reloading are further explored in Chapter 10.

Muscle Injury and Repair

Muscle can be damaged by a direct injury, such as a laceration or contusion, or indirectly by a sudden forceful contraction causing a muscle or tendon tear; damage may also be due to a chronic overuse injury (Kellett 1986). Whatever the mechanism of injury, the effect on muscle tissue is similar (Hurme et al. 1991) and can be considered in three phases: inflammatory or lag phase, regeneration phase and remodelling phase (Jarvinen & Lehto 1993).

The inflammatory or lag phase is characterized by haematoma formation, tissue necrosis and an inflammatory reaction. Necrosis of muscle tissue occurs with retraction of the muscle fibres on either side of the necrotic zone. It is generally accepted that treatment for the first 48–72 hours of a muscle injury is summarized by RICE: rest, ice, compression and elevation (Evans 1980; Kellett 1986). This has more recently been revised to the acronym POLICE (Bleakley et al. 2012), which stands for protection, optimal loading, ice, compression, elevation, with the emphasis now being more on returning the injury to loading in a controlled manner (see Chapter 10).

During the regeneration phase there is phagocytosis of damaged tissue, and production of connective scar tissue. Capillary growth satellite cells migrate into the necrotic area. Muscle fibres regenerate by differentiation into myoblasts and then into myotubes, which link the two stumps on either side of the necrotic region. The connective tissue within muscle is also damaged and undergoes healing with subsequent scar formation (Jarvinen & Lehto 1993). Following a short period of immobilization – more than 3–5 days for rats (Jarvinen & Lehto 1993) – it is considered beneficial to mobilize the muscle, within the limits of symptoms. Early mobilization is thought to enhance tensile strength, orientation of the regenerating muscle fibres, resorption of connective scar tissue and blood flow to the damaged area and to avoid atrophy brought about by immobilization (Jarvinen & Lehto 1993). The tensile strength of a tendon has been found to increase as a result of 60 repetitions per day of manual wrist and finger flexion/extension following a primary repair (Takai et al. 1991).

The remodelling phase is characterized by the maturation of regenerated muscle (Jarvinen & Lehto 1993). There is contraction and reorganization of scar tissue and a gradual recovery of the functional capacity of the muscle.

Treatment of a muscle injury may include soft-tissue mobilization, frictions, controlled exercises, lengthening, tape and electrotherapy. The reader is directed to relevant texts for further information. Careful consideration is needed when applying any of these passive modalities to muscle of how much and when, as they all add load to the tissue and the priority for muscle injury treatment will always be exercise.

Alongside damage to muscle and connective tissue, neural tissue may also be damaged. It is worth mentioning here that a patient presenting with classical signs of a hamstring tear may, in fact, have a neurodynamic component to the problem. In Australian Rules football, players with signs of a hamstring tear had a positive slump test and when this was addressed in treatment there was a better result than with more traditional muscle treatment techniques (Kornberg & Lew 1989). This highlights the need for a full and comprehensive examination of a patient.

Delayed-Onset Muscle Soreness

Muscle strain injury occurs with eccentric exercise, producing DOMS (Friden et al. 1983; Jones et al. 1986). Pain, weakness and muscle stiffness are felt after unaccustomed eccentric exercise. There is breakdown of collagen (Brown et al. 1997) and disruption of the Z band, predominantly in type II fibres, with repair largely completed by 6 days (Friden et al. 1983; Jones et al. 1986). The reason for DOMS following eccentric contraction may be that eccentric actions produce more force within the muscle than other types of muscle contraction, resulting in greater damage and inflammation (Kanda et al. 2013).

Tendon Injury and Repair

Tendons can tear in the middle region, by avulsion of bone and, more rarely, at the insertion site. The myotendinous region is the weakest part of the tendon–muscle unit and is the region most susceptible to strain injuries (Garrett et al. 1989; Garrett 1990; Tidball 1991). Healing of tendon is similar to that of other soft tissues and consists of three phases: lag or inflammation phase (1–7 days), regeneration or proliferation phase (7–21 days) and remodelling or maturation phase (21 days to 1 year) (Jozsa & Kannus 1997).

Repetitive strain may alter the collagenous structure of tendon with resultant inflammation, oedema and pain (Jozsa & Kannus 1997). Overuse injury occurs where this repetitive strain causing tissue damage is greater than the natural repair and healing process (Archambault et al. 1995; Jozsa & Kannus 1997). Conditions including tendinopathies may lead, with further strain, to partial or complete rupture of the tendon. Eccentric exercises have been advocated for chronic Achilles tendinopathy (Alfredson et al. 1998); however it is the high load which is important here as the tendon cannot differentiate between types of muscle action.

In work-related upper-limb tendon injuries, the repetitive nature of the task may be sufficient to cause change in the tissue. It is proposed that, initially, in the first 5 days, there is ischaemia, metabolic disturbance and cell membrane damage leading to inflammation (Jozsa & Kannus 1997). The increase in tissue pressure further impairs the circulation and enhances the ischaemic changes. In the proliferation phase (5–21 days) there is fibrin clotting, and fibroblast, synovial cell and capillary proliferation followed by the maturation phase (<21 days) in which adhesions and thickening of the tenosynovium and paratenon occur (Kvist & Kvist 1980; Jozsa & Kannus 1997).

Treatment of a tendon injury may include soft-tissue mobilization, frictions, controlled exercises, lengthening, tape and electrotherapy. The reader is directed to relevant texts for further information.

Choice of Muscle Treatment

The choice of treatment depends on the assessment of the patient, whether the patient has a dysfunction of muscle and, if so, what that dysfunction is. Treatment may be to increase muscle strength, power and/or endurance, increase muscle length, alter motor control (increase muscle activation, reduce muscle activation, increase time of onset) and reduce symptoms. The overall aim of treatment is to normalize a dysfunction, that is, to eradicate the abnormal signs and symptoms.

Modification, Progression and Regression of Treatment

The continuous monitoring of the patient's subjective and physical status guides the entire treatment and management programme of the patient. The clinician judges the degree of change with treatment and relates this to the expected rate of change from the prognosis and normal physiological responses, and decides whether or not a treatment needs to be altered in some way. The nature of this alteration can be to modify the technique in some way, to progress or regress the treatment. Regardless of which alteration is made, the clinician makes every effort to determine what effect this alteration has on the patient's subjective and physical status. In order to do this, the clinician alters one aspect of treatment at a time, and reassesses immediately to determine the value of the alteration.

Modification of Treatment

The clinician may modify the treatment given to a patient by altering an existing treatment, adding a new treatment or stopping a treatment. At all times the treatment should have the functional goals of the patient in mind. Altering an existing treatment involves altering some aspect of the treatment dose (outlined earlier). The immediate and more long-term effect of the alteration is then evaluated by reassessment of the subjective and physical characteristics (Fig. 5.6). The clinician then decides whether, overall, the patient is better, the same or worse, relating this to the prognosis. For instance,

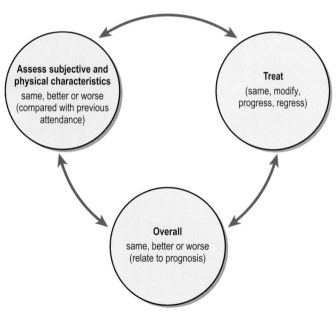

FIG. 5.6 ■ Modification, progression and regression of treatment.

if a quick improvement was expected but only some improvement occurred, the clinician may progress treatment. If the patient is worse after treatment, the dose may be regressed in some way, and if the treatment made no difference at all then a more substantial modification may be made. Before discarding a treatment it is worth making sure that it has been fully utilized, as it may be that a much stronger or much weaker treatment dose may be effective.

Progression and Regression of Treatment

A treatment is progressed or regressed by altering appropriate aspects of the treatment dose in such a way that more treatment, or less treatment, is applied to the tissues.

Fig. 5.7 shows typical load progression for a muscle injury. It starts with midrange isometric contractions; once these have been performed without symptoms and with symmetrical strength (within 10%), the patient progresses to multiangle isometric contractions (mid to inner to outer range). From there eccentric concentric contractions would be performed in the midrange, before progressing (once these have been performed without symptoms and with symmetrical strength [within 10%]) to outer-range eccentric and concentric contractions. When undertaking eccentric and concentric

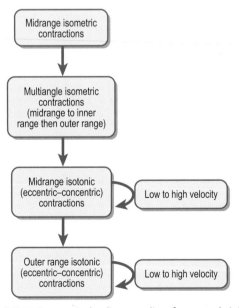

FIG. 5.7 ■ Progressive loading paradigm for a muscle injury.

contractions the velocity of contraction along the rate of force development would need to be considered and progressively applied.

SUMMARY

This chapter has outlined the principles of muscle treatment. Treatment is only a part of the overall management of a patient; the reader is therefore encouraged to go now to Chapter 10, where the principles of management are discussed.

REFERENCES

Alexander, C.M., Stynes, S., Thomas, A., et al., 2003. Does tape facilitate or inhibit the lower fibres of trapezius? Man. Ther. 8, 37–41.

Alfredson, H., Pietila, T., Jonsson, P., et al., 1998. Heavy load eccentric calf muscle training for the treatment of chronic achilles tendinosis. Am. J. Sports Med. 26, 360–366.

American College of Sports Medicine (ACSM), 2013. Resource manual for guidelines for exercise testing and prescription, seventh ed. Williams & Wilkins, Baltimore.

Andersen, J.L., Aagaard, P., 2000. Myosin heavy chain IIX overshoot in human skeletal muscle. Muscle Nerve 23, 1095–1104.

Archambault, J.M., Wiley, J.P., Bray, R.C., 1995. Exercise loading of tendons and the development of overuse injuries, a review of current literature. Sports Med. 20, 77–89.

Augustsson, J., Esko, A., Thomee, R., et al., 1998. Weight training of the thigh muscles using closed vs open kinetic chain exercises: a comparison of performance enhancement. J. Orthop. Sports Phys. Ther. 27, 3–8.

Bandy, W.D., Irion, J.M., Briggler, M., 1997. The effect of time and frequency of static stretching on flexibility of the hamstring muscles. Phys. Ther. 77, 1090–1096.

Barcroft, H., Edholm, O.G., 1943. The effect of temperature on blood flow and deep temperature in the human forearm. J. Physiol. 102, 5–20.

Behm, D.G., Sale, D.G., 1993. Intended rather than actual movement velocity determines velocity-specific training response. J. Appl. Physiol. 74, 359–368.

Blackburn, J.R., Morrissey, M.C., 1998. The relationship between open and closed kinetic chain strength of the lower limb and jumping performance. J. Orthop. Sports Phys. Ther. 27, 430–435.

Bleakley, C., Glasgow, P., MacAuley, D., 2012. PRICE needs updating, should we call the POLICE? Br. J. Sports Med. 46, 220–221.

Borg, G.A.V., 1982. Psychophysical bases of perceived exertion. Med. Sci. Sports Exerc. 14, 377–381.

Brosseau, L., Pelland, L., Wells, G., et al., 2004. Efficacy of aerobic exercises for osteoarthritis (part II): a meta-analysis. Phys Ther Rev 9, 125–145.

Brown, S.J., Child, R.B., Day, S.H., et al., 1997. Indices of skeletal muscle damage and connective tissue breakdown following eccentric muscle contractions. Eur. J. Appl. Physiol. 75, 369–374.

Bruton, A., 2002. Muscle plasticity: response to training and detraining. Physiotherapy 88, 398–408.

Chaitow, L., 2013. Muscle energy techniques, fourth ed. Churchill Livingstone, Edinburgh.

Chaitow, L., 2015. Positional release techniques, fourth ed. Churchill Livingstone, Edinburgh.

Cormie, P., McGuigan, M.R., Newton, R.U., 2010. Influence of strength on magnitude and mechanisms of adaptation to power training. Med. Sci. Sports Exerc. 42, 1566–1568.

Cormie, P., McGuigan, M.R., Newton, R.U., 2011. Developing maximal neuromuscular power: part 2 – training considerations for improving maximal power production. Sports Med. 41, 125–146.

Cowan, S.M., Bennell, K.L., Crossley, K.M., et al., 2002. Physical therapy alters recruitment of the vasti in patellofemoral pain syndrome. Med. Sci. Sports Exerc. 34, 1879–1885.

Craig, K.D., 1999. Emotions and psychobiology. In: Wall, P.D., Melzack, R. (Eds.), Textbook of pain, fourth ed. Churchill Livingstone, Edinburgh, pp. 331–343.

Cyriax, J., 1984. Textbook of orthopaedic medicine, vol. 2. Baillière Tindall, London.

DeLateur, B., Lehmann, J.F., Warren, C.G., et al., 1972. Comparison of effectiveness of isokinetic and isotonic exercise in quadriceps strengthening. Arch. Phys. Med. Rehabil. 53, 60–64.

DeMichele, P.L., Pollock, M.L., Graves, J.E., et al., 1997. Isometric torso rotation strength: effect of training frequency on its development. Arch. Phys. Med. Rehabil. 78, 64–69.

Demirel, H.A., Powers, S.K., Naito, H., et al., 1999. Exercise-induced alterations in skeletal muscle myosin heavy chain phenotype: dose–response relationship. J. Appl. Physiol. 86, 1002–1008.

deVries, H.A., Housh, T.J., 1994. Physiology of exercise for physical education, athletics and exercise science, fifth ed. Brown & Benchmark, Madison, WI.

DiNubile, N.A., 1991. Strength training. Clin. Sports Med. 10, 33–62.

Earp, J.E., Newton, R.U., Cormie, P., et al., 2015. Inhomogeneous quadriceps femoris hypertrophy in response to strength and power training. Med. Sci. Sports Exerc. 47, 2389–2397.

Eldred, E., Hagbarth, K.E., 1954. Facilitation and inhibition of gamma efferents by stimulation of certain skin areas. J. Neurophysiol. 17, 59–65.

Enoka, R.M., 1988. Muscle strength and its development: new perspectives. Sports Med. 6, 146–168.

Evans, P., 1980. The healing process at cellular level: a review. Physiotherapy 66, 256–259.

Fanselow, M.S., 2007. The midbrain periaqueductal gray as a coordinator of action in response to fear and anxiety. In: Depaulis, A., Bandler, R. (Eds.), The midbrain periaqueductal gray matter. Plenum Press, New York, pp. 151–173.

Feigenbaum, M.S., Pollock, M.L., 1999. Prescription of resistance training for health and disease. Med. Sci. Sports Exerc. 31, 38–45.

Fields, H.L., Basbaum, A.I., 1999. Central nervous system mechanisms of pain modulation. In: Wall, P.D., Melzack, R. (Eds.), Textbook of pain, fourth ed. Churchill Livingstone, Edinburgh, pp. 309–329.

Friden, J., Sjostrom, M., Ekblom, B., 1983. Myofibrillar damage following intense eccentric exercise in man. Int. J. Sports Med. 4, 170–176.

Garnett, R., Stephens, J.A., 1981. Changes in the recruitment threshold of motor units produced by cutaneous stimulation in man. J. Physiol. 311, 463–473.

Garrett, W.E., 1990. Muscle strain injuries: clinical and basic aspects. Med. Sci. Sports Exerc. 22, 436–443.

Garrett, W.E., Rich, F.R., Nikolaou, P.K., et al., 1989. Computed tomography of hamstring muscle strains. Med. Sci. Sports Exerc. 21, 506–514.

Gea, J.G., 1997. Myosin gene expression in the respiratory muscles. Eur. Respir. J. 10, 2404–2410.

Gerhart, K.D., Yezierski, R.P., Giesler, G.J., et al., 1981. Inhibitory receptive fields of primate spinothalamic tract cells. J. Neurophysiol. 46, 1309–1325.

Gilleard, W., McConnell, J., Parsons, D., 1998. The effect of patellar taping on the onset of vastus medialis obliquus and vastus lateralis muscle activity in persons with patellofemoral pain. Phys. Ther. 78, 25–32.

Gregory, M.A., Deane, M.N., Mars, M., 2003. Ultrastructural changes in untraumatised rabbit skeletal muscle treated with deep transverse friction. Physiotherapy 89, 408–416.

Grimby, G., 1995. Muscle performance and structure in the elderly as studied cross-sectionally and longitudinally. J. Gerontol. 50A (special issue), 17–22.

Haff, G.G., Nimphius, S., 2012. Training principles for power. Strength Cond. J. 34, 2–12.

Hainan, Y., Kristi, R., Pierre, C., et al., 2016. The effectiveness of physical agents for lower-limb soft tissue injuries: a systematic review. J. Orthop. Sports Phys. Ther. 46, 523–554.

Hakkinen, K., Newton, R.U., Gordon, S.E., et al., 1998. Changes in muscle morphology, electromyographic activity, and force production characteristics during progressive strength training in young and older men. J. Gerontol. 53A, B415–B423.

Harris, N.K., Cronin, J.B., Hopkins, W.G., et al., 2008. Squat jump training at maximal power loads vs. heavy loads: effect on sprint ability. J. Strength Cond. Res. 22, 1742–1749.

Haskell, W.L., Lee, I.M., Pate, R.R., et al., 2007. Physical activity and public health: updated recommendation for adults from the American College of Sports Medicine and the American Heart Association. Med. Sci. Sports Exerc. 39, 1423–1434.

Heinricher, M.M., Fields, H.L., 2013. Central nervous system mechanisms of pain modulation. In: Wall, P.D., Melzack, R. (Eds.), Textbook of pain, sixth ed. Churchill Livingstone, Edinburgh, pp. 129–142.

Hill, A.V., 1938. The heat of shortening and the dynamic constants of muscle. Proceedings of the Royal Society of London (Biology) 126, 136–195.

Hill, A.V., 1950. The series elastic component of muscle. Proc. R. Soc. Lond., B, Biol. Sci. 137, 273–280.

Hodges, P.W., Richardson, C.A., 1996. Inefficient muscular stabilization of the lumbar spine associated with low back pain. A motor control evaluation of transversus abdominis. Spine 21, 2640–2650.

Holloszy, J.O., 1976. Adaptations of muscular tissue to training. Prog. Cardiovasc. Dis. 18, 445–458.

Hortobagyi, T., Dempsey, L., Fraser, D., et al., 2000. Changes in muscle strength, muscle fibre size and myofibrillar gene expression after immobilization and retraining in humans. J. Physiol. 524, 293–304.

Hortobagyi, T., Hill, J.P., Houmard, J.A., et al., 1996. Adaptive responses to muscle lengthening and shortening in humans. J. Appl. Physiol. 80, 765–772.

Housh, D.J., Housh, T.J., Johnson, G.O., et al., 1992. Hypertrophic response to unilateral concentric isokinetic resistance training. J. Appl. Physiol. 73, 65–70.

Hunter, G., 1998. Specific soft tissue mobilization in the management of soft tissue dysfunction. Man. Ther. 3, 2–11.

Hurme, T., Kalimo, H., Lehto, M., et al., 1991. Healing of skeletal muscle injury: an ultrastructural and immunohistochemical study. Med. Sci. Sports Exerc. 23, 801–810.

Ingjer, F., 1979. Capillary supply and mitochondrial content of different skeletal muscle fiber types in untrained and endurance-trained men. A histochemical and ultrastructural study. Eur. J. Appl. Physiol. Occup. Physiol. 40, 197–209.

Izquierdo, M., Hakkinen, K., Anton, A., et al., 2001. Maximal strength and power, endurance performance, and serum hormones in middle-aged and elderly men. Med. Sci. Sports Exerc. 33, 1577–1587.

Izquierdo, M., Ibanez, J., Gonzalez-Badillo, J.J., et al., 2006. Differential effects of strength training leading to failure versus not to failure on hormonal responses, strength, and muscle power gains. J. Appl. Physiol. (1985) 100, 1647–1656.

Jarvinen, M.J., Lehto, M.U.K., 1993. The effects of early mobilisation and immobilisation on the healing process following muscle injuries. Sports Med. 15, 78–89.

Jenner, J.R., Stephens, J.A., 1982. Cutaneous reflex responses and their central nervous system pathways studied in man. J. Physiol. 333, 405–419.

Jones, D.A., Newham, D.J., Round, J.M., et al., 1986. Experimental human muscle damage: morphological changes in relation to other indices of damage. J. Physiol. 375, 435–448.

Jozsa, L., Kannus, P., 1997. Human tendons: anatomy, physiology and pathology. Human Kinetics, Champaign, IL.

Kanda, K., Sugama, K., Hayashida, H., et al., 2013. Eccentric exercise-induced delayed-onset muscle soreness and changes in markers of muscle damage and inflammation. Exerc. Immunol. Rev. 19, 72–85.

Kaneko, M., Fuchimoto, T., Toji, H., et al., 1983. Training effect of different loads on the force–velocity relationship and mechanical power output in human muscle. Scand. J. Med. Sci. Sports 5, 50–55.

Kaser, L., Mannion, A.F., Rhyner, A., et al., 2001. Active therapy for chronic low back pain: part 2. Effects on paraspinal muscle cross-sectional area, fiber type size, and distribution. Spine 26, 909–919.

Kawakami, Y., Abe, T., Fukunaga, T., 1993. Muscle-fiber pennation angles are greater in hypertrophied than in normal muscles. J. Appl. Physiol. 74, 2740–2744.

Kawakami, Y., Abe, T., Kuno, S.-Y., et al., 1995. Training-induced changes in muscle architecture and specific tension. Eur. J. Appl. Physiol. 72, 37–43.

Kellett, J., 1986. Acute soft tissue injuries – a review of the literature. Med. Sci. Sports Exerc. 18, 489–500.

Knight, K.L., 1985. Guidelines for rehabilitation of sports injuries. Clin. Sports Med. 4, 405–416.

Komi, P.V., 1986. Training of muscle strength and power: interaction of neuromotoric, hypertrophic, and mechanical factors. Int. J. Sports Med. 7 (Suppl.), 10–15.

Kornberg, C., Lew, P., 1989. The effect of stretching neural structures on grade one hamstring injuries. J. Orthop. Sports Phys. Ther. 6, 481–487.

Kuraishi, Y., 1990. Neuropeptide-mediated transmission of nociceptive information and its regulation. Novel mechanisms of analgesics. Yakugaku Zasshi 110, 711–726.

Kuraishi, Y., Harada, Y., Aratani, S., et al., 1983. Separate involvement of the spinal noradrenergic and serotonergic systems in morphine analgesia: the differences in mechanical and thermal algesic tests. Brain Res. 273, 245–252.

Kvist, H., Kvist, M., 1980. The operative treatment of chronic calcaneal paratenonitis. J. Bone Joint Surg. Br. 62B, 353–357.

Labarque, V.L., Eijnde, B., Van Leemputte, M., 2002. Effect of immobilization and retraining on torque–velocity relationship of human knee flexor and extensor muscles. Eur. J. Appl. Physiol. 86, 251–257.

Leggett, S.H., Graves, J.E., Pollock, M.L., et al., 1991. Quantitative assessment and training of isometric cervical extension strength. Am. J. Sports Med. 19, 653–659.

Lehmann, J.F., DeLateur, B.J., Silverman, D.R., 1966. Selective heating effects of ultrasound in human beings. Arch. Phys. Med. Rehabil. 47, 331–339.

Lehmann, J.F., Masock, A.J., Warren, C.G., et al., 1970. Effect of therapeutic temperature on tendon extensibility. Arch. Phys. Med. Rehabil. 51, 481–487.

Lovick, T., 2007. Interactions between descending pathways from the dorsal and ventrolateral periaqueductal gray matter in the rat. In: Depaulis, A., Bandler, R. (Eds.), The midbrain periaqueductal gray matter. Plenum Press, New York, pp. 101–120.

Macdonald, R., 2004. Taping techniques, second ed. Butterworth-Heinemann, Oxford.

Mannion, A.F., Taimela, S., Muntener, M., et al., 2001. Active therapy for chronic low back pain. Part I. Effects on back muscle activation, fatigability, and strength. Spine 26, 897–908.

McConnell, J., 2002. Recalcitrant chronic low back and leg pain – a new theory and different approach to management. Man. Ther. 7, 183–192.

Melissa, L., MacDougall, J.D., Tarnopolsky, M.A., et al., 1997. Skeletal muscle adaptations to training under normobaric hypoxic versus normoxic conditions. Med. Sci. Sports Exerc. 29, 238–243.

Melzack, R., 1975. Prolonged relief of pain by brief, intense transcutaneous somatic stimulation. Pain 1, 357–373.

Melzack, R., Wall, P.D., 1965. Pain mechanisms: a new theory. Science 150, 971–979.

Mense, S., Meyer, H., 1985. Different types of slowly conducting afferent units in cat skeletal muscle and tendon. J. Physiol. 363, 403–417.

Millard, J.B., 1961. Effect of high-frequency currents and infra-red rays on the circulation of the lower limb in man. Ann. Phys. Med. 6, 45–66.

Moore, S.P., Marteniuk, R.G., 1986. Kinematic and electromyographic changes that occur as a function of learning a time-constrained aiming task. J. Mot. Behav. 18, 397–426.

Moritani, T., DeVries, H.A., 1979. Neural factors versus hypertrophy in the time course of muscle strength gain. Am. J. Phys. Med. 58, 115–130.

Mulligan, B.R., 1995. Manual therapy 'nags', 'snags', 'MWM' etc., third ed. Plane View Services, New Zealand.

Narici, M.V., Hoppeler, H., Kayser, B., et al., 1996. Human quadriceps cross-sectional area, torque and neural activation during 6 months strength training. Acta Physiol. Scand. 157, 175–186.

Nelson, M.E., Rejeski, W.J., Blair, S.N., et al., 2007. Physical activity and public health in older adults: recommendation from the American College of Sports Medicine and the American Heart Association. Med. Sci. Sports Exerc. 39, 1435–1445.

Newham, D.J., Hurley, M.V., Jones, D.W., 1989. Ligamentous knee injuries and muscle inhibition. J. Orthop. Rheumatol. 2, 163–173.

Pollock, M.L., Graves, J.E., Bamman, M.M., et al., 1993. Frequency and volume of resistance training: effect on cervical extension strength. Arch. Phys. Med. Rehabil. 74, 1080–1086.

Quintner, J.L., Cohen, M.L., 1994. Referred pain of peripheral nerve origin: an alternative to the 'myofascial pain' construct. Clin. J. Pain 10, 243–251.

Rigby, B.J., 1964. The effect of mechanical extension upon the thermal stability of collagen. Biochim. Biophys. Acta 79, 634–636.

Rohter, F.D., Rochelle, R.H., Hyman, C., 1963. Exercise blood flow changes in the human forearm during physical training. J. Appl. Physiol. 18, 789–793.

Sady, S.P., Wortman, M., Blanke, D., 1982. Flexibility training: ballistic, static or proprioceptive neuromuscular facilitation? Arch. Phys. Med. Rehabil. 63, 261–263.

Sale, D.G., 1988. Neural adaptation to resistance training. Med. Sci. Sports Exerc. 20, S135–S145.

Sale, D.G., MacDougall, J.D., Upton, A.R.M., et al., 1983. Effect of strength training upon motor neurone excitability in man. Med. Sci. Sports Exerc. 15, 57–62.

Sapega, A.A., Quedenfield, T.C., Moyer, R.A., et al., 1981. Biophysical factors in range-of-motion exercise. Phys. Sportsmed. 9, 57–65.

Scott, W., Stevens, J., Binder-Macleod, S.A., 2001. Human skeletal muscle fiber type classifications. Phys. Ther. 81, 1810–1816.

Seynnes, O.R., de Boer, M., Narici, M.V., 2007. Early skeletal muscle hypertrophy and architectural changes in response to high-intensity resistance training. J. Appl. Physiol. 102, 368–373.

Simoneau, J.A., Lortie, G., Boulay, M.R., et al., 1986. Inheritance of human skeletal muscle and anaerobic capacity adaptation to high-intensity intermittent training. Int. J. Sports Med. 7, 167–171.

Staron, R.S., Karapondo, D.L., Kraemer, W.J., et al., 1994. Skeletal muscle adaptations during early phase of heavy-resistance training in men and women. J. Appl. Physiol. 76, 1247–1255.

Sterling, M., Jull, F., Wright, A., 2001. Cervical mobilisation: concurrent effects on pain, sympathetic nervous system activity and motor activity. Man. Ther. 6, 72–81.

Suetta, C., Aagaard, P., Rosted, A., et al., 2004. Training-induced changes in muscle CSA, muscle strength, EMG, and rate of force development in elderly subjects after long-term unilateral disuse. J. Appl. Physiol. (1985) 97, 1954–1961.

Takai, S., Woo, S.L.-Y., Horibe, S., et al., 1991. The effects of frequency and duration of controlled passive mobilization on tendon healing. J. Orthop. Res. 9, 705–713.

Talishev, F.M., Fedina, T.I., 1976. Influence of muscle viscoelastic characteristics on the accuracy of movement control. In: Komi, P.V. (Ed.), Biomechanics V-A. Baltimore: University Park, pp. 124–128.

Taylor, D.C., Dalton, J.D., Seaber, A.V., et al., 1990. Viscoelastic properties of muscle–tendon units: the biomechanical effects of stretching. Am. J. Sports Med. 18, 300–309.

Taylor, N.F., Dodd, K.J., Shields, N., et al., 2007. Therapeutic exercise in physiotherapy practice is beneficial: a summary of systematic reviews 2002–2005. Aust. J. Physiother. 53, 7–16.

Terrados, N., Jansson, E., Sylven, C., et al., 1990. Is hypoxia a stimulus for synthesis of oxidative enzymes and myoglobin? J. Appl. Physiol. 68, 2369–2372.

Tidball, J.G., 1991. Myotendinous junction injury in relation to junction structure and molecular composition. Exerc. Sport Sci. Rev. 19, 419–445.

Tobin, S., Robinson, G., 2000. The effect of McConnell's vastus lateralis inhibition taping technique on vastus lateralis and vastus medialis obliquus activity. Physiotherapy 86, 173–183.

Todd, J.S., Shurley, J.P., Todd, T.C., Thomas, L., 2012. DeLorme and the science of progressive resistance exercise. J. Strength Cond. Res. 26, 2913–2923.

Toji, H., Kaneko, M., 2004. Effect of multiple-load training on the force–velocity relationship. J. Strength Cond. Res. 18, 792–795.

Toji, H., Suei, K., Kaneko, M., 1997. Effects of combined training loads on relations among force, velocity, and power development. Can. J. Appl. Physiol. 22, 328–336.

Vanderhoof, E.R., Imig, C.J., Hines, H.M., 1961. Effect of muscle strength and endurance development on blood flow. J. Appl. Physiol. 16, 873–877.

Vicenzino, B., 2003. Lateral epicondylalgia: a musculoskeletal physiotherapy perspective. Man. Ther. 8, 66–79.

Vicenzino, B., Paungmali, A., Buratowski, S., et al., 2001. Specific manipulative therapy treatment for chronic lateral epicondylalgia produces uniquely characteristic hypoalgesia. Man. Ther. 6, 205–212.

Vlaeyen, J.W.S., Crombez, G., 1999. Fear of movement/(re)injury, avoidance and pain disability in chronic low back pain patients. Man. Ther. 4, 187–195.

Waddell, G., 2004. Diagnostic triage. In: Waddell, G. (Ed.), The back pain revolution, second ed. Churchill Livingstone, Edinburgh, p. 9.

Waddell, G., Main, C.J., 2004. Beliefs about back pain. In: Waddell, G. (Ed.), The back pain revolution, second ed. Churchill Livingstone, Edinburgh, pp. 187–202.

Waters-Banker, C., Dupont-Versteegden, E.E., Kitzman, P.H., et al., 2014. Investigating the mechanisms of massage efficacy: the role of mechanical immunomodulation. J. Athl. Train. 49, 266–273.

Watson, T., 2000. The role of electrotherapy in contemporary physiotherapy practice. Man. Ther. 5, 132–141.

Yaksh, T.L., Elde, R.P., 1981. Factors governing release of methionine enkephalin-like immunoreactivity from mesencephalon and spinal cord of the cat in vivo. J. Neurophysiol. 46, 1056–1075.

6

FUNCTION AND DYSFUNCTION OF NERVE

KIERAN BARNARD ■ COLETTE RIDEHALGH

CHAPTER CONTENTS

Patients presenting with musculoskeletal dysfunction present with vastly differing problems. In neurological terms this may range from central nervous system pathology through to nerve root pathology and peripheral nerve pathology. The thoughtful clinician must clinically reason to differentiate between such pathologies and establish a suitable management plan accordingly. The patient with signs and symptoms of cauda equina syndrome (CES), myelopathy or an acute flaccid foot drop, for example, needs appropriate referral onwards as a matter of urgency (see clinical examples of nerve pathology, on page 167), whilst patients with arm/leg pain and dermatomal numbness without strength or reflex change may require close monitoring of their neurological status and careful evaluation of their response to treatment. In order for the clinician to manage the patient appropriately, it is important to have a thorough understanding of nerve function and dysfunction.

NERVE FUNCTION

The nervous system can be broadly divided into the central nervous system (brain and spinal cord), autonomic nervous system (which will be discussed under nerve movement) and peripheral nervous system (cranial nerves and spinal nerves with their branches).

The following aspects of nerve function will be considered:

- anatomy and physiology of the spinal cord and nerve roots
- tracts of the spinal cord
- anatomy and physiology of peripheral nerves
- biomechanics of peripheral nerves
- movement of the nervous system.

Anatomy and Physiology of the Spinal Cord

The human spinal cord extends from the foramen magnum to the conus medullaris around the level of the first lumbar vertebra. From the conus medullaris, the roots of the cauda equina (horse's tail) project inferiorly (Fig. 6.1). Three layers of connective tissue, collectively known as the meninges, surround and protect the delicate brain and the spinal cord; they are the dura mater, arachnoid mater and pia mater (Fig. 6.2). The pia mater, the innermost meningeal layer, is a thin, highly vascular structure that blends and intimately follows the contours of the underlying brain and spinal cord. Cerebrospinal fluid and larger blood vessels fill the subarachnoid space which lies between the pia mater and the overlying arachnoid mater. The outermost meningeal layer, the dura mater, is a tough fibrous structure. The subdural space between the arachnoid mater and the dura mater contains no cerebrospinal fluid and few blood vessels. In the cranium the dura mater is continuous with the periosteum. The space between the dura mater of the spinal cord and the vertebral periosteum is known as the epidural space. The epidural space extends to the level of the second sacral vertebra and contains the spinal nerve roots, fat and the epidural venous plexus. The epidural space may be injected with anaesthetic and steroid which may provide pain relief and improved function in some patients with a symptomatic lumbar disc herniation (Manchikanti et al. 2015).

Blood is supplied to the spinal cord segmentally from the aorta and other adjacent arteries, including the vertebral, cervical, intercostal, lumbar and sacral arteries. As a consequence, spinal cord ischaemia may occur in up to 20% of patients undergoing aortic aneurysm surgery and paraplegia may be a devastating consequence in some cases (Wynn & Acher 2014). Each segmental artery passes through the intervertebral foramina and divides into the dorsal (posterior) and ventral (anterior) radicular arteries. The ventral radicular arteries supply the anterior spinal artery, which runs in the midline down the ventral aspect of the cord. The anterior artery provides 75% of the cord's vascularity. The dorsal radicular arteries feed the two posterior spinal arteries, which supply the remainder of the cord (Fig. 6.3). As well as the arterial system, which envelops the spinal cord from the anterior and posterior arteries, venous drainage occurs via an extensive venous plexus.

Spinal rootlets project from the spinal cord both dorsally and ventrally. These rootlets unite to form the dorsal and ventral roots. The dorsal roots contain sensory

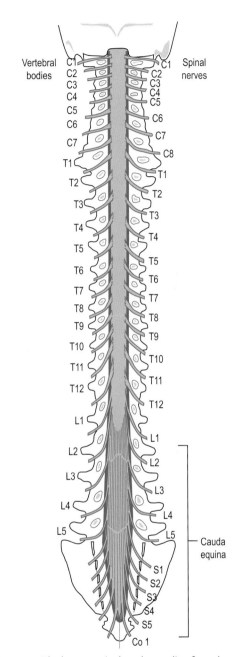

FIG. 6.1 ■ The human spinal cord extending from the occiput to the conus medullaris, from where the roots of the cauda equina project inferiorly. (From Palastanga & Soames 2012, with permission.)

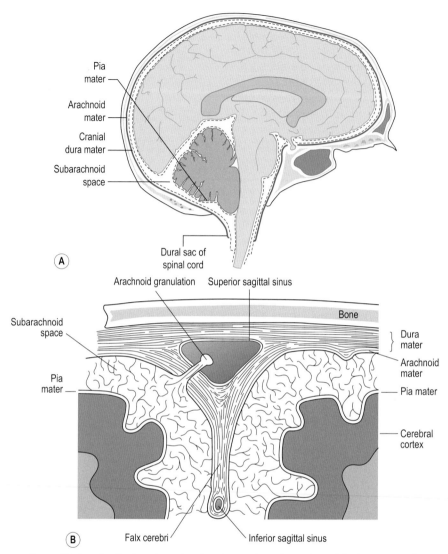

Pia
mater

Arachnoid
mater

Cranial
dura mater

Subarachnoid
space

Dural sac of
spinal cord

(A)

Arachnoid granulation   Superior sagittal sinus

Subarachnoid
space

Bone

Dura
mater

Arachnoid
mater

Pia mater

Pia
mater

Cerebral
cortex

(B)   Falx cerebri   Inferior sagittal sinus

FIG. 6.2 ■ The meninges. (A) Longitudinal section, showing the meningeal covering of the brain. (B) The meningeal covering at the falx cerebri. *(From Palastanga & Soames 2012, with permission.)*

fibres whilst the ventral roots contain motor fibres (Fig. 6.4). The cell bodies of the ventral nerve axons lie in the grey matter of the ventral horn within the spinal cord whilst the cell bodies of the dorsal axons lie outside the spinal cord in the dorsal root ganglion (DRG). The dorsal and ventral roots are enveloped by an extension of the dura mater known as the dural sleeve. The dorsal and ventral roots soon converge to form the roots of the spinal nerves, which contain the sensory and motor nerve fibres responsible for the innervation of a segment

of the body. The dural sleeve becomes the epineurium (Fig. 6.5).

The spinal nerve roots descend within the spinal canal by varying amounts and then exit the intervertebral foramina, as shown in Fig. 6.1. The nerve roots are named according to the level of the spine from which they emerge. There are eight pairs of cervical roots (the first of which emerges above the level of C1), 12 pairs of thoracic roots, five pairs of lumbar roots, five pairs of sacral roots and one pair of coccygeal roots. The sensory

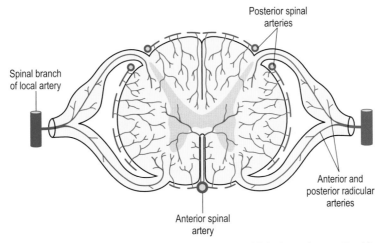

FIG. 6.3 ■ Arterial blood supply to the spinal cord. *(From Middleditch & Oliver 2005, with permission.)*

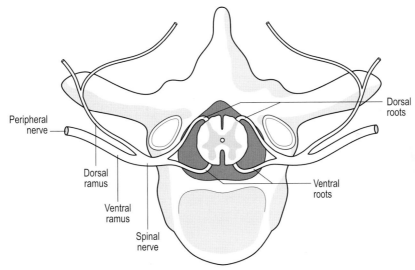

FIG. 6.4 ■ A horizontal cross-section of the spinal cord demonstrating the dorsal and ventral roots. *(After Palastanga & Soames 2012, with permission.)*

nerve fibres within each nerve root supply a specific segment of skin known as a dermatome. Similarly, the motor fibres within each nerve root supply a given muscle known as a myotome (shown in Fig. 4.27). Although dermatomal and myotomal innervation is not exact, as there is some cross-over in the dermatomal fields and muscles are typically supplied by more than one nerve root, clinically, this arrangement can be very useful in determining the site of a lesion. It is worth noting, however, that not all root lesions are the same

in clinical terms. The patient with an L3–L4 nerve root problem, for example, may present with isolated discomfort and numbness over the anterior aspect of the thigh without weakness, if mild, or may present, if more severe with pain, numbness, an absent knee jerk reflex and a knee that buckles due to quadriceps weakness. An acute quadriceps palsy should be seen as a neurosurgical emergency and should be referred on appropriately and urgently. It is worth noting that, with concurrent pain, weakness may be the result of pain inhibition. If there

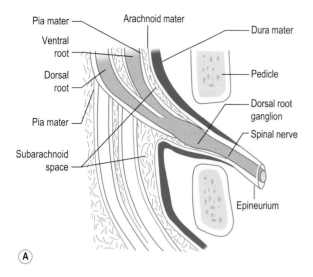

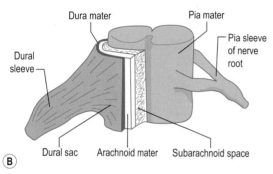

FIG. 6.5 ■ (A) The relationship of the meningeal layers to the dorsal and ventral roots. (B) The roots are enveloped by an extension of the dura mater to form the dural sleeve. *(From Palastanga & Soames 2012, with permission.)*

is painfree giving way, or weakness with corresponding sensory and reflex change, the clinician should suspect myotomal dysfunction.

Because of the anatomical difference between the nerve root and a peripheral nerve, the root may be more susceptible to mechanical injury. As shown in Fig. 6.5A, the nerve sheath is relatively thin. The perineurium, which importantly acts as a diffusion barrier to protect the delicate endoneurial environment (Peltonen et al. 2013) and helps to maintain resting tension, is poorly developed and the epineurium is also not well developed when compared to the peripheral nerve, where it tends to be thickened to provide protection when passing over bony prominences. The dura and

arachnoid mater together with the cerebrospinal fluid are therefore almost solely responsible for protecting the nerve root as it exits the intervertebral foramen. The connective tissue covering of peripheral nerves is discussed later in this chapter.

On exiting the intervertebral foramina, the spinal nerve divides into two branches: the dorsal and ventral rami. The dorsal rami supply the zygapophyseal joints, muscles and skin overlying the head, neck and spine. The ventral rami supply the anterior and lateral trunk, and the upper and lower limbs. The ventral rami, which become the peripheral nerves, join in the cervical region to form the cervical and brachial plexi and in the lumbar and sacral regions to form the lumbar, lumbosacral and sacral plexi (Fig. 6.6). A branch from the ventral rami together with an autonomic branch from the grey ramus communicans forms the sinuvertebral nerve, which passes into the intervertebral foramen. On entering the canal, the sinuvertebral nerve branches to form a complex neural network that innervates the posterior longitudinal ligament, the dura mater and outer third of the annulus fibrosus of the disc at the level of entry but also the disc one level above (Adams et al. 2006; Baron & Tunstall 2015) (Fig. 6.7).

Tracts of the Spinal Cord

Information is continually relayed to and from the peripheries along a series of well-organized tracts within the white matter of the spinal cord. An ascending nerve signal must however first enter the spinal cord. This occurs via a given axon that enters the dorsal horn and terminates in the grey matter. In cross-section, the grey matter conforms to a pattern of lamination known as Rexed's laminae (Fig. 6.8). The ascending nerve signal must therefore cross one or more synapses to pass into the appropriate ascending tract within the white matter. The distinct tracts which convey ascending and descending information are represented in Fig. 6.9. A nerve signal may synapse several times en route to the cortex and may move into different tracts within the white matter at different stages of its journey. The ascending signal eventually reaches the thalamus, from where it is projected to the cortex. For a descending nerve signal, the converse is true. The signal travels down a descending tract within the white matter before synapsing, passing into the grey matter and exiting the spinal cord via the ventral horn.

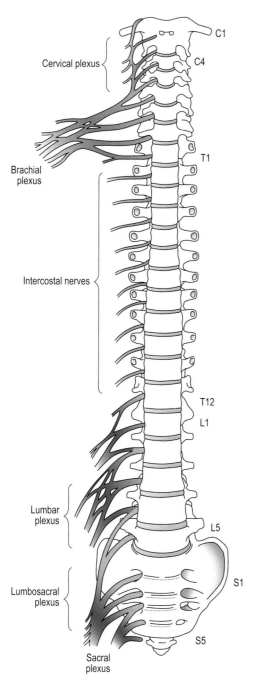

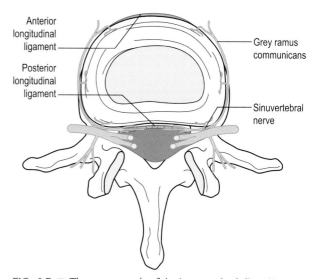

FIG. 6.7 ■ The nerve supply of the intervertebral disc. *(From Baron & Tunstall 2015, with permission.)*

FIG. 6.6 ■ Spinal nerves exit the intervertebral foramina to form the cervical, brachial, lumbar, lumbosacral and sacral plexi. *(From Palastanga & Soames 2012, with permission.)*

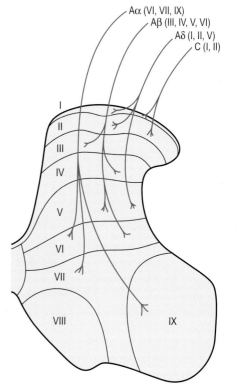

FIG. 6.8 ■ Laminae of Rexed and the termination of afferent fibres. *(After Todd & Koerber 2006.)*

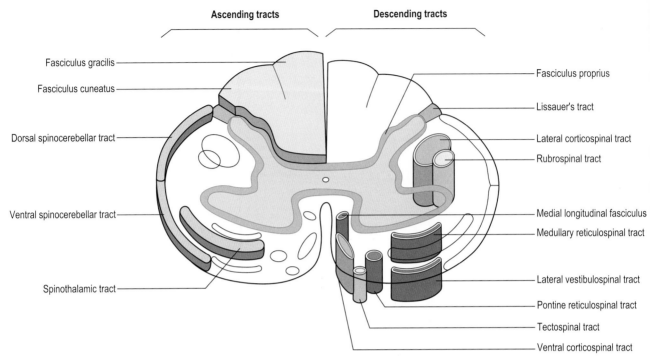

FIG. 6.9 ■ Transverse section of the spinal cord showing the ascending and descending tracts. *(From Crossman & Neary 2015, with permission.)*

It is outside the scope of this book to describe the ascending and descending tracts of the spinal cord in detail. For further detail, the reader is directed to Crossman and Neary (2015) and Mtui et al. (2015).

Anatomy and Physiology of Peripheral Nerves

Sensory and Motor Fibres

Peripheral nerves typically consist of sensory and motor nerve fibres surrounded by connective tissue. A typical sensory nerve fibre consists of dendrites at its distal end (peripheral axon), a cell body lying in the DRG in the intervertebral foramen and a central axon to the dorsal horn in the spinal cord (Fig. 6.10A). A typical motor nerve fibre consists of dendrites, a cell body in the ventral horn of the spinal cord and an axon (Fig. 6.10B). Each sensory or motor nerve fibre is a single, extremely elongated cell which may run from the spinal cord as far as the toe or finger.

The fascicles (nerve fibres enclosed by the endoneurium; see later in this chapter) do not have a straight course along a nerve; rather, they repeatedly join and divide to form a complex plexus (Fig. 6.11). The number of fascicles seen on cross-section of a nerve increases where a nerve crosses a joint, increasing its tensile strength (Sunderland 1990).

Most axons are myelinated, that is, they are surrounded by a myelin sheath; some, however, do not have this covering and are said to be unmyelinated. The myelin sheath is formed by Schwann cells wrapped a number of times around part of an axon (Fig. 6.12A). Longitudinally along the axon, gaps occur between the Schwann cells, and these are known as nodes of Ranvier. Impulses travel along the nerve and 'jump' from one node of Ranvier to the next, a process known as saltatory conduction, which increases the speed of nerve conduction (Schmid 2015). Unmyelinated nerve fibres are also covered in Schwann cells but they have no myelin sheath (Fig. 6.12B). Impulses travel in a continuous manner along an unmyelinated nerve fibre; there is

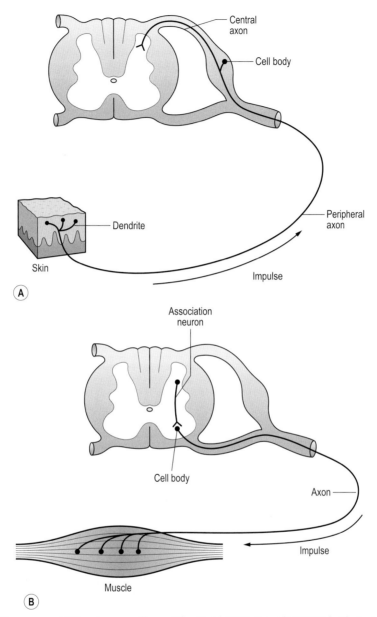

FIG. 6.10 ■ Typical (A) sensory and (B) motor nerve fibres. *(After Marieb 1995. Copyright © 1995 by The Benjamin/Cummings Publishing Company, Inc. Reprinted by permission of Pearson Education, Inc.)*

no 'jumping', which reduces the speed of conduction. Large myelinated Aβ nerve fibres conduct the sense of touch, vibration, pressure and sense of position. Aδ nerve fibres conduct pressure, pain and temperature, while the small unmyelinated C nerve fibres conduct dull diffuse pain, temperature and pressure (Palastanga & Soames 2012).

Peripheral nerve fibres (sensory, motor and autonomic) are classified according to their conduction velocities (Table 6.1). Afferent fibres can be classified

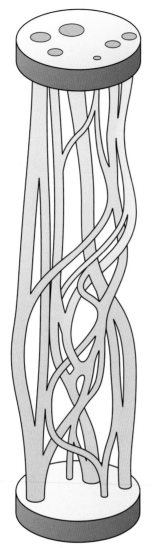

FIG. 6.11 ■ Fascicular plexus within a nerve. *(From Sunderland 1990, with permission.)*

in a variety of ways (Palastanga & Soames 2012). In this text the following terms only are used:

- Aα, which is the same as group I afferent
- Aβ, which is the same as group II afferent
- Aδ, which is the same as group III afferent
- C fibres, which are the same as group IV fibres.

Efferent fibres, that is, motor fibres supplying muscle, can be broadly classified as Aα and Aγ (or fusimotor)

fibres, both of which are fast-conducting myelinated fibres (Palastanga & Soames 2012).

The sensory nerves end distally in various types of receptor in almost all the tissues of the body. The sensory receptors in joint and muscle have been covered in the relevant chapters on joint and muscle. What remains to be clarified here are the receptors found in skin, which will clearly have relevance for all types of nerve, muscle and joint treatments.

Cutaneous Sensory Receptors

There is a variety of sensory receptors in the skin (Fig. 6.13); these are briefly outlined below:

- Free nerve endings. These lie in the dermis and at the root of hair follicles. They respond to low-threshold mechanical stimuli such as touch, pressure and temperature, and high-threshold noxious mechanical stimuli; they thus act as nociceptors.
- Merkel's discs. These lie in the epidermis in hairless skin, particularly the fingertips, and are low-threshold mechanical receptors providing the sense of touch.
- Meissner's corpuscles. These are surrounded by a fibrous capsule and lie in the dermis. They respond to touch.
- Krause end-bulbs. These are also surrounded by a fibrous capsule and lie in the dermis. They are low-threshold mechanical receptors, and so respond to touch.
- Ruffini corpuscles. These lie within a covering of collagen fibres and lie in the dermis. They respond to pressure.
- Pacinian corpuscles. These are covered in layers of modified Schwann cells encased in a fibrous capsule. They lie in the dermis and respond to pressure.

Free nerve endings responding to noxious mechanical and thermal stimuli are supplied by fast myelinated Aδ and slow unmyelinated C fibres. All the other skin receptors are supplied by fast-conducting myelinated Aβ fibres (Palastanga et al. 2002).

Axonal Transport

Nerve cells contain axoplasm (synonymous with cytoplasm) which, as in all cells, plays a vital role in

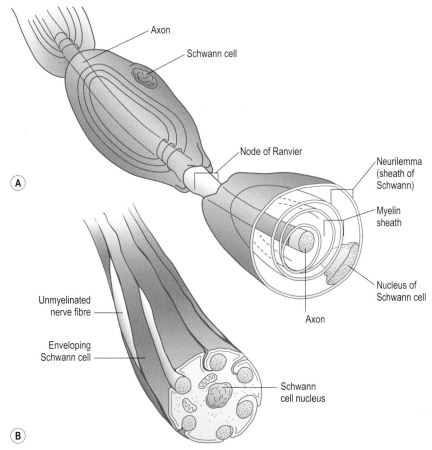

FIG. 6.12 ■ Nerve fibres: (A) myelinated and (B) unmyelinated. *(From Marieb 1995. Copyright © 1995 by The Benjamin/Cummings Publishing Company, Inc. Reprinted by permission of Pearson Education, Inc.)*

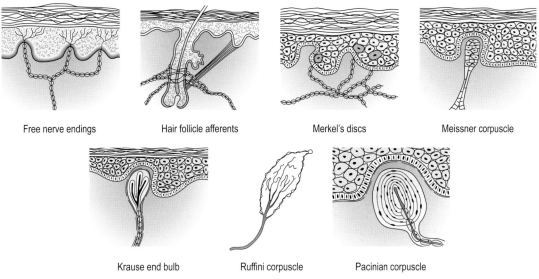

FIG. 6.13 ■ Sensory receptors in the skin. *(From Palastanga & Soames 2012, with permission.)*

TABLE 6.1
Classification of Peripheral Nerve Fibres (Williams & Warwick 1980)

Characteristics of fibre						
Type of sheath	Myelinated					Non-myelinated
Fibre diameter	22 μm				1.5 μm	2.0–0.1 μm
Conduction speed (metres/second)	120	60	50	30	4	0.5
Classification		A				
1. Erlanger and Gasser: All fibres				B		C
Subclasses: Efferent	Aα Skeletomotor	Aβ Fusimotor collaterals of A fibres	Aγ Fusimotor	B Preganglionic autonomic		C Postganglionic autonomic
Afferent	Aα and smaller. Muscle and tendon; cutaneous			Aβ Cutaneous muscle, visceral, etc.		C Cutaneous muscle, visceral, etc.
2. Lloyd Afferent – skeletal muscle and articular	I (a) Primary spindle ending (b) Tendon ending	II Secondary spindle ending		III Free ending (nociceptor etc.), paciniform ending?		IV Free ending (nociceptor, etc.)

It should be noted that the scale for conduction velocities is not arithmetical.

cell function. Nerve cells (cell body and axon) can be extremely long structures, running, for example, from the lumbar spine to the toe, or from the cervical spine to the finger. Because of these long distances, a special method is required to transport substances from the cell body to the end of the axon and back (Crossman & Neary 2015; Mtui et al. 2015; Schmid 2015). It is now understood that this process is active and involves the utilization of molecular 'motors' which drive contents along hollow microtubules within the axon. For this reason the process is now known as axonal transport rather than the previously termed axoplasmic flow (Schmid 2015). There are three methods of axonal transport: fast anterograde (forward moving to the end of the axon, to the periphery), slow anterograde and fast retrograde (backward moving towards the cell body) (Mtui et al. 2015).

1. Fast anterograde axonal transport moves synaptic vesicles, transmitter substances and mitochondria to the terminal of the nerve. Axoplasmic flow occurs at a rate of approximately 300–400 mm/day (Dahlin & Lundborg 1990; Mtui et al. 2015).
2. Slow anterograde axonal transport is the method by which the majority of axoplasm moves. Fibrous

and soluble proteins and enzymes are transported slowly along the axon at a rate of 5–10 mm/day (Mtui et al. 2015).
3. Fast retrograde axonal transport moves materials from the end of the axon to the cell body. These materials can be degraded or recycled, or inform the cell body about events at the end of the axon (Bisby 1982; Dahlin & Lundborg 1990). For example, where nerve growth factor is released to stimulate growth of neurons, this is transported back to inform the cell body (Schwartz 1991). The rate of flow is about 150–200 mm/day (Mtui et al. 2015).

Immune Cells

The perineurium provides a blood–nerve diffusion barrier (discussed in the next section) which protects the delicate endoneurial environment (Peltonen et al. 2013). Because of this barrier, immune cells cannot freely enter the peripheral nervous system to counter an attack from infectious pathogens. For this reason a small number of immune cells such as lymphocytes, macrophages and mast cells reside within the endoneurium to allow an immune response (Schmid 2015).

These immune cells have an inflammatory effect once activated, releasing inflammatory mediators such as cytokines. Furthermore, other cells such as glial cells which support neural tissue but are not directly involved in synaptic interaction and Schwann cells which produce myelin may have the potential to develop an immunomodulatory function within the dorsal root ganglia (Schmid et al. 2013; Schmid 2015).

Connective Tissue Covering of Peripheral Nerves

Nerve fibres are organized into a bundle (or fascicle) by a layer of connective tissue called the endoneurium; this makes up the functional unit of a nerve. The endoneurium surrounding individual nerve fibres is made up of collagen and fibroblasts. The pressure within the endoneurium is slightly more than in the tissues surrounding a nerve (Rydevik et al. 1989). A number of fascicles are surrounded by another layer of connective tissue called the perineurium. The perineurium acts as a diffusion barrier between the adjacent tissues (Rydevik & Lundborg 1977; Sunderland 1990) and is considered by Sunderland (1990) to be mostly responsible for providing nerves with tensile strength and elasticity. The outermost layer of connective tissue of a peripheral nerve is called the epineurium (Fig. 6.14). The epineurium consists of loose connective tissue which helps to protect the nerve during movement. The epineurium

rather than the perineurium is considered by Haftek (1970) to be mostly responsible for providing nerves with tensile strength and elasticity.

Blood Supply of Peripheral Nerves

Peripheral nerves are well vascularized (Fig. 6.15). Blood vessels running alongside nerves send regional feeding vessels to the epineurium which then divide and supply the deep and superficial layers of the epineurium, perineurium and endoneurium (Lundborg et al. 1987). The blood vessels are coiled, which allows a certain amount of lengthening to occur without affecting blood flow (Fig. 6.16). Vessels lie obliquely in the perineurium, and it is thought that increased endoneurial pressure will therefore close these vessels (Lundborg 1975). This is supported by the fact that a small increase in endoneurial pressure results in a reduction in blood flow within the endoneurium (Lundborg et al. 1983). For example, if a nerve is elongated by more than 8%, the intraneural blood flow is reduced, and at 15% the vessels are completely occluded, causing nerve ischaemia (Lundborg & Rydevik 1973).

Nerve Supply of Peripheral Nerves

The connective tissue sheaths surrounding peripheral nerves are innervated by the nervi nervorum (Fig. 6.17) (Hromada 1963; Bove & Light 1995). The epineurium,

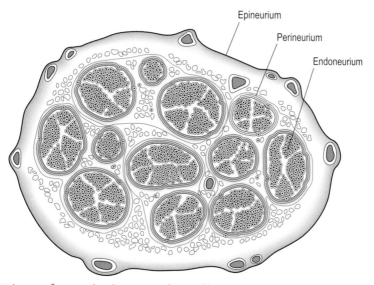

FIG. 6.14 ▪ Layers of connective tissue around nerve fibres. *(After Lundborg et al. 1987, with permission.)*

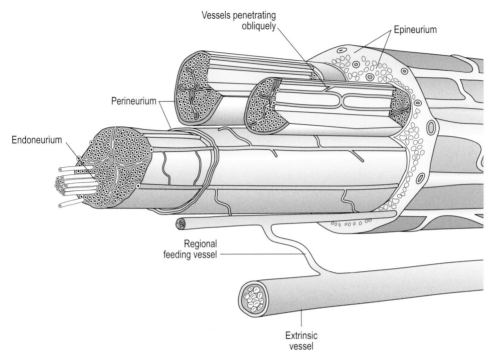

FIG. 6.15 ■ Intraneural microcirculation. *(After Lundborg et al. 1987, with permission.)*

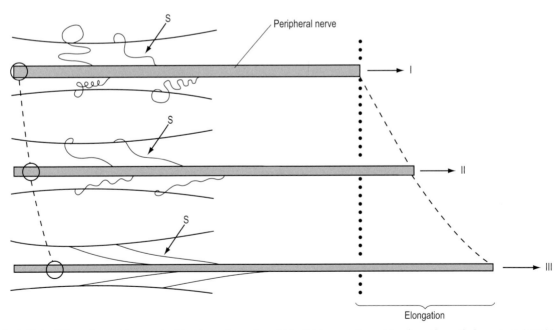

FIG. 6.16 ■ Effect of stretching on the blood supply to the rabbit tibial nerve. Stage I is where the coiled segmental (S) blood vessels are unaffected by nerve lengthening. Stage II is where further increase in nerve lengthening begins to stretch the blood vessels and impair flow. Stage III is where the cross-sectional area of the nerve (circled) is reduced, which further impairs blood flow. *(From Rydevik et al. 1989, with permission.)*

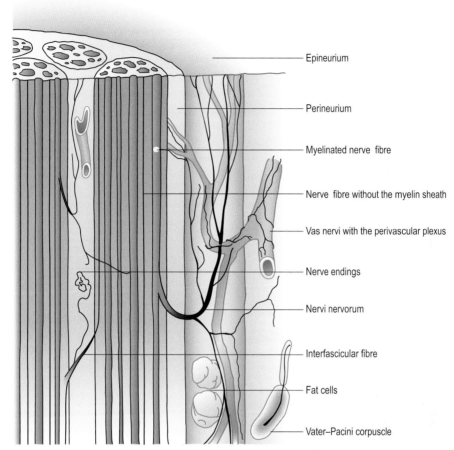

FIG. 6.17 ▪ A longitudinal schematic drawing demonstrating the nervi nervorum and nerve endings within the connective tissue sheath of a peripheral nerve. (After Hromada 1963, with permission from the publisher, S. Karger AG, Basel.)

perineurium and endoneurium contain both free nerve endings and encapsulated endings, and the afferent fibres are mostly unmyelinated C fibres with some thinly myelinated fibres (Hromada 1963). The nerve supply originates from the axons within the sheath and from the blood vessels that supply the nerve (Hromada 1963; Bahns et al. 1986; Bove & Light 1995). The nerve endings respond to high-threshold mechanical stimuli as well as chemical stimuli (capsaicin, bradykinin, hypertonic sodium chloride or potassium chloride) and thermal stimuli, and are therefore considered to have a nociceptive function (Bahns et al. 1986; Bove & Light 1995). The connective tissue of nerve can therefore be a direct source of pain, by mechanical deformation or chemicals released with inflammation.

The epineurium covering the ventral and dorsal roots is also innervated, as are the spinal and sympathetic ganglia (Hromada 1963).

Biomechanics of Peripheral Nerves

Because peripheral nerves lie on either side of joints they must shorten and lengthen with movement. The connective tissue surrounding nerves contains elastin. This therefore enables nerves to return to a shortened position following lengthening; for example, the median nerve has to shorten by about 15% on elbow flexion (Zoech et al. 1991).

There are three main mechanical events occurring with joint movement which causes the nerve bed to elongate. First of all the nerve, which sits uncoiled in the nerve bed, starts to uncoil, followed by excursion (sliding) of the nerve with a gradual increase in nerve strain (percentage change in length) as the nerve bed continues to lengthen. The direction of nerve movement will follow the direction of the moving joint (Boyd et al. 2005; Ridehalgh et al., 2014). When lengthening occurs, tensile (longitudinal) force is transmitted along the length of a nerve. Nerves have considerable tensile strength to withstand this tensile force. The tensile properties of nerve roots, compared with bone, cartilage, ligament, muscle and tendon, are given in Table 6.2 (Panjabi & White 2001).

Peripheral nerve is viscoelastic and, as such, has a force–displacement (or stress–strain) curve similar to that of other tissues (Sunderland & Bradley 1961). The load–displacement curve is dependent on the rate of lengthening (Sunderland 1990): the faster the lengthening, the greater the resistance. A typical force–displacement curve of a rabbit tibial nerve demonstrates

an early toe region (Fig. 6.18) where a small force causes a relatively large displacement (Haftek 1970). During the toe region, the undulation of the nerve is straightened out (Haftek 1970), accounting for about 75% of the total change in length (Zoech et al. 1991). Resistance then increases to produce the linear part of the curve until the limit of elasticity is reached. During this phase, all of the nerve, but particularly the epineurium and perineurium, resists the movement until, at the limit of elasticity, the epineurium ruptures (Haftek 1970). Generally this occurs at about 20% elongation, although it can occur as low as 8% (Sunderland & Bradley 1961). Resistance then decreases as elongation continues. Complete rupture generally occurs at about 30% of elongation, although there is a wide variation between nerves (Sunderland & Bradley 1961).

Like all viscoelastic materials, nerve undergoes stress relaxation. A 6% strain held for 1 hour causes a 57% reduction in tension (Wall et al. 1992), an 8% strain held for 30 minutes causes a 50% reduction in tension (Clark et al. 1992), while a 12% strain held for 1 hour causes a 50% reduction in tension (Wall et al. 1992) and a 15% strain held for 30 minutes causes a 40% reduction in tension (Clark et al. 1992). There is no structural damage to the nerve after a 12% strain held for 1 hour (Wall et al. 1992), although there could be a change in function if the blood supply to the nerve is affected.

Elongation of a nerve will lead to a reduction in the cross-sectional area of the nerve, which results in increased pressure to the endoneurium (Topp & Boyd 2006). Such compression may lead to changes in the microcirculation to the nerve (Sunderland 1990). Hence in clinical situations where the nerve is already subject to compression, seen in some entrapment neuropathies

TABLE 6.2

Tensile Properties of Nerve Roots Compared With Bone, Cartilage, Ligament, Muscle and Tendon (Panjabi & White 2001)

Tissue	Stress at Failure (MPa)	Strain at Failure (%)
Nerve roots	15	19
Cortical bone	100–200	1–3
Cancellous bone	10	5–7
Cartilage	10–15	80–120
Ligament	10–40	30–45
Muscle (passive)	0.17	60
Tendon	55	9–10

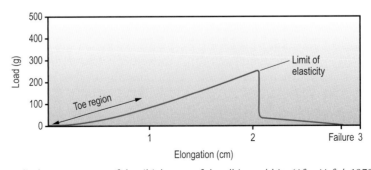

FIG. 6.18 ■ Force-displacement curve of the tibial nerve of the albino rabbit. *(After Haftek 1970, with permission.)*

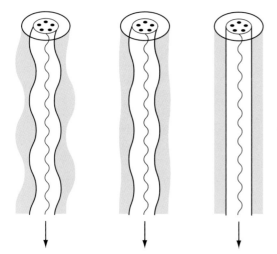

FIG. 6.19 ▪ Changes to nerve when it is lengthened. *(From Sunderland 1990, with permission.)*

such as carpal tunnel syndrome (CTS), it is possible that movement which elongates the nerve could place further pressure on to the nerve, resulting in greater ischaemic changes.

Whether the resistance to lengthening a nerve is provided mainly by the perineurium (Sunderland 1990) or by the epineurium (Haftek 1970), it seems clear that it is the connective tissue in nerve that resists the lengthening, and not the nerve fibres (Fig. 6.19). It can be seen that, under normal physiological lengthening, the nerve fibres remain undulated and thus protected (Sunderland 1990).

The number of fascicles and thus the amount of connective tissue may vary between nerves. It had been suggested that where a nerve requires greater protection there is an increase in the number of the fascicles (Sunderland & Bradley 1961: Sunderland 1978). However, Phillips et al. (2004) found a greater number of fascicles in the non-joint region of the sciatic nerve compared to the joint region. Greater compliance was found at the joint regions. The reason for greater compliance in the joint regions is not established, although it has been postulated that, in some cases, the thinness of the collagen fibrils may account for this (Ottani et al. 2001). Indeed, Mason and Phillips (2011) found the joint regions of the median nerve to have thinner fibrils than the non-joint regions in rats, but this was not the case for the sciatic nerve, despite being more compliant. Nerve roots, on the other hand, exiting

from the spinal cord, lack an epineurium and perineurium and are less protected from a traction or compression injury (Sunderland 1990).

Movement of the Nervous System

During normal functional movements the nervous system moves as a continuum. Movement of the brain, spinal cord, nerve roots and peripheral nerves will be discussed in relation to both normal functional movements and during tests which explore the mechanosensitivity of the nervous system, and enable the clinician to identify nerves as a potential source of symptoms – neurodynamic tests.

Movement of the Brain

As mentioned previously, three layers of connective tissue, collectively known as the meninges, surround the brain and spinal cord; they are the dura mater, arachnoid mater and pia mater. The dura mater covering the brain is referred to as cerebral dura mater, and that around the spinal cord is spinal dura mater.

The cerebral dura mater is the outermost layer and is attached to the inner aspect of the cranium. The pia mater is adherent to the outside of the brain. The dura mater, arachnoid and pia mater in the cranium are all innervated and therefore can be a source of symptoms. The cranial nerves are covered in connective tissue and lie close to the cerebral dura mater (Williams et al. 1995). Movements of the head are thought to cause sliding, elongation and compression of the dura mater, falx cerebri, tentorium cerebelli and the cranial nerves (Breig 1978; von Piekartz & Bryden 2001). Upper cervical flexion and contralateral lateral flexion have been found to cause 5–7 mm of movement in the trigeminal, hypoglossal, facial and accessory cranial nerves (Breig 1978). Fig. 6.20 demonstrates the effect of cervical flexion on the spinal cord and branches of the mandibular nerve.

Movement of the Spinal Cord

The spinal cord is covered in dura mater, arachnoid mater and pia mater (Fig. 6.21). The outermost layer of spinal dura mater forms a tube known as the dural theca, which contains the spinal cord. Twenty-one pairs of fibrous denticulate ligaments (or ligamentum denticulatum) lie between the level of the foramen magnum and the T12–L1 level and attach to the pia mater and

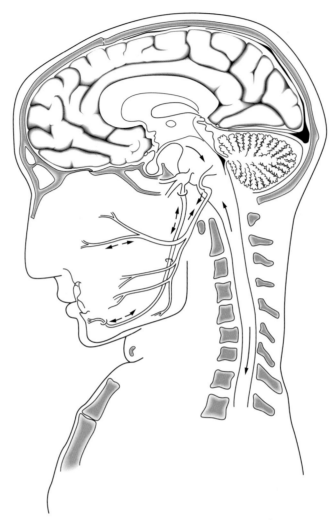

FIG. 6.20 ■ Effect of cervical flexion on the spinal cord and branches of the mandibular nerve. *(From von Piekartz & Bryden 2001, with permission.)*

the dural sac (Fig. 6.22). They keep the spinal cord central in the dural theca, and they deform and move during spinal movements (Epstein 1966). The dura mater is innervated anteriorly by the sinuvertebral nerve, but not posteriorly. The pia mater and arachnoid are also innervated (Williams et al. 1995). Thus the dura mater, arachnoid and pia mater may transmit nociception and thus be a source of pain.

The autonomic nervous system must also adapt with movement, and of particular interest is the sympathetic trunk that is closely related to the vertebral column (Fig. 6.23). It can be seen that the trunk lies anterior

to the axis of movement in the cervical region and posterior to the axis in the thoracic and lumbar regions. Consequently, the trunk will be lengthened when the cervical spine is extended and when the thoracic and lumbar regions are flexed. From the anterior view of the vertebral column it can be seen that the trunk lies to one side and will therefore be lengthened on contralateral lateral flexion. It is perhaps also worth highlighting the close position of the sympathetic trunk to the costotransverse joints; movement at this joint will cause movement of the trunk. The close anatomical arrangement of the pre- and postganglionic axons of

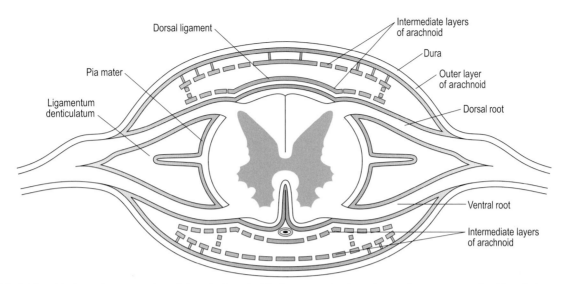

FIG. 6.21 ■ Horizontal cross-section of the spinal cord with the connective tissue layers, dura mater, arachnoid and pia mater. *(From Williams et al. 1995, with permission.)*

the grey and white rami communicans (Fig. 6.24) demonstrates that movements that affect the spinal nerve roots will also affect the sympathetic nervous system.

Cervical flexion in isolation has been shown to move and tension the spinal dura in the cervical spine in particular, but also in the thoracic and lumbar regions (Breig & Marions 1963; Tencer et al. 1985). With whole-spine movements, from full extension to full flexion, the spinal canal lengthens by about 5–9 cm (Inman & Saunders 1942; Breig 1978; Louis 1981). The axis of flexion and extension movements lies in the vertebral bodies, which are anterior to the spinal canal. For this reason, during flexion, the posterior wall lengthens more than the anterior wall. During flexion the neuraxis (all the nervous tissue and meninges in the skull and vertebral canal) elongates and moves anteriorly in the spinal canal (Breig 1978). The movement, however, is not even throughout: little movement occurs at C6, T6 and L4 (Louis 1981). Butler (1991) referred to these regions as 'tension points' (Fig. 6.25). It should be noted that the neuraxis moves relative to its meningeal covering: they do not move as one (Louis 1981). During extension the spinal cord uncoils and rests in a wrinkled position (Breig 1960, 1978; Breig & Marions 1963).

Movements of the spine also affect the size of the intervertebral foramen, where the nerve root lies. In the lumbar spine, from a neutral start position, lumbar spine flexion has been found to increase the size of the intervertebral foramen by 12%, and extension decreases it by 15% (Inufusa et al. 1996). Flexion would therefore potentially reduce compression on the exiting nervous tissue, while extension could increase compression (Adams et al. 2006).

The spinal arachnoid and pia mater are continuous with the perineurium of a peripheral nerve, and the spinal dura mater is continuous with the epineurium of a peripheral nerve (Williams et al. 1995). Thus, the cerebral meninges, spinal meninges, and perineurium and epineurium of peripheral nerves are one continuous structure, and this is the principle behind the concept of neurodynamic tests, and the continuity of the nervous system.

Movement of the Nerve Roots

Both trunk (Breig 1960; Breig & Marions 1963) and limb movements (Goddard & Reid 1965; Smith et al. 1993; Gilbert et al. 2007) have been shown to have an impact on the motion or strain of the lumbosacral nerve roots, and more recently upper-limb movements on the cervical nerve roots (Lohman et al. 2015). Trunk flexion appears to induce tensile stress through the lumbosacral nerve roots and cervical flexion may induce small amounts of nerve root excursion (1–2 mm) (Breig

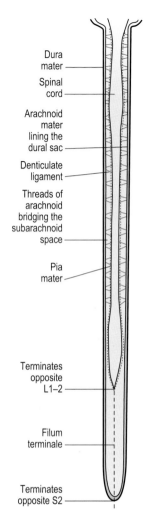

Dura mater

Spinal cord

Arachnoid mater lining the dural sac

Denticulate ligament

Threads of arachnoid bridging the subarachnoid space

Pia mater

Terminates opposite L1–2

Filum terminale

Terminates opposite S2

FIG. 6.22 ■ Longitudinal section of the spinal cord. *(From Palastanga et al. 2002, with permission.)*

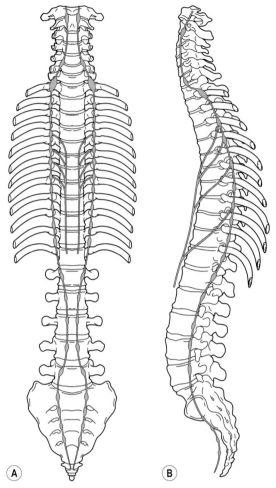

FIG. 6.23 ■ Relationship of the sympathetic trunk and the vertebral column: (A) anterior view and (B) lateral view. *(From Butler 1991, with permission.)*

1960; Breig & Marions 1963). However, methods used may be subject to high error, since observational methods were used to estimate excursion and tension was measured by resistance encountered whilst lifting a piece of thread wrapped around the nerve root.

During straight-leg raise (SLR) (Fig. 6.26), excursion of the lumbosacral nerve roots has been found to vary between 5 mm at S1 in cadavers from younger age groups (Goddard & Reid 1965) to 0.48 mm at L5 in older cadavers (Gilbert et al. 2007). Strain levels have also been found to vary between studies from 3.4% at

S1 (Smith et al. 1993) to negligible strain, found by Gilbert et al. (2007), although this increased to 1.89% with the addition of ankle dorsiflexion, a component thought to sensitize the tibial nerve during the SLR test (Shacklock 2005). The main finding from these studies is that the evidence suggests that manoeuvres which lengthen the nerve bed of the nerve root, lumbosacral plexus and extensions into the sciatic nerve do produce biomechanical changes at the nerve root.

More recently, the impact of the upper-limb neurodynamic test (ULNT) (median nerve bias, Fig. 6.27)

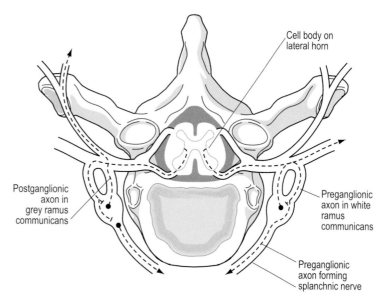

FIG. 6.24 ■ Cross-section of the spinal cord demonstrating the pre- and postganglionic axons of the white and grey rami communicans. *(From Palastanga et al. 2002, with permission.)*

Cell body on lateral horn

Postganglionic axon in grey ramus communicans

Preganglionic axon in white ramus communicans

Preganglionic axon forming splanchnic nerve

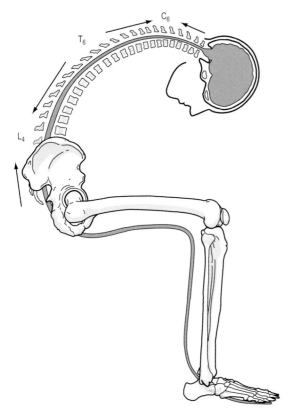

FIG. 6.25 ■ Tension points in the neuraxis where little movement occurs. *(From Butler 1991, with permission.)*

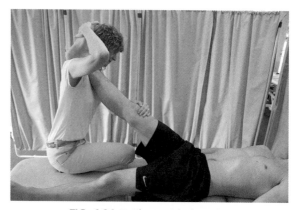

FIG. 6.26 ■ The straight-leg raise.

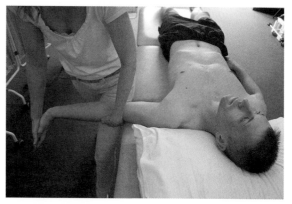

FIG. 6.27 ■ The upper-limb neurodynamic test 1.

on excursion and strain of the cervical nerve roots has been explored (Lohman et al. 2015) in unembalmed cadavers. The range of excursion varied dependent on whether the nerve root was measured within the intravertebral foramen, or distal to the foramen, and mean inferolateral excursion ranged from 2.16 (C5) to 2.29 mm (C7) within the intravertebral foramen, and from 3.15 (C5) to 4.14 mm (C7) distal to the intravertebral foramen. Strain levels also varied between levels, but most greatly between C5 (6.8%) and C6 (11.87%). The confidence interval for strain at C6 suggested that, 95% of the time, the strain was not less than 9.28%, which may be above the level previously found to have a detrimental effect on blood flow (Lundborg & Rydevik 1973; Driscoll et al. 2002). However, it must be remembered that strain would not be held at this level for sustained periods of time during most neurodynamic treatment interventions, and therefore any detrimental effects to blood flow are likely to be transient.

Taken together these studies support the use of neurodynamic tests for the examination of neural tissue mechanosensitivity of the cervical and lumbosacral nerve roots.

Movement of Peripheral Nerves

Peripheral nerves are covered with a conjunctiva-like adventitia that allows extraneural gliding with adjacent tissues; there is also gliding between the fascicles (intraneural gliding) (Rempel et al. 1999). There is a great deal of data available on peripheral nerve movement. Nerve movement has been measured in cadavers and more recently in vivo utilizing real-time ultrasound imaging (USI) (Hough et al. 2000a, b; Dilley et al. 2001; Erel et al. 2003; Coppieters et al. 2009, 2015: Ellis et al. 2012; Ridehalgh et al. 2012, 2014, 2015). Whilst USI enables better estimates of the in vivo situation, the lack of ability to see larger areas of the nerve due to the small field of view offered by the transducers and current inability to measure strain has its limitations. Nonetheless it has provided a unique opportunity to investigate in vivo nerve motion in a number of areas.

Movement of the fingers causes movement of the median nerve in the forearm and wrist. From full flexion of the index finger to 30° extension at the interphalangeal joints, the median nerve in the forearm moves longitudinally between 1.6 and 4.5 mm (Dilley et al. 2001). Under the flexor retinaculum at the wrist joint, index finger extension causes the median nerve to glide up to 2 mm in an ulnar direction (Nakamichi & Tachibana 1995). Such changes to excursion of the median nerve in the hand during these movements support the use of nerve gliding exercises seen in some programmes for people with CTS (Akalin et al. 2002; Bardak et al. 2009).

Movement of the wrist also causes movement of the median nerve at the wrist and at the elbow. Wrist movement from 30° flexion to 30° extension causes the median nerve at the wrist to move approximately 3–5 mm in an ulnar direction (Greening et al. 2001) and 2 mm in an anterior direction (Greening et al. 2001). With rather more wrist movement, from 55° flexion to 55° extension, the median nerve at the elbow has been found to move distally between 10 and 21 mm (Hough et al. 2000a).

Median nerve movement and tension have been measured in the upper limb in five cadavers (Wright et al. 1996). As might be expected, finger hyperextension and wrist extension caused distal movement and increased tension at the wrist. Shoulder abduction to 110° caused proximal movement and increased tension of the median nerve at both the wrist and elbow. Supination caused proximal movement at both the wrist and elbow, with increased tension at the wrist and reduced tension at the elbow; all changes in movement and tension were small. It should be remembered that these values are based on five cadavers, and greater variation might have been found if a larger number had been used. In addition, cadaveric measurements may be rather different from in vivo measurements. Nevertheless, the study provides useful information about nerve movement and provides support for some of the movements used in ULNT1 and 2a to assess nerve mechanosensitivity.

Differences in longitudinal excursion in people with peripheral neuropathic pain of the upper limb have varied in their results. Erel et al. (2003) did not find any differences in longitudinal excursion of the median nerve in patients with CTS measured at the forearm compared to asymptomatic participants. However, in contrast, Hough et al. (2007) and Korstanje et al. (2012) found reduced longitudinal excursion at the wrist in this population. Differences may be explained by the location of the imaging (one might imagine greater impact at the site of the potential entrapment), and the methods of scanning and offline analysis.

More recently, movement of the nerves has been assessed during ULNTs to establish the difference biomechanically of techniques which aim to increase the excursion of the nerve whilst minimizing nerve strain (nerve sliders) and those which increase nerve strain (tensioners), and the details of these studies can be found in Chapter 7.

With respect to the lower limb, sciatic nerve excursion and strain have been examined both in cadaveric studies (Coppieters et al. 2006; Gilbert et al. 2007; Boyd et al. 2013) and in studies utilizing USI (Ellis et al. 2012; Ridehalgh et al. 2012, 2014, 2015; Coppieters et al. 2015).

Strain values have varied between 6.6 and 8% in the sciatic nerve measured around the ischial tuberosity during the SLR in cadaveric studies (Coppieters et al. 2006; Boyd et al. 2013). Excursion values vary from around 4 mm (Goddard & Reid 1965) to 28 mm (Coppieters et al. 2006), but this is dependent on the location of where the nerve was studied, the exact number of joint components added and the methods used to measure. It is not useful to compare these values directly because of these factors, but the trends are the same in each study; that is, the nerve moves towards the moving joint, and most nerve movement occurs around the moving joint.

Ranges of nerve excursion found between USI studies also vary dependent on the exact range and choice of joint movements used, and the position of the participants. Most studies looking at the sciatic nerve have used the posterior thigh as the best location for viewing the sciatic nerve (Ellis et al. 2012; Ridehalgh et al. 2014, 2015; Coppieters et al. 2015). All follow the same trends as discussed above. Recently, Ellis et al. (2016) found no difference in sciatic nerve excursion during a knee extension in sitting between an upright and a slumped position. It would be expected that the slumped position would reduce nerve excursion since the trunk flexion component would increase the nerve bed length of the neuraxis (Breig 1960, 1978), resulting in greater amounts of nerve elongation with resultant reduction in excursion. Indeed, this has been found in a number of studies comparing nerve sliding and tensioner activities (Coppieters et al. 2009, 2015; Ellis et al. 2012).

The amount of nerve excursion which occurred was not discussed, and as such with error measures (smallest detectable differences) calculated from the data found to be 0.69 mm for the slump position, differences greater than these would have been needed to show significant differences. In a previous study using the same seated position (Ellis et al. 2012), mean ranges of excursion were in the region of 2–3 mm of movement. Hence there may be insufficient amounts of excursion occurring in this position to be able to establish conclusively a difference larger than error between the two positions.

Differences in nerve excursion between asymptomatic and symptomatic populations have yet to be established in the lower limb. Ridehalgh et al. (2015) found no significant differences in sciatic nerve excursion between participants with radicular pain and those without. However, measurements were taken at the posterior thigh, some distance from the lumbosacral nerve roots, and therefore it is possible that alterations in movement may exist at the site of dysfunction, which were not of sufficient magnitude to detect further away. Certainly nerve mechanics have been found to be altered after disc herniation (Kobayashi et al. 2003). Nerve root restriction was found to be greatest at the same point in range as the symptomatic SLR, which returned to normal after surgery.

The studies looking at biomechanical events occurring to the nervous system during normal limb and trunk movements demonstrate the connectivity between the nervous system as well as enabling a better understanding of the impact of movement to nerve dynamics. The adaptation of the nervous system after nerve dysfunction is not clear. In certain conditions, such as nerve entrapment neuropathies, it may be expected that mechanics would be altered. However, at present more research is required to establish this in more conditions using high-quality methods.

Summary of Nerve Function

The central and peripheral nervous systems are anatomically, biomechanically and physiologically linked as part of one whole system. This highly complex system not only produces movement of the body, through the coordinated activation of numerous muscles, but is also adapted to cope with the physical stresses applied to it during these very movements.

NERVE DYSFUNCTION

As highlighted at the beginning of this chapter, patients with musculoskeletal dysfunction present with vastly different problems. When the patient with signs and symptoms of nerve dysfunction attends the clinic, an appreciation of normal nerve function is firstly necessary before the clinician can clinically reason what the nature of the dysfunction might be. The remainder of this chapter will discuss dysfunction of nerves and draw upon clinical examples in order for the reader to contextualize the theory.

The following aspects of nerve dysfunction will be considered in this section:

- neuropathic pain
- mechanisms of local dysfunction
- mechanisms of central dysfunction
- summary of local and central mechanisms
- clinical examples of nerve pathology
- nerve regeneration and repair
- reduced nerve movement
- summary of nerve dysfunction.

Neuropathic Pain

The International Association for the Study of Pain (IASP) defines peripheral neuropathic pain as pain emanating from a 'lesion or disease of the peripheral somatosensory nervous system' (IASP 2014). This rather wide-ranging definition described a continuum from a mild ankle sprain causing bruising to the common peroneal nerve to severe radiculopathic pain caused by nerve root compromise as a result of, for example a herniated intervertebral disc. It is important that the reader understands the distinction between referred pain, radicular pain and radiculopathy. Pain emanating from musculoskeletal tissue has the potential to spread (or refer) from its source. Chapters 2 and 4 describe referral patterns from joint and muscle tissue. Often referral from musculoskeletal tissue is described as 'somatic referral' in that it arises from somatic tissue and is distinct from referral from visceral structures or radicular pain, which emanates from the dorsal root or its ganglion. Radiculopathy encompasses the signs and symptoms of altered nerve conductivity, namely pins and needles, numbness, weakness and reflex changes. The reader is directed to an excellent review by Bogduk (2009) which expands on these definitions.

TABLE 6.3	
Comparative Typical Presentation of Somatic Referred Vs. Radicular Pain	
Somatic Referred Pain	Radicular Pain
Dull, diffuse, deep	Sharp, lancinating, linear, superficial
Central pain tends to be worse than leg/arm pain	Leg/arm pain tends to be worse than central pain
Not tending to refer below the knee or elbow from a central source	May refer to the foot or hand (depending on the level affected)
No signs or symptoms of radiculopathy (pins and needles, numbness, weakness, reflex changes)	± signs of symptoms of radiculopathy (pins and needles, numbness, weakness, reflex changes)

As well as the common clinical indicators which may help to identify neuropathic from non-neuropathic pain (Table 6.3), other tools such as the PainDETECT questionnaire have been validated to identify components of neuropathic pain (Cappelleri et al. 2014).

Mechanisms of Local Dysfunction

It is well established that there are local mechanisms which lead to nerve dysfunction, although our understanding of these underlying mechanisms is continually evolving. More recently it has become apparent that there are subcortical and cortical processes at play also in the generation of nerve dysfunction. This section will discuss the local mechanisms of dysfunction, including detrimental mechanical effects and inflammatory and immunological change. The following section will discuss central mechanisms.

Detrimental Mechanical Effects

Detrimental mechanical effects can be broadly categorized as adverse effects emanating from compression and strain.

Compression. Large compressive force may result in major disruption to nerve function. Smaller levels of pressure can however cause ischaemic or mechanical changes to the nerve. Whilst compression of a normal nerve may cause sensory change initially but no pain (Lundborg et al. 1982), sustained ischaemic change may lead to increasing symptoms due to disruption in the

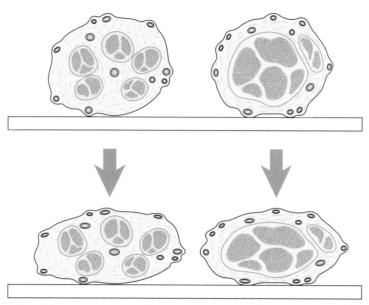

FIG. 6.28 ▪ Smaller fascicles within larger amounts of epineurium are less vulnerable than large fascicles in less epineurium. *(From Lundborg 2004, with permission.)*

diffusion barrier and intraneural oedema leading to microenvironmental and fibrotic change (Rydevik & Lundborg 1977; Lundborg 2004). Experimental studies have investigated the effects of compression on animal peripheral nerves and have demonstrated mechanical injury to the blood vessels and endoneurial oedema (Lundborg et al. 1983; Yoshii et al. 2010), and direct injury to the nerve fibres (Dyck et al. 1990; Rempel et al. 1999; Rempel & Diao 2004; Topp & Boyd 2006). Whilst mechanical injury may alter the conductivity of the nerve, ischaemic change, as well as causing detrimental intraneural change, may also lead to demyelination which may in turn lead to increased ectopic nerve signal discharge (Schmid et al. 2013).

Nerves are susceptible to compression predominantly because of their superficial arrangement, location close to nerve interfaces (e.g. bone or passing through tight tunnels, for example the carpal tunnel), and their response to changes in circulation and alterations in intraneural pressure (Sunderland 1978; Rempel et al. 1999). The effects of such compression will depend on the magnitude and duration of the compression (Rydevik & Lundborg 1977; Dahlin & McLean 1986) and to some extent the make-up of the nerve. For example, a nerve which has fewer, larger fascicles, embedded therefore in less connective tissue, will be

more vulnerable to compression than a nerve which has numerous fascicles and therefore more connective tissue (Fig. 6.28) (Sunderland 1978; Lundborg 2004). In addition, certain sections of the same nerve are more vulnerable to compression than others, depending on their location; nerve fibres located on the periphery of the nerve are more susceptible to compressive forces than those in the middle of the nerve (Lundborg 2004).

Nerve can be broadly compressed in one of two ways, either a circumferential pressure or a lateral pressure. As the name suggests, circumferential pressure is where the compression is applied circumferentially around the nerve, for example, with CTS or spinal stenosis. The forces applied to the nerve and the alteration in shape of the nerve are demonstrated in Fig. 6.29. The main effect is at the edge of the compressed segment and is referred to as the 'edge effect' (Ochoa et al. 1972).

A lateral pressure is where something presses on the side of a nerve, causing deformation of the nerve, such as a posterolateral disc protrusion compressing an exiting nerve root (Fig. 6.30). It has been speculated that this lengthening of the nerve fibre membrane may alter its permeability and conductivity, which could trigger nociception (Rydevik et al. 1989).

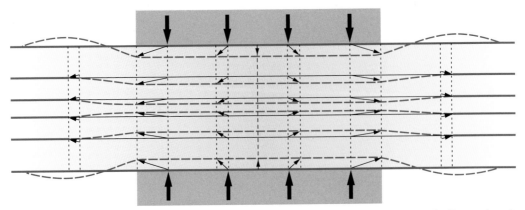

FIG. 6.29 ■ The 'edge effect' whereby circumferential pressure is applied to a nerve with maximal effect at the edge of the compression. *(From Rydevik et al. 1984, with permission.)*

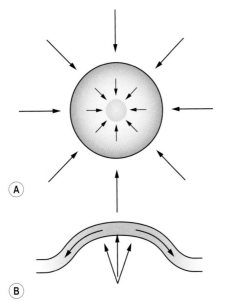

FIG. 6.30 ■ (A) Circumferencial pressure, such as spinal stenosis. (B) Lateral pressure on a nerve – from a prolapsed intervertebral disc, for example – causing nerve deformation. *(From Rydevik et al. 1984, with permission.)*

The blood vessels within the epineurium of the nerve are the parts most sensitive to compression injuries (Rydevik & Lundborg 1977; Lundborg et al. 1983). Compression injury of the blood vessels results in increased permeability of the vessel walls, with oedema formation within the epineural space (Rydevik & Lundborg 1977). The perineurium provides an important barrier to oedema, protecting the endoneurial space and therefore the nerve fibres themselves; however, more severe compression can lead to damage of the endoneurial vessels, resulting in oedema within the endoneurium (Rydevik & Lundborg 1977; Rydevik et al. 1981). Interestingly, it appears that the failure of the blood–nerve barrier function of the perineurium is more susceptible to direct trauma from the compression itself rather than ischaemia (Lundborg 1970). It is important to note that much higher pressures (above 200 mmHg) are necessary for endoneurial oedema to be present (Rydevik & Lundborg 1977) compared with 50 mmHg for epineurial oedema, and the authors suggest that this is more to do with endoneurial vessel leakage than failure of the perineurial barrier. Another important response to compression of the vessels is a reduction in blood flow (Ogata & Naito 1986). Pressures as low as 20–30 mmHg can reduce the blood flow to the epineurium (Rydevik et al. 1981).

Mechanical injury to the nerve, including a sustained insult, as seen in entrapment neuropathies such as CTS, may cause disruption to Schwann cell function, demyelination distal to the area of compression and dysfunction to axonal transportation which is essential for optimum neuronal health (Lundborg et al. 1983; Dahlin & McLean 1986; Powell & Myers 1986; Schmid 2015).

Pressure of about 30 mmHg held for 8 hours can cause a reduction in the slow and fast axonal transport systems (Dahlin & McLean 1986). Such changes to the axonal transport systems could result in the distal axon being depleted of certain structures essential for repair and maintenance of the cell structure and transmitter substances needed to allow synaptic function (Lundborg 2004). In addition, retrograde axonal transport is inhibited at pressures as low as 20 mmHg (Lundborg & Dahlin 1992) and this results in the suspension in provision of specific neurotrophic factors to the cell body. A depletion of these factors at the cell body has been suggested to activate the cell death programme in nerve cells (Kandel et al. 2000).

Pressures of 50 mmHg held for 2 minutes (Dyck et al. 1990), 30 mmHg for 2 hours (Powell & Myers 1986) and 80 mmHg for 4 hours (Lundborg et al. 1983) have been shown to cause demyelination of nerve fibres and axonal damage. Fibrosis between the epineurium and adjacent muscles has been observed following a compression injury (Powell &Myers 1986); such fibrosis is likely to disrupt the normal movement of nerve through the interface.

In summary, nerve compression of above 20 mmHg may cause widespread mechanical and ischaemic changes to nerves. These changes may include endoneural oedema, damage to the blood–nerve barrier, disruption to conductivity and impaired axonal transportation, which in turn may impede the nerve's normal reparative processes.

Strain. Lengthening a nerve beyond its normal resting length can also cause dysfunction of the nerve by both mechanical and ischaemic means. In animal studies increasing strain by as little as 5–10% can reduce the blood flow in a nerve and alter nerve function (Lundborg & Rydevik 1973; Clark et al. 1992). The nerve injury at the limit of elasticity (see Fig. 6.18) would correspond to a neuropraxia (temporary interruption of conduction, with or without segmental demyelination, but no structural damage to the axon) or an axonotmesis (structural damage to axon and myelin sheath but intact connective tissue) (Haftek 1970). Beyond the limit of elasticity the injury would correspond to a neurotmesis (structural damage to axon, myelin sheath and surrounding connective tissue) (Haftek 1970). The effects of excessive nerve stretch on one fasciculus are depicted in Fig. 6.31.

It has been suggested that neurodynamic tests and techniques could lengthen the nerve beyond normal

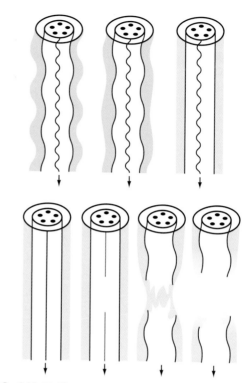

FIG. 6.31 ■ Changes to one fasciculus in a nerve as it is stretched to structural failure. *(From Sunderland 1990, with permission.)*

resting length and therefore be responsible for changes in nerve function, particularly in individuals with an already-present neuropathy. However there is very little evidence to support this theory. Ridehalgh et al. (2005) found no change to vibration thresholds after the application of the SLR test and treatment using ankle movements in the SLR position thought to load the common peroneal nerve. The subjects used were asymptomatic runners and non-runners. It has been postulated that runners may be more susceptible to changes in nerve function due to the repetitive nature of running (Colak et al. 2005), and therefore this study suggests that SLR does not alter function even in potentially susceptible individuals. More recently, no detrimental changes to vibration thresholds were found after the same treatment dose in participants with spinally referred leg pain, including those with radiculopathy (Ridehalgh et al. 2015).

Inflammatory and Immunological Change

Whilst oedematous change in the presence of nerve dysfunction has been recognized for some years (Rydevik & Lundborg 1977; Lundborg 2004), the extent to which immune cells and inflammatory mediators drive the production of symptoms has only recently begun to be elucidated. Immune cells such as mast cells, neutrophils, macrophages and T cells are recruited to the area of peripheral nerve injury and release inflammatory mediators such as proinflammatory cytokines, which have been implicated in neuropathic pain by lowering the threshold at which nociceptive neurons fire and by generating ectopic impulses (Thacker et al. 2007; Grossmann et al. 2009; Schmid et al. 2013). The degradation of the diffusion barrier by mechanical or chemical means and the immunomodulatory role adopted by resident satellite glial cells and Schwann cells may accelerate the immune response by further recruiting immune cells to the area (Schmid et al. 2013; Schmid 2015) (Fig. 6.32).

Radicular pain emanating from a disc prolapse highlights the immunological role in the generation of neuropathic pain. It was once thought that nerve root pain was purely a compressive phenomenon. Animal and human studies have demonstrated that the nucleus pulposus has autoimmune properties and that cytokine activation following an immune response to a disc prolapse is an important component in the generation of symptoms (Geiss et al. 2009). Interestingly, animal studies show that cytokine inhibitors may have a positive effect on nerve injury and conduction velocity (Olmarker 2011). The use of such interventions may therefore prove beneficial in the future management of neuropathic arm or leg pain.

Mechanisms of Central Dysfunction

As well as a local mechanism, there are central mechanisms which may also play a role in the generation of symptoms in response to nerve injury. This section will briefly discuss changes to the DRG and dorsal horn, as well as subcortical and cortical changes.

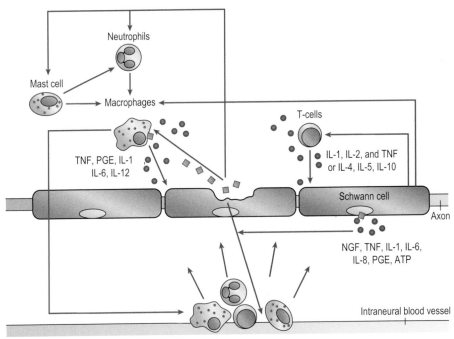

FIG. 6.32 ■ Inflammatory and immunological change in response to peripheral nerve injury. Resident immune cells and those recruited to the area release inflammatory mediators. Schwann cells also adopt an immunomodulatory role. *ATP*, adenosine triphosphate; *IL-1β*, interleukin-1β; *PGE*, prostaglandin E; *TNF*, tumour necrosis factor. *(From Schmid et al. 2013, with permission.)*

Changes to the Dorsal Root Ganglion and Dorsal Horn

As well as the local immune and inflammatory response to peripheral nerve injury, immune cells are also found in the DRG and even at the level of the dorsal horn in response to peripheral nerve compression (Schmid et al. 2013; Schmid 2015). As in the periphery, the release of inflammatory mediators here may result in a reduced firing threshold of nociceptive neurons and the production of ectopic discharges.

It has been hypothesized that inflammatory mediators within the DRG, for example, may affect adjacent nerves, which may explain the spread of symptoms in entrapment neuropathies (Schmid et al. 2013). Indeed, Nora et al. (2005) found that CTS confirmed with electrophysiological studies is rarely restricted to the cutaneous distribution of the median nerve and is often felt in the fourth or fifth digits, or proximal to the wrist. From a clinical perspective therefore it is important not to discount entrapment pathology as a clinical hypothesis purely on the basis of the symptoms not conforming to a given cutaneous distribution.

The presence of inflammatory mediators at the dorsal horn further complicates the picture. Because first-order afferent neurons entering the dorsal horn may ascend or descend before synapsing with a second-order neuron in the same way that inflammatory mediators may affect adjacent nerves in the DRG, the same is true in the dorsal horn. Theoretically, inflammatory mediators may affect neurons at multiple levels and even bilaterally (Schmid et al. 2013). An appreciation of such diverse neurophysiological processes will help the clinician make sense of widespread and varied symptoms which may not necessary follow a well-defined sensory distribution.

Subcortical and Cortical Changes

As well as local mechanical and immunoinflammatory effects of nerve dysfunction, and changes to the DRG and dorsal horn, there may be changes at subcortical and cortical levels. It is known that the nociceptive system can become sensitized as a result of a particularly noxious or repeated nociceptive stimulus (Latremoliere & Woolf 2009) and that entrapment neuropathies can cause changes to cortical representations in the brain (Maeda et al. 2014). There is also emerging evidence to suggest that severe nerve injuries may cause glial cell activity change in the midbrain and thalamus and the resultant 'sensory relay' may result in widespread symptoms (Schmid et al. 2013, p. 452).

Summary of Local and Central Mechanisms

As can be seen, the complexity of the local and central responses to nerve injury has the potential for the same pathology to produce significantly differing symptoms in different individuals. CTS may produce classic paraesthesia in the median nerve distribution in one individual but more diffuse and widespread symptoms, possibly bilateral, in someone else. To some extent this may be dependent upon the degree of insult to the nerve tissue but it must be acknowledged that psychosocial factors may also play a significant role in how symptoms are experienced and expressed (Carlino & Benedetti 2016). Fig. 6.33 summarizes the mechanisms of local and central nerve dysfunction.

Clinical Examples of Nerve Pathology

The above mechanisms of local and central nerve dysfunction will now be contextualized with some specific examples of nerve pathology in relation to the spine. The clinical presentations will be highlighted rather than the pathophysiology but the reader is encouraged to consider the local and central mechanism discussed above.

Canal, Lateral Recess and Foraminal Stenosis

Whilst cord compression may produce widespread neurological disturbance if severe, other types of compressive pathologies may produce subtly different clinical presentations. In the lumbar spine, if the entire spinal canal becomes narrowed in the presence of degenerative disc disease, hypertrophy to the zygapophyseal joints and thickening to the ligamentum flavum, numerous roots of the cauda equina may be affected. This is a condition known as spinal canal stenosis (narrowing). Canal stenosis is commonly a degenerative condition but the canal can become narrowed in more acute cases also, for example, in the presence of a large disc prolapse. Canal stenosis typically causes 'claudicant' unilateral or bilateral leg pain (Maus 2012). Claudication describes leg pain which occurs on standing and walking (caused by a reduction in the cross-sectional area of the canal) which is relieved on sitting. The most common

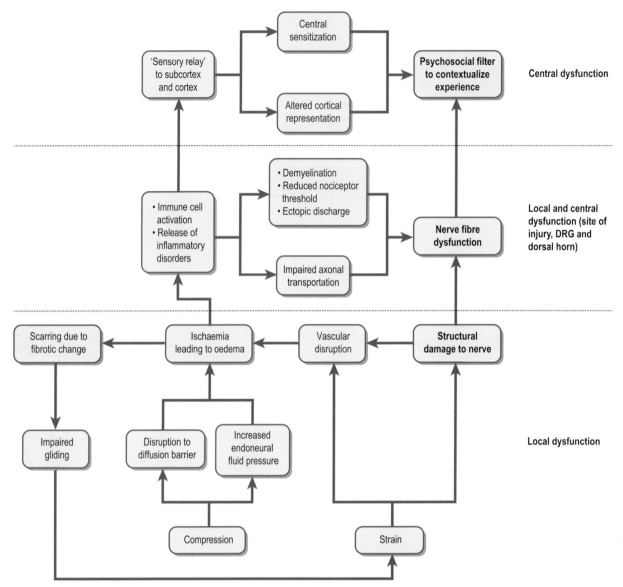

FIG. 6.33 ■ Summary of mechanisms of local and central nerve dysfunction. *DRG*, dorsal root ganglion.

symptoms of canal stenosis include back pain (95%), claudication (91%), leg pain (71%), weakness (33%) and bladder/bowel disturbance (12%, Amundsen et al. 1995). Fig. 6.34A depicts the cross-sectional anatomy of the spinal canal, lateral recess and intervertebral foramen. Fig. 6.34B shows canal stenosis on a magnetic resonance imaging (MRI) axial image at the level of L5.

Stenosis of the lateral recess is a common presentation in the patient presenting with a posterolateral disc prolapse (Fig. 6.34C). In lateral recess stenosis the descending nerve root may be compressed in isolation or in combination with the exiting nerve root at that level. For example, at the level of L5–S1, the L5 nerve root is located in the intervertebral foramen and the S1 nerve root is located in the lateral recess on its journey

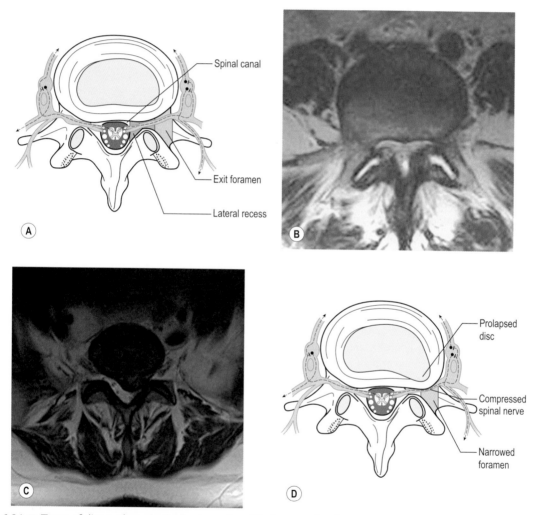

FIG. 6.34 ■ Types of disc prolapse in the lumbar spine. (A) Cross-sectional anatomy of the spinal canal. *DRG*, dorsal root ganglion. (B) Spinal canal stenosis. (C) Lateral recess stenosis. (D) Exit foramen stenosis. *(A and D adapted from Palastanga & Soames 2012, B from Resnick & Kransdorf 2005, C from McNair & Breakwell 2010, reproduced with permission.)*

caudally to leave the spinal canal at the level of S1. For this reason, patients with L5–S1 lateral recess stenosis may experience signs and symptoms emanating from the L5 and S1 levels. A lateral disc prolapse however produces narrowing to the intervertebral foramen (Fig. 6.34D). At the level of L5–S1, these patients may experience L5 signs and symptoms only as only the L5 root is mechanically affected.

Cauda Equina Syndrome

CES is characterized by dysfunction of two of more of the roots that comprise the cauda equina (see Fig. 6.1). Signs and symptoms of CES include unilateral or bilateral leg pain, progressive neurological deficit, perianal and genital numbness, sexual dysfunction, reduced anal sphincter tone and bladder and bowel disturbance, including a loss of desire to urinate, straining and a loss of awareness that the bladder is full (Greenhalgh & Selfe 2015). The most common cause of CES is a prolapsed intervertebral disc (Fig. 6.35). The condition is a neurosurgical emergency and, if suspected, the patient should be advised to attend Accident & Emergency immediately as prompt MRI imaging is required. Signs and symptoms of CES together with significant canal stenosis involving the roots of the cauda equina on MRI confirm the diagnosis. The consequences of delay to treatment can be catastrophic as the patient may be left with significant neurological problems in one or both legs and/or permanent bladder, bowel and sexual dysfunction. Some sources recommend surgical decompression within 24 hours of onset if feasible (Nater

& Fehlings 2015), although it is generally agreed that decompression within 48 hours optimizes recovery (Greenhalgh & Selfe 2015).

Cord Compression

Spinal cord compression is a potentially serious nerve pathology which may, for example, be caused by an acute injury, e.g. fracture, infection, degenerative spondylitic change or metastatic disease where there is either a vertebral body collapse or direct compression to the cord from a tumour (Greenhalgh & Selfe 2015). Cord compression may also be caused by cysts and benign tumours which are often intradural. These include meningiomas, nerve sheath tumours, epidermoid cysts and arachnoid cysts (Seidenwurm & Expert Panel on Neurologic Imaging 2008). The term myelopathy is often used to describe neurological deficit resulting from cord compression.

Potentially, cord compression can result in irreversible neurological dysfunction so it is important that the clinician is able to identify myelopathy, or at least the possibility thereof. Although myelopathy may be mild and stable, acute and/or progressive myelopathy is a neurosurgical emergency. The diagnosis is confirmed on MRI. Theoretically cord compression can cause widespread neurological dysfunction below the level of the lesion. Signs and symptoms may include scattered and bilateral sensory disturbance which does not correspond to a dermatomal or peripheral nerve distribution, multilevel weakness, problems with coordination and disturbance to bladder and bowel function: The

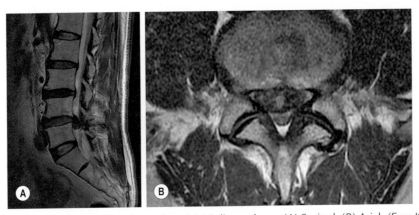

FIG. 6.35 ■ Cauda equina syndrome arising from a large L4–L5 disc prolapse. (A) Sagittal. (B) Axial. *(From Kusakabe 2013, with permission.)*

higher the lesion, the more profound the potential disability. There are physical tests which may indicate upper motor neuron pathology such as the Babinski test or Hoffman's sign, but the clinician is encouraged to look at the entire clinical picture rather than focus on the results of one or two specific tests (see Petty & Ryder 2017).

Degenerative cervical myelopathy is the most common cause of cord dysfunction in the elderly and may result from spondylitic change, degenerative disc disease and ossification to the posterior longitudinal ligament and the ligamentum flavum (Nouri et al. 2015). Fig. 6.36 shows sagittal and axial images of the cord compression at C4 in a patient with features of cervical myelopathy.

Nerve Regeneration and Repair

Following nerve injury the distal portion of the nerve undergoes Wallerian degeneration. Distal to the site of injury, the Schwann cells proliferate and the myelin and axoplasm disintegrate and are reabsorbed by macrophagic activity. Proximal to the site of injury axons grow a large number of sprouts, which grow at approximately 1 mm/day towards the distal segment. If the Schwann cell columns remain intact the sprouting axons will be guided to reinnervate the target organ. If the Schwann cell columns have been destroyed by the injury

then sprouting axons may grow and innervate inappropriate areas, giving a poorer clinical result.

The reinnervation and sensory restoration following a myocutaneous skin flap have been investigated and highlight the clinical outcome of nerve regeneration. Some axons were found to sprout into Schwann cell columns, whereas a number of axons were found to be unmyelinated and associated with blood vessels (Turkof et al. 1993; Terenghi 1995). The degree of sensory restoration varied widely between individuals; some flaps were totally numb while others had moderate sensation (Turkof et al. 1993). From this research it seems that there is a wide variation in the functional regeneration of sensory nerves, from very poor to moderately good.

An additional effect in regeneration of nerve axons occurs at the dorsal horn within 2 weeks of a nerve injury (Doubell & Woolf 1997). C fibres, which synapse in lamina II of the dorsal horn, atrophy and leave vacant synaptic spaces (Fig. 6.37). Large myelinated A fibres sprout into these spaces, altering the processing of mechanoreceptor input from A fibres (Woolf et al. 1992; Doubell & Woolf 1997).

The repair process of the connective tissue around nerves is similar to that of ligament. Following a nerve injury, there is an increase in the collagen tissue within the perineurium and endoneurium, indicative of scar

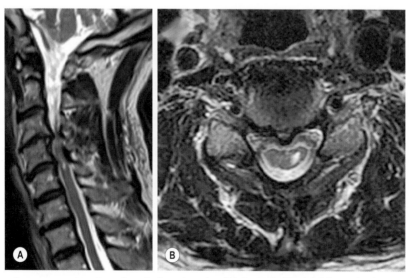

FIG. 6.36 ■ Magnetic resonance imaging of cervical myelopathy. (A) Sagittal. (B) Axial (note the increased signal within the cord indicating possible oedematous change). *(From Maus 2012, with permission.)*

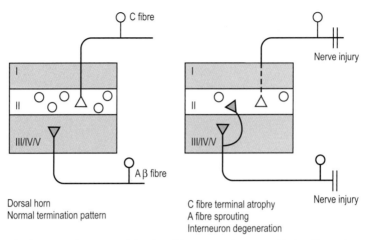

FIG. 6.37 ■ Sprouting of A fibres into lamina II of the dorsal horn to replace atrophied C fibres. *(From Doubell et al. 1999, with permission.)*

formation (Starkweather et al. 1978; Salonen et al. 1985). Additionally, it has been demonstrated in rat sciatic nerves that, 3 weeks after a nerve injury, there is a 28% reduction in nerve length (Clark et al. 1992). Common musculoskeletal injuries may also have an element of nerve dysfunction to them. Ankle sprains commonly affect not only the ligamentous structures but also either the common peroneal nerve or sural nerve (Nitz et al. 1985; Johnston & Howell 1999). Indeed, footdrop also is a rare complication of an ankle inversion sprain (Brief et al. 2009). This could be either due to the direct inversion sprain causing a sudden increase in length of the nerve or secondary to healing and scar tissue formation of structures close to the nerve. Sunderland (1978) termed these conditions friction fibrosis. In such conditions it may be that the nerve loses its ability to slide and glide through its interface (Butler 2000). Another example of restricted interface movement is the adhesion formation between lumbar nerve roots and the intervertebral foramina that can reduce the ability of the nerve to move (Goddard & Reid 1965; Kobayashi et al., 2003). This can be caused by local pathological changes or may occur as a result of normal age-related changes (Goddard & Reid 1965).

Reduced Nerve Movement

Upper-limb neural mobility in response to movement is well documented. Studies examining the median nerve have shown that not only does the nerve move longitudinally in asymptomatic subjects (McLellan & Swash 1976; Hough et al. 2000c; Dilley et al. 2003; Lai et al. 2014), but there is also a small amount of transverse gliding of the median nerve beneath the flexor retinaculum during flexion/extension of the wrist (Nakamichi & Tachibana 1995; Greening et al. 1999; Wang et al. 2014).

The increasing use of USI is increasing the accessibility of studying nerve function in vivo (Ridehalgh et al. 2012, 2014; Boyd & Dilley 2014). It has been suggested that injury or pathology affecting peripheral neural tissue may lead to a reduced neural compliance (Elvey 1986) and thereby an alteration in the patterns of normal nerve movement. Limited data exist however on the response of nerve dysfunction on the mechanical properties of the nerve. Data which do exist appear contradictory. For example, Yoshii et al. (2013) found transverse movement of the median nerve at the wrist to be reduced in the presence of CTS, Yang et al. (2013) found increased movement of the ulnar nerve at the elbow in the presence of cubital tunnel syndrome, whilst Ridehalgh et al. (2015) found there was no difference in sciatic nerve excursion at the posterior thigh between participants with spinally referred leg pain and the asymptomatic population.

Whilst reduced neural mobility, therefore, including an impaired ability of a nerve to lengthen and move relative to adjacent tissues, has been assumed to contribute to peripheral nerve dysfunction, further research is needed to understand the relationship between peripheral nerve dysfunction and nerve mechanics.

Carpal Tunnel Syndrome – a Clinical Example

Even though the relationship between nerve mechanics and nerve dysfunction is not fully understood, the pathophysiology of CTS has been extensively investigated.

The development of signs and symptoms of CTS has been linked to the effects of circumferential nerve compression of the median nerve. Early signs are intermittent paraesthesia and alteration in sensation, particularly at night; this may be due to changes in the intraneural circulation, with some oedema accumulating at night and disappearing during the day (Lundborg et al. 1983; Chammas et al. 2014). Later in the progression of nerve compression there is increased numbness and paraesthesia, impaired dexterity and muscle weakness. These symptoms may be present during the day as well as at night and may be related to altered circulation and the presence of epineural and intrafascicular oedema (Fuchs et al. 1991; Chammas et al. 2014). Compression and the resulting oedematous change may disrupt the diffusion barrier, impair axonal transportation and cause demyelination, leading to disruption of conductivity and ectopic discharge (Schmid et al. 2013). Minor mechanical irritation can lead to radiating pain (Smyth & Wright 1958; MacNab 1972; Howe et al. 1977; Rydevik et al. 1984). At this stage, once compression has been removed, symptoms resolve rapidly as intraneural circulation is restored (Chammas et al. 2014). Finally, there is constant pain, atrophy of the thenar muscles and permanent sensory changes; this may be due to a neuropraxia caused by lesions of the myelin sheath of the nerve fibres (Lundborg & Dahlin 1996). Clinical measurement of nerve conduction velocity and latency can be carried out objectively; however, there is a 20% false-negative response in patients with CTS (Spindler & Dellon 1982). Following the resolution of severe compression, recovery is variable and may depend upon an individual's potential for axonal regeneration (Chammas et al. 2014). Maximal recovery after the removal of compression may take some months and may indeed be incomplete (Chammas et al. 2014).

The pressure within the carpal tunnel is generally increased in patients with CTS. Carpal pressures exceeding 40 mmHg are thought to be sufficient to impair venous return and therefore intraneural circulation

(Chammas et al. 2014). It appears that pressures increase substantially in the carpal tunnel during maximal wrist flexion and extension in both asymptomatic and symptomatic subjects. A study by Gelberman et al. (1981) recorded mean flexion pressures of 94 mmHg in symptomatic patients, compared with 42 mmHg in asymptomatic patients, and extension pressures of 110 mmHg in symptomatic patients, compared with 33 mmHg in asymptomatic patients. Research examining more functional tasks has also demonstrated significant rises in carpal tunnel pressure. Making a fist with the hand, for example, has been shown to increase carpal tunnel pressure from 24 to 234 mmHg (Seradge et al. 1995); this is almost a 10-fold increase.

Environmental factors may also play a role in the development of CTS. The increasing use of computer keyboards, for example, has been postulated for a rise in CTS (Keir et al. 1999). Keir et al. (1999) found that a marked rise in carpal tunnel pressure occurred during dragging and pointing tasks using a mouse. Such studies should however be treated with caution as a systematic review examining CTS and the use of a computer and mouse found insufficient epidemiological evidence to postulate that computer use caused CTS (Thomsen et al. 2008). There is however strong evidence that tasks requiring 'repetition and forceful exertion', and moderate evidence that exposure to vibration tools, may increase the risk of developing CTS (Kozak et al. 2015). Indeed, individuals with CTS who are regularly exposed to hand-held vibration tools have been found to have demyelination and incomplete regeneration of the dorsal interosseous nerve at the wrist (Stromberg et al. 1997). This suggests that, in some patients, CTS may be caused by two mechanisms: nerve compression and nerve vibration (Stromberg et al. 1997).

Experimental compression of nerves in normal subjects provides valuable information on the effect of nerve compression on clinical neurological testing. A catheter inserted into the carpal tunnel allows for controlled and accurate increases in carpal pressure to 30, 40, 50, 60, 70 and 90 mmHg (Lundborg et al. 1982; Gelberman et al. 1983; Szabo et al. 1983). The earliest signs of nerve impairment are the subjective reporting of numbness, tingling or paraesthesia in the distribution of the median nerve (Gelberman et al. 1983; Szabo et al. 1983). At 40–50 mmHg sensation is completely blocked (Gelberman et al. 1983), and in hypertensive subjects with a higher neural arteriole pressure, sensory block occurs at 60–70 mmHg (Szabo et al. 1983). This suggests that patients with raised or lowered blood pressure may respond differently to a given amount of nerve compression (Szabo et al. 1983). At 90 mmHg paraesthesia in the hand was felt after 20 minutes, after 30–50 minutes there was a complete sensory block and after a further 10–30 minutes there was a complete motor block (Lundborg et al. 1982).

Nerve conduction studies are the gold standard in diagnosis of CTS (Bueno-Gracia et al. 2015); however, in the absence of electrophysiological testing, it is useful to be able to test the function of the peripheral nerves in individuals with suspected minor nerve pathology clinically. The most sensitive physical tests of large-diameter nerve impairment are vibration sensibility (Gelberman et al. 1983; Szabo et al. 1983) using a 256 cycles-per-second tuning fork (Dellon 1980, 1981) or vibrameter (Goldberg & Lindblom 1979; Martina et al. 1998) and mechanical threshold testing (Gelberman et al. 1983; Szabo et al. 1983) using von Frey monofilaments (Levin et al. 1978). These sensory changes occurred before any motor changes (Gelberman et al. 1983; Szabo et al. 1983). More recently the use of quantitative sensory testing focusing on small fibres has been advocated as small fibres may degenerate earlier or to a greater extent than large axons in people with minor entrapment neuropathy (Tamburin et al. 2011; Schmid et al. 2013). Such tests include warm detection thresholds and cold detection thresholds.

As well as the physiological changes described, reduced median nerve mobility in CTS may further compromise nerve function. Reduced transverse (Nakamichi & Tachibana 1995; Allmann et al. 1997; Erel et al. 2003; Yoshii et al. 2013; Kang et al. 2016) and longitudinal (Hough et al. 2007; Korstanje et al. 2012; Filius et al. 2015) median nerve mobility has been observed in subjects with CTS. An impaired ability of the median nerve to lengthen and move relative to adjacent tissue therefore appears to be a factor in the development and maintenance of CTS.

Production of Symptoms

Pain from a peripheral nerve can arise from its innervated connective tissue covering or from the axon itself. Where pain arises from the connective tissue it can be considered similar to pain arising from ligament or muscle, in the sense that nociceptors lying in the tissue can provoke symptoms. The pain coming from the connective tissue is therefore classified in the same way as joint and muscle pain, as mechanical or chemical pain, with chemical pain being further subdivided into inflammatory and ischaemic (Gifford 1998). The effects of nerve compression and CTS, discussed earlier, are examples of peripheral neurogenic or neuropathic pain. For further details on pain, the reader is advised to refer to Chapter 8.

Summary of Nerve Dysfunction

For a nerve to function optimally, there must be normal functioning of the relevant joints and muscles. Conversely, nerve dysfunction may in turn adversely affect joints and muscles. The physiological and mechanical mechanisms leading to nerve dysfunction have been explored. Chapter 7 discusses nerve treatment.

REFERENCES

Adams, M.A., Burton, K., Dolan, P., et al., 2006. The biomechanics of back pain, second ed. Churchill Livingstone, Edinburgh.

Akalin, E., El, O., Peker, O., et al., 2002. Treatment of carpal tunnel syndrome with nerve and tendon gliding exercises. Am. J. Phys. Med. Rehabil. 81, 108–113.

Allmann, K.H., Horch, R., Uhl, M., et al., 1997. MR imaging of the carpal tunnel. Eur. J. Radiol. 25, 141–145.

Amundsen, T., Weber, H., Lilleas, F., et al., 1995. Lumbar spinal stenosis: clinical and radiologic features. Spine 20, 1178–1186.

Bahns, E., Ernsberger, U., Janig, W., et al., 1986. Discharge properties of mechanosensitive afferents supplying the retroperitoneal space. Pflügers Archives 407, 519–525.

Bardak, A.N., Alp, M., Erhan, B., et al., 2009. Evaluation of the clinical efficacy of conservative treatment in the management of carpal tunnel syndrome. Adv. Ther. 26, 108–113.

Baron, E.M., Tunstall, R., 2015. Standring, S. Gray's anatomy: the anatomical basis of clinical practice. Elsevier Health Sciences, Edinburgh.

Bisby, M.A., 1982. Functions of retrograde axonal transport. Fed. Proc. 41, 2307–2311.

Bogduk, N., 2009. On the definitions and physiology of back pain, referred pain, and radicular pain. Pain 15, 17–19.

Bove, G.M., Light, A.R., 1995. Unmyelinated nociceptors of rat paraspinal tissues. J. Neurophysiol. 73, 1752–1762.

Boyd, B.S., Dilley, A., 2014. Altered tibial nerve biomechanics in patients with diabetes mellitus. Muscle Nerve 50, 216–223.

Boyd, B.S., Puttlitz, C., Jerylin, G., et al., 2005. Strain and excursion in the rat sciatic nerve during a modified straight leg raise are altered after traumatic nerve injury. J. Orthop. Res. 23, 764–770.

Boyd, B.S., Topp, K.S., Coppieters, M.W., 2013. Impact of movement sequencing on sciatic and tibial nerve strain and excursion during the straight leg raise test in embalmed cadavers. J. Orthop. Sports Phys. Ther. 43, 398–403.

Breig, A., 1960. Biomechanics of the central nervous system: some basic normal and pathologic phenomena. Almqvist & Wiksell, Stockholm.

Breig, A., 1978. Adverse mechanical tension in the central nervous system. Almqvist & Wiksell, Stockholm.

Breig, A., Marions, O., 1963. Biomechanics of the lumbosacral nerve roots. Acta Radiol. 1, 1141–1160.

Brief, J.M., Brief, R., Ergas, E., et al., 2009. Peroneal nerve injury with foot drop complicating ankle sprain. Bull. NYU Hosp. Jt. Dis. 67, 374–377.

Bueno-Gracia, E., Tricás-Moreno, J.M., Fanlo-Mazas, P., et al., 2015. Validity of the upper limb neurodynamic test 1 for the diagnosis of carpal tunnel syndrome. The role of structural differentiation. Man. Ther. 22, 190–195.

Butler, D.S., 1991. Mobilisation of the nervous system. Churchill Livingstone, Melbourne.

Butler, D.S., 2000. The sensitive nervous system. Noigroup, Adelaide.

Cappelleri, J.C., Bienen, E.J., Koduru, V., et al., 2014. Measurement properties of painDETECT by average pain severity. Clinicoecon. Outcomes Res. 6, 497–504.

Carlino, E., Benedetti, F., 2016. Different contexts, different pains, different experiences. Neuroscience 338, 19–26.

Chammas, M., Boretto, J., Burmann, L.M., et al., 2014. Carpal tunnel syndrome – part I (anatomy, physiology, etiology and diagnosis). Rev. Bras. Ortop. 49, 429–436.

Clark, W.L., Trumble, T.E., Swiontkowski, M.F., et al., 1992. Nerve tension and blood flow in a rat model of immediate and delayed repairs. J. Hand Surg. Am. 17A, 677–687.

Colak, T., Bamaç, B., Gönener, A., et al., 2005. Comparison of nerve conduction velocities of lower extremities between runners and controls. J. Sci. Med. Sport 8, 403–410.

Coppieters, M.W., Alshami, A.M., Babri, A.S., et al., 2006. Strain and excursion of the sciatic, tibial, and plantar nerves during a modified straight leg raising test. J. Orthop. Res. 24, 1883–1889.

Coppieters, M.W., Hough, A.D., Dilley, A., 2009. Different nerve-gliding exercises induce different magnitudes of median nerve longitudinal excursion: an in vivo study using dynamic ultrasound imaging. J. Orthop. Sports Phys. Ther. 39, 164–171.

Coppieters, M.W., Crooke, J.L., Lawrenson, P.R., et al., 2015. A modified straight leg raise test to differentiate between sural nerve pathology and Achilles tendinopathy. A cross-sectional cadaver study. Man. Ther. 20, 587–591.

Crossman, A., Neary, D., 2015. Neuroanatomy: an illustrated colour text, fifth ed. Elsevier Health Sciences, London.

Dahlin, L.B., Lundborg, G., 1990. The neurone and its response to peripheral nerve compression. J. Hand Surg. Am. 15B, 5–10.

Dahlin, L.B., McLean, W.G., 1986. Effects of graded experimental compression on slow and fast axonal transport in rabbit vagus nerve. J. Neurol. Sci. 72, 19–30.

Dellon, A.L., 1980. Clinical use of vibratory stimuli to evaluate peripheral nerve injury and compression neuropathy. Plast. Reconstr. Surg. 65, 466–476.

Dellon, A.L., 1981. Evaluation of sensibility and re-education of sensation in the hand. Williams and Wilkins, Baltimore.

Dilley, A., Greening, J., Lynn, B., et al., 2001. The use of cross-correlation analysis between high-frequency ultrasound images to measure longitudinal median nerve movement. Ultrasound Med. Biol. 27, 1211–1218.

Dilley, A., Lynn, B., Greening, J., et al., 2003. Quantitative in vivo studies of median nerve sliding in response to wrist, elbow, shoulder and neck movements. Clin. Biomech. (Bristol, Avon) 18, 899–907.

Doubell, T.P., Woolf, C.J., 1997. Growth-associated protein 43 immunoreactivity in the superficial dorsal horn of the rat spinal cord is localized in atrophic C-fiber, and not in sprouted A-fiber, central terminals after peripheral nerve injury. J. Comp. Neurol. 386, 111–118.

Doubell, T.P., Mannion, R.J., Woolf, C.J., 1999. The dorsal horn: state-dependent sensory processing, plasticity and the generation of pain. In: Wall, P.D., Melzack, R. (Eds.), Textbook of pain, fourth ed. Churchill Livingstone, Edinburgh, pp. 165–181.

Driscoll, P.J., Glasby, M.A., Lawson, G.M., 2002. An in vivo study of peripheral nerves in continuity: biomechanical and physiological responses to elongation. J. Orthop. Res. 20, 370–375.

Dyck, P.J., Lais, A.C., Giannini, C., et al., 1990. Structural alterations of nerve during cuff compression. Proc. Natl. Acad. Sci. USA 87, 9828–9832.

Ellis, R.F., Hing, W.A., McNair, P.J., 2012. Comparison of longitudinal sciatic nerve movement with different mobilization exercises: an in vivo study utilizing ultrasound imaging. J. Orthop. Sports Phys. Ther. 42, 667–675.

Ellis, R., Osborne, S., Whitfield, J., et al., 2016. The effect of spinal position on sciatic nerve excursion during seated neural mobilisation exercises: an in vivo study using ultrasound imaging. J. Man. Manip. Ther. doi:10.1179/2042618615Y.0000000020.

Elvey, R.L., 1986. Treatment of arm pain associated with abnormal brachial plexus tension. Aust. J. Physiother. 32, 224–229.

Epstein, B.S., 1966. An anatomic, myelographic and cinemyelographic study of the dentate ligaments. Am. J. Roentgenol. Radium Ther. Nucl. Med. 98, 704–712.

Erel, E., Dilley, A., Greening, J., et al., 2003. Longitudinal sliding of the median nerve in patients with carpal tunnel syndrome. J. Hand Surg. Br. 28, 439–443.

Filius, A., Thoreson, A.R., Wang, Y., et al., 2015. The effect of tendon excursion velocity on longitudinal median nerve displacement: differences between carpal tunnel syndrome patients and controls. J. Orthop. Res. 33, 483–487.

Fuchs, P.C., Nathan, P.A., Myers, L.D., 1991. Synovial histology in carpal tunnel syndrome. J. Hand Surg. Am. 16A, 753–758.

Geiss, A., Larsson, K., Junevik, K., et al., 2009. Autologous nucleus pulposus primes T cells to develop into interleukin-4-producing effector cells: an experimental study on the autoimmune properties of nucleus pulposus. J. Orthop. Res. 27, 97–103.

Gelberman, R.H., Hergenroeder, P.T., Hargens, A.R., et al., 1981. The carpal tunnel syndrome. A study of carpal canal pressures. J. Bone Joint Surg. Am. 63, 380–383.

Gelberman, R.H., Szabo, R.M., Williamson, R.V., et al., 1983. Sensibility testing in peripheral-nerve compression syndromes, an experimental study in humans. J. Bone Joint Surg. Am. 65A, 632–638.

Gifford, L., 1998. Pain. In: Pitt-Brooke, J., Reid, H., Lockwood, J. (Eds.), Rehabilitation of movement, theoretical basis of clinical practice. W.B. Saunders, London, pp. 196–232.

Gilbert, K.K., Brismée, J.M., Collins, D.L., et al., 2007. 2006 Young Investigator Award winner: lumbosacral nerve root displacement and strain: part 2. A comparison of 2 straight leg raise conditions in unembalmed cadavers. Spine 32, 1521–1525.

Gillard, D.M., 2014. The lumbar MRI page. Available at: http://www.chirogeek.com/MRI%20READING/MRI-reading.html. (Accessed 30 October 2016).

Goddard, M.D., Reid, J.D., 1965. Movements induced by straight leg raising in the lumbo-sacral roots, nerves and plexus, and in the intrapelvic section of the sciatic nerve. J. Neurol. Neurosurg. Psychiatry 28, 12–18.

Goldberg, J.M., Lindblom, U., 1979. Standardised method of determining vibratory perception thresholds for diagnosis and screening in neurological investigation. J. Neurol. Neurosurg. Psychiatry 42, 793–803.

Greenhalgh, S., Selfe, J., 2015. Masqueraders. In: Jull, G., Moore, A.P., Falla, D., et al. (Eds.), Grieve's modern musculoskeletal physiotherapy. Churchill Livingstone, Edinburgh.

Greening, J., Smart, S., Leary, R., et al., 1999. Reduced movement of median nerve in carpal tunnel during wrist flexion in patients with non-specific arm pain. Lancet 354, 217–218.

Greening, J., Lynn, B., Leary, R., et al., 2001. The use of ultrasound imaging to demonstrate reduced movement of the median nerve during wrist flexion in patients with non-specific arm pain. J. Hand Surg. Am. 26B, 401–406.

Grossmann, L., Gorodetskaya, N., Baron, R., et al., 2009. Enhancement of ectopic discharge in regenerating A-and C-fibers by inflammatory mediators. J. Neurophysiol. 101, 2762–2774.

Haftek, J., 1970. Stretch injury of peripheral nerve, acute effects of stretching on rabbit nerve. J. Bone Joint Surg. Am. 52B, 354–365.

Hough, A.D., Moore, A.P., Jones, M.P., 2000a. Peripheral nerve motion measurement with spectral Doppler sonography: a reliability study. J. Hand Surg. Am. 25B, 585–589.

Hough, A.D., Moore, A.P., Jones, M.P., 2000b. Measuring longitudinal nerve motion using ultrasonography. Man. Ther. 5, 173–180.

Hough, A., Moore, A., Jones, M., 2000c. Doppler ultrasound measurement of median nerve motion 62 56 International Federation of Orthopaedic Manipulative Therapists 7th Scientific Conference Proceedings, abstract.

Hough, A.D., Moore, A.P., Jones, M.P., 2007. Reduced longitudinal excursion of the median nerve in carpal tunnel syndrome. Arch. Phys. Med. Rehabil. 88, 569–576.

Howe, J.F., Loeser, J.D., Calvin, W.H., 1977. Mechanosensitivity of dorsal root ganglia and chronically injured axons: a physiological basis for the radicular pain of nerve root compression. Pain 3, 25–41.

Hromada, J., 1963. On the nerve supply of the connective tissue of some peripheral nervous system components. Acta Anat. (Basel) 55, 343–351.

Inman, V.T., Saunders, J.B., 1942. The clinico-anatomical aspects of the lumbosacral region. Radiology 38, 669–678.

International Association for the Study of Pain 2014 IASP taxonomy. Available online at: http://www.iasp-pain.org/Taxonomy#Peripheralneuropathicpain. (Accessed 4 December 2016).

Inufusa, A., An, H.S., Lim, T.-H., et al., 1996. Anatomic changes of the spinal canal and intervertebral foramen associated with flexion–extension movement. Spine 21, 2412–2420.

Johnston, E.C., Howell, S.J., 1999. Tension neuropathy of the superficial peroneal nerve: associated conditions and results of release. Foot Ankle Int. 20, 576–582.

Kandel, E.R., Schwarz, J.H., Jessel, T.M., 2000. Principles of neural science, fourth ed. McGraw-Hill, New York.

Kang, S., Yang, S.N., Joon, J.S., et al., 2016. Effect of carpal tunnel syndrome on the ulnar nerve at the wrist sonographic and electrophysiologic studies. J. Ultrasound Med. 35, 37–42.

Keir, P.J., Bach, J.M., Rempel, D., 1999. Effects of computer mouse design and task on carpal tunnel pressure. Ergonomics 42, 1350–1360.

Kobayashi, S., Shizu, N., Suzuki, Y., et al., 2003. Changes in nerve root motion and intraradicular blood flow during an intraoperative straight leg raise test. Spine 28, 1427–1434.

Korstanje, J.W., Scheltens-De Boer, M., Blok, J.H., et al., 2012. Ultrasonographic assessment of longitudinal median nerve and hand flexor tendon dynamics in carpal tunnel syndrome. Muscle Nerve 45, 721–729.

Kozak, A., Schedlbauer, G., Wirth, T., et al., 2015. Association between work-related biomechanical risk factors and the occurrence of carpal tunnel syndrome: an overview of systematic reviews and a meta-analysis of current research. BMC Musculoskelet. Disord. 16, 231.

Kusakabe, T., 2013. (iv) Cauda equina syndrome. Orthop. Trauma 27, 215–219.

Lai, W.K., Chiu, Y.T., Law, W.S., 2014. The deformation and longitudinal excursion of median nerve during digits movement and wrist extension. Man. Ther. 19, 608–613.

Latremoliere, A., Woolf, C., 2009. Central sensitization: a generator of pain hypersensitivity by central neural plasticity. J. Pain 10, 895–926.

Levin, S., Pearsell, G., Ruderman, R.J., 1978. Von Frey's method of measuring pressure sensibility in the hand: an engineering analysis of the Weinstein–Semmes pressure aesthesiometer. J. Hand Surg. Am. 3, 211–216.

Lohman, C.M., Gilbert, K.K., Sobczak, S., et al., 2015. Young Investigator Award Winner: cervical nerve root displacement and strain during upper limb neural tension testing: part 2: role of foraminal ligaments in the cervical spine. Spine 40, 801–808.

Louis, R., 1981. Vertebroradicular and vertebromedullar dynamics. Anatomica Clinica 3, 1–11.

Lundborg, G., 1970. Ischaemic nerve injury. Scand. J. Plast. Reconstr. Surg. (Suppl. 6).

Lundborg, G., 1975. Structure and function of the intraneural microvessels as related to trauma, edema formation, and nerve function. J. Bone Joint Surg. Am. 57A, 938–948.

Lundborg, G., 2004. Nerve injury and repair. Regeneration, reconstruction and cortical remodelling, second ed. Churchill Livingstone, Edinburgh.

Lundborg, G., Dahlin, L.B., 1992. The pathophysiology of nerve compression. Hand Clin. 8, 215–227.

Lundborg, G., Dahlin, L.B., 1996. Anatomy, function, and pathophysiology of peripheral nerves and nerve compression. Hand Clin. 12, 185–193.

Lundborg, G., Rydevik, B., 1973. Effects of stretching the tibial nerve of the rabbit. A preliminary study of the intraneural circulation and the barrier function of the perineurium. J. Bone Joint Surg. Am. 55B, 390–401.

Lundborg, G., Gelbermann, R.H., Minteer-Convery, M., et al., 1982. Median nerve compression in the carpal tunnel: functional response to experimentally induced controlled pressure. J. Hand Surg. Am. 7, 252–259.

Lundborg, G., Myers, R., Powell, H., 1983. Nerve compression injury and increased endoneurial fluid pressure: a 'miniature compartment syndrome'. J. Neurol. Neurosurg. Psychiatry 46, 1119–1124.

Lundborg, G., Rydevik, B., Manthorpe, M., et al., 1987. Peripheral nerve: the physiology of injury and repair. In: Woo, S.L.-Y., Buckwalter, J.A. (Eds.), Injury and repair of the musculoskeletal soft tissues. American Academy of Orthopaedic Surgeons, Park Ridge, IL, pp. 295–352.

MacNab, I., 1972. The mechanism of spondylogenic pain. In: Hirsch, C., Zotterman, Y. (Eds.), Cervical pain. Pergamon Press, Oxford, pp. 89–95.

Maeda, Y., Kettner, N., Holden, J., et al., 2014. Functional deficits in carpal tunnel syndrome reflect reorganization of primary somatosensory cortex. Brain 137, 1741–1752.

Manchikanti, L., Benyamin, R.M., Falco, F.J., et al., 2015. Do epidural injections provide short-and long-term relief for lumbar disc herniation? A systematic review. Clin. Orthop. Relat. Res. 473, 1940–1956.

Marieb, E.N., 1995. Human anatomy and physiology, third ed. Benjamin/Cummings, San Francisco, CA.

Martina, I.S.J., van Koningsveld, R., Schmitz, P.I.M., et al., 1998. Measuring vibration threshold with a graduated tuning fork in normal aging and in patients with polyneuropathy. J. Neurol. Neurosurg. Psychiatry 65, 743–747.

Mason, S., Phillips, J.B., 2011. An ultrastructural and biochemical analysis of collagen in rat peripheral nerves: the relationship between fibril diameter and mechanical properties. J. Peripher. Nerv. Syst. 16, 261–269.

Maus, T., 2012. Imaging of spinal stenosis: neurogenic intermittent claudication and cervical spondylotic myelopathy. Radiol. Clin. North Am. 50, 651–679.

McLellan, D.L., Swash, M., 1976. Longitudinal sliding of the median nerve during movements of the upper limb. J. Neurol. Neurosurg. Psychiatry 39, 566–570.

McNair, C., Breakwell, L.M., 2010. Disc degeneration and prolapse. Orthop. Trauma 24, 430–434.

Middleditch, A., Oliver, J., 2005. Functional anatomy of the spine, second ed. Butterworth Heinemann, Edinburgh.

Mtui, E., Gruener, G., Dockery, P., et al., 2015. Fitzgerald's clinical neuroanatomy and neuroscience. Elsevier Health Sciences, Philadelphia.

Nakamichi, K., Tachibana, S., 1995. Restricted motion of the median nerve in carpal tunnel syndrome. J. Hand Surg. Am. 20B, 460–464.

Nater, A., Fehlings, M.G., 2015. The timing of decompressive spinal surgery in cauda equina syndrome. World Neurosurg. 83, 19–22.

Nitz, A.J., Dobner, J.J., Kersey, D., 1985. Nerve injury and grades II and III ankle sprains. Am. J. Sports Med. 13, 177–182.

Nora, D.B., Becker, J., Ehlers, J.A., et al., 2005. What symptoms are truly caused by median nerve compression in carpal tunnel syndrome? Clin. Neurophysiol. 116, 275–283.

Nouri, A., Tetreault, L., Singh, A., et al., 2015. Degenerative cervical myelopathy: epidemiology, genetics, and pathogenesis. Spine 40, E675–E693.

Ochoa, J., Fowler, T.J., Gilliatt, R.W., 1972. Anatomical changes in peripheral nerves compressed by a pneumatic tourniquet. J. Anat. 113, 433–455.

Ogata, K., Naito, M., 1986. Blood flow of peripheral nerve effects of dissection, stretching and compression. J. Hand Surg. Am. 11B, 10–14.

Olmarker, K., 2011. Combination of two cytokine inhibitors reduces nucleus pulposus-induced nerve injury more than using each inhibitor separately. Open Orthop. J. 28, 151–153.

Ottani, V., Raspanti, M., Ruggeri, A., 2001. Collagen structure and functional implications. Micron 32, 251–260.

Palastanga, N., Soames, R., 2012. Anatomy and human movement, structure and function, sixth ed. Churchill Livingstone, Edinburgh.

Palastanga, N., Field, D., Soames, R., 2002. Anatomy and human movement: structure and function, fourth ed. Butterworth-Heinemann, Oxford.

Panjabi, M.M., White, A.A., 2001. Biomechanics in the musculoskeletal system. Churchill Livingstone, New York.

Peltonen, S., Alanne, M., Peltonen, J., 2013. Barriers of the peripheral nerve. Tissue Barriers 1, e24956.

Petty, N.J., Ryder, D., 2017. Musculoskeletal examination and assessment: a handbook for therapists, fourth ed. Churchill Livingstone, Edinburgh.

Phillips, J.B., Smit, X., Zoysa, N.D., et al., 2004. Peripheral nerves in the rat exhibit localized heterogeneity of tensile properties during limb movement. J. Physiol. 557, 879–887.

Powell, H.C., Myers, R.R., 1986. Pathology of experimental nerve compression. Lab. Invest. 55, 91–100.

Rempel, D.M., Diao, E., 2004. Entrapment neuropathies: pathophysiology and pathogenesis. J. Electromyogr. Kinesiol. 14, 71–75.

Rempel, D., Dahlin, L., Lundborg, G., 1999. Pathophysiology of nerve compression syndromes: response of peripheral nerves to loading. J. Bone Joint Surg. Am. 81A, 1600–1610.

Resnick, D., Kransdorf, M.J., 2005. Degenerative disease of the spine. In: Bone and joint imaging. Elsevier, Richmond, VA, (Chapter 30).

Ridehalgh, C., Greening, J., Petty, N.J., 2005. Effect of straight leg raise examination and treatment on vibration thresholds in the lower limb: a pilot study in asymptomatic subjects. Man. Ther. 10, 136–143.

Ridehalgh, C., Moore, A., Hough, A., 2012. Repeatability of measuring sciatic nerve excursion during a modified passive straight leg raise test with ultrasound imaging. Man. Ther. 17, 572–576.

Ridehalgh, C., Moore, A., Hough, A., 2014. Normative sciatic nerve excursion during a modified straight leg raise test. Man. Ther. 19, 59–64.

Ridehalgh, C., Moore, A., Hough, A., 2015. Sciatic nerve excursion during a modified passive straight leg raise test in asymptomatic participants and participants with spinally referred leg pain. Man. Ther. 20, 564–569.

Rydevik, B., Lundborg, G., 1977. Permeability of intraneural microvessels and perineurium following acute, graded experimental nerve compression. Scand. J. Plast. Reconstr. Surg. 11, 179–187.

Rydevik, B., Lundborg, G., Bagge, U., 1981. Effects of graded compression on intraneural blood flow. An in vivo study on rabbit tibial nerve. J. Hand Surg. Am. 6, 3–12.

Rydevik, B., Brown, M.D., Lundborg, G., 1984. Pathoanatomy and pathophysiology of nerve root compression. Spine 9, 7–15.

Rydevik, B., Lundborg, G., Skalak, R., 1989. Biomechanics of peripheral nerves. In: Nordin, M., Frankel, V.H. (Eds.), Basic biomechanics of the musculoskeletal system, second ed. Lea & Febiger, Philadelphia, pp. 75–87.

Salonen, V., Lehto, M., Vaheri, A., et al., 1985. Endoneurial fibrosis following nerve transection. Acta Neuropathol. (Berlin) 67, 315–321.

Schmid, A., 2015. The peripheral nervous system and its compromise in entrapment neuropathies. In: Jull, G., Moore, A.P., Falla, D., et al. (Eds.), Grieve's modern musculoskeletal physiotherapy. Churchill Livingstone, Edinburgh.

Schmid, A.B., Nee, R.J., Coppieters, M.W., 2013. Reappraising entrapment neuropathies – mechanisms, diagnosis and management. Man. Ther. 18, 449–457.

Schwartz, J.H., 1991. Synthesis and trafficking of neuronal proteins. In: Kandel, E.R., Schwartz, J.H., Jessell, T.M. (Eds.), Principles of neural science, third ed. Elsevier, New York, pp. 49–65.

Seidenwurm, D.J., Expert Panel on Neurologic Imaging, 2008. Myelopathy. AJNR Am. J. Neuroradiol. 29, 1032–1034.

Seradge, H., Jia, Y.-C., Owens, W., 1995. In vivo measurement of carpal tunnel pressure in the functioning hand. J. Hand Surg. Am. 20A, 855–859.

Shacklock, M., 2005. Clinical neurodynamics: a new system of musculoskeletal treatment. Elsevier Health Sciences, London.

Smith, S.A., Massie, J.B., Chestnut, R., et al., 1993. Straight leg raising: anatomical effects 424 on the spinal nerve root without and with fusion. Spine 18, 992–999.

Smyth, M.J., Wright, V., 1958. Sciatica and the intervertebral disc, an experimental study. J. Bone Joint Surg. Am. 40A, 1401–1418.

Spindler, H.A., Dellon, A.L., 1982. Nerve conduction studies and sensibility testing in carpal tunnel syndrome. J. Hand Surg. Am. 7, 260–263.

Starkweather, R.J., Neviaser, R.J., Adams, J.P., et al., 1978. The effect of devascularization on the regeneration of lacerated peripheral nerves: an experimental study. J. Hand Surg. Am. 3, 163–167.

Stromberg, T., Dahlin, L.B., Brun, A., et al., 1997. Structural nerve changes at wrist level in workers exposed to vibration. Occup. Environ. Med. 54, 307–311.

Sunderland, S., 1978. Nerves and nerve injuries, second ed. Churchill Livingstone, Edinburgh, pp. 39–680.

Sunderland, S., 1990. The anatomy and physiology of nerve injury. Muscle Nerve 13, 771–784.

Sunderland, S., Bradley, K.C., 1961. Stress–strain phenomena in human peripheral nerve trunks. Brain 84, 102–119.

Szabo, R.M., Gelberman, R.H., Williamson, R.V., et al., 1983. Effects of increased systemic blood pressure on the tissue fluid pressure threshold of peripheral nerve. J. Orthop. Res. 1, 172–178.

Tamburin, S., Cacciatori, C., Praitano, M.L., et al., 2011. Median nerve small- and large-fiber damage in carpal tunnel syndrome: a quantitative sensory testing study. J. Pain 12, 205–212.

Tencer, A.F., Allen, B.L., Ferguson, R.L., 1985. A biomechanical study of thoracolumbar spine fractures with bone in the canal, part III, mechanical properties of the dura and its tethering ligaments. Spine 10, 741–747.

Terenghi, G., 1995. Peripheral nerve injury and regeneration. Histol. Histopathol. 10, 709–718.

Thacker, M.A., Clark, A.K., Marchand, F., et al., 2007. Pathophysiology of peripheral neuropathic pain: immune cells and molecules. Anesth. Analg. 105, 838–847.

Thomsen, J.F., Gerr, F., Atroshi, I., 2008. Carpal tunnel syndrome and the use of computer mouse and keyboard: a systematic review. BMC Musculoskelet. Disord. 9, 134.

Todd, A.J., Koerber, R., 2006. Neuroanatomical substrates of spinal nociception. Wall and Melzack's textbook of pain, fifth ed. Churchill Livingstone, Edinburgh.

Topp, K.S., Boyd, B.S., 2006. Structure and biomechanics of peripheral nerves: nerve responses to physical stresses and implications for physical therapist practice. Phys. Ther. 86, 92–109.

Turkof, E., Jurecka, W., Sikos, G., et al., 1993. Sensory recovery in myocutaneous, noninnervated free flaps: a morphologic, immunohistochemical, and electron microscopic study. Plast. Reconstr. Surg. 92, 238–247.

von Piekartz, H., Bryden, L., 2001. Craniofacial dysfunction and pain: manual therapy, assessment and management. Butterworth-Heinemann, Oxford.

Waldman, S.D., 2011. Facet arthropathy of the lumbar spine. In: Waldman, S.D., Campbell, R.S.D. (Eds.), Imaging of pain. Elsevier, Philadelphia, (Chapter 55).

Wall, E.J., Massie, J.B., Kwan, M.K., et al., 1992. Experimental stretch neuropathy. Changes in nerve conduction under tension. J. Bone Joint Surg. Am. 74B, 126–129.

Wang, Y., Zhao, C., Passe, S.M., et al., 2014. Transverse ultrasound assessment of median nerve deformation and displacement in the human carpal tunnel during wrist movements. Ultrasound Med. Biol. 40, 53–61.

Williams, P.L., Warwick, R., 1980. Gray's anatomy, thirty-sixth ed. Churchill Livingstone, Edinburgh.

Williams, P.L., Bannister, L.H., Berry, M.M., et al., 1995. Gray's anatomy, thirty-eighth ed. Churchill Livingstone, New York.

Woolf, C.J., Shortland, P., Coggeshall, R.E., 1992. Peripheral nerve injury triggers central sprouting of myelinated afferents. Nature 355, 75–77.

Wright, T.W., Glowczewskie, F., Wheeler, D., et al., 1996. Excursion and strain of the median nerve. J. Bone Joint Surg. Am. 78A, 1897–1903.

Wynn, M.M., Acher, C.W., 2014. A modern theory of spinal cord ischemia/injury in thoracoabdominal aortic surgery and its implications for prevention of paralysis. J. Cardiothorac. Vasc. Anesth. 28, 1088–1099.

Yang, S.N., Yoon, J.S., Kim, S.J., et al., 2013. Movement of the ulnar nerve at the elbow: a sonographic study. J. Ultrasound Med. 32, 1747–1752.

Yoshii, Y., Nishiura, Y., Terui, N., et al., 2010. The effects of repetitive compression on nerve conduction and blood flow in the rabbit sciatic nerve. J. Hand Surg. Eur. 35, 269–278.

Yoshii, Y., Ishii, T., Tung, W.L., et al., 2013. Median nerve deformation and displacement in the carpal tunnel during finger motion. J. Orthop. Res. 31, 1876–1880.

Zoech, G., Reihsner, R., Beer, R., et al., 1991. Stress and strain in peripheral nerves. Neuro-orthopaedics 10, 73–82.

7

PRINCIPLES OF NERVE TREATMENT

COLETTE RIDEHALGH ■ KIERAN BARNARD

CHAPTER CONTENTS

Management of patients with nerve dysfunction consists of a multimodal approach, utilizing a variety of techniques designed to enhance function, reduce pain and optimize health and well-being. No one technique can result in such changes; rather, it is the careful detailed examination of the patient, meticulous clinical reasoning processes and shared management planning and goal setting that produce a detailed, comprehensive and, most importantly, individualized management plan. The focus of this chapter is on the principles underlying nerve treatment and specific techniques available to the clinician, but it is important to note that these techniques should never be considered in isolation, but together with an overall management strategy to maximize outcomes.

Over the past 30 years, management strategies for patients with nerve dysfunction have evolved as

knowledge and understanding of neurophysiology have progressed. Interestingly, the specific techniques have not really changed in that time, but the use of the techniques and understanding of potential treatment effects have advanced. The main focus of nerve treatment is to normalize nerve function (both in terms of reducing heightened sensitivity as well as restoring nerve conduction where possible and feasible), enhancing normal range of motion (both of the nerve itself and as a consequence to physiological ranges of joint motion) and restoring a normal healthy nerve environment (reducing oedema and inflammatory mediators). A summary of the aims and types of nerve techniques can be found in Table 7.1 and some specific techniques are illustrated in Figs 7.1–7.5. The reader is referred to the accompanying examination book for a full description of the neurodynamic tests (Petty & Ryder 2017).

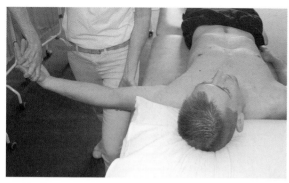

FIG. 7.1 ■ Upper-limb neurodynamic test 1 (ULNT1) slider technique.

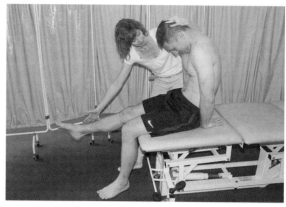

FIG. 7.4 ■ Slump tensioner technique.

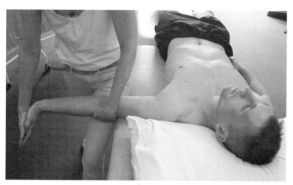

FIG. 7.2 ■ Upper-limb neurodynamic test 1 (ULNT1) tensioner technique.

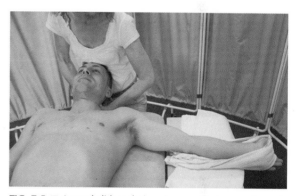

FIG. 7.5 ■ Lateral glide technique in upper-limb neurodynamic test 1 (ULNT1) position.

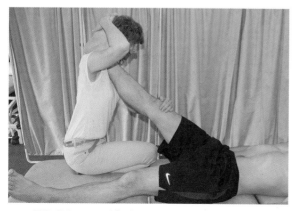

FIG. 7.3 ■ Straight-leg raise tensioner technique.

OVERVIEW OF TYPES OF NERVE TREATMENT

There are predominantly two main types of nerve treatment technique: those which influence the nerve directly (moving the nerve through the tissues, most commonly referred to as sliders or tensioners) or those which aim to alter the structures which the nerve passes through or close to (interface techniques). During normal limb motion, nerves move longitudinally and to some degree medially or laterally and superficially or deep (see Chapter 6). Certain joint movements will influence particular nerves to undergo a series of biomechanical events, including uncoiling, excursion, strain and compression (see Chapter 6), and these are termed neurodynamic tests (Figs 7.1–7.4). These movements can be converted into treatment techniques, by

TABLE 7.1
Aims of Nerve Treatment

Nerve Treatment Technique	Aim of Treatment	Examples of Treatment
Direct slider or tensioner	■ Restore normal movement ■ Improve circulation ■ Improve axonal transport ■ Reduce oedema ■ Reduce pain ■ Reduce fear of movement	■ Straight-leg raise ■ Slump ■ Femoral nerve mobilization (side-lying slump) ■ ULNT1 median nerve ■ ULNT2a median nerve or 2b radial nerve ■ ULNT3 ulnar nerve
Indirect interface	■ Reduce pain ■ Improve circulation ■ Restore normal biomechanics of the nerve–nerve interface ■ Reduce oedema	■ Fibular head mobilizations for common peroneal nerve ■ Supinator soft-tissue mobilizations for posterior interosseous nerve ■ Piriformis hold/relax for sciatic nerve ■ Carpal bone mobilizations for median nerve

ULNT, upper-limb neurodynamic test.

repeatedly oscillating one joint to produce an overall nerve mobilization. The terms sliders and tensioners were developed to consider further the biomechanical effects of applying different combinations of joint movements within a neurodynamic test either to lengthen the nerve or to increase the excursion of the nerve (Shacklock 2005; Coppieters et al. 2009, 2015). A slider is a combination of a series of joint movements which lengthen one end of the nerve bed whilst simultaneously shortening the other end. An example would be that, during upper-limb neurodynamic test 1 (ULNT1), the cervical spine is contralaterally side flexed whilst the wrist is flexed. A tensioner is described as a technique where the two ends of the system are simultaneously lengthened. An example of this would be that, in ULNT1 the cervical spine is contralaterally side flexed whilst the wrist is extended (see further details of these in biomechanical effects below and Fig. 7.6).

The choice of technique will relate to the severity (the patient is unable to tolerate the symptom being produced), irritability (once symptoms are provoked they take some time to ease) and nature (including elements such as pathology, red flags and yellow flags) of the condition as well as the potential source of symptoms and contributing factors. In a situation where the patient's symptoms are severe and irritable, a slider may be preferable to a tensioner as less strain is produced. Where an obvious interface is suspected, it may be useful to consider treatment of this structure first in order to restore a normal relationship between the nerve and the interfacing tissue. This may be helpful

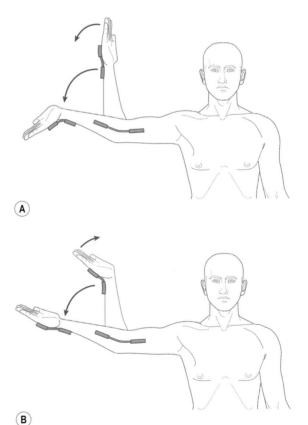

FIG. 7.6 ■ Tensioning (A) and sliding (B) upper-limb neurodynamic test 1 (ULNT1) mobilization techniques. (From Coppieters & Butler 2008, with permission.)

for a number of reasons, such as relieving nerve compression, aiding blood supply to the nerve as well as potentially activating hypoalgesic pathways (see Chapter 8). The postulated effects of such treatments will be discussed later in this chapter. An example of such a technique may be mobilization of the fibular head to influence the common peroneal nerve or a soft-tissue technique to supinator muscle to influence the radial nerve. A combination of both an interface treatment with a direct nerve mobilizing technique may also be considered to target the affected tissue, for example, mobilizing the fibular head whilst the leg is in a straight-leg raise (SLR) position.

The following aspects of nerve treatment will be considered in this chapter:

- neurophysiological effects of nerve treatment
- biomechanical effects of nerve treatment
- effectiveness of nerve treatment
- worked clinical example.

NEUROPHYSIOLOGICAL EFFECTS OF NERVE TREATMENT

Traditionally, nerve treatments focused on the biomechanical effects (Butler 1991), but a growing body of evidence has demonstrated a number of important and clinically relevant neurophysiological changes which occur after neurodynamic treatments, and it is arguable these effects will have a greater influence on restoring the healthy nerve environment in patients with painful peripheral neuropathy than the biomechanical effects. However, it must be remembered that the stimulus for such change is through the biomechanical events that occur during the neurodynamic treatment positions or techniques. The details of these biomechanical events can be found in Chapter 6.

Oedema

As described in Chapter 6, the structure of the peripheral nerve with its peripheral nerve sheaths ensures a strong, adaptable system to convey afferent and efferent stimulus through the body. The perineurium not only provides the most tensile strength to the nerve, but also provides an efficient diffusion barrier (Lundborg & Rydevik 1973; Lundborg 2004). This means that larger molecules and subsequently fluid migrate less easily into the endoneurium, providing some protection from oedema (Lundborg & Rydevik 1973). In addition the blood vessels within the endoneurium have an efficient diffusion barrier. However the endoneurial vessels at the nerve root and dorsal root ganglion have a less effective barrier and as such may be more susceptible to oedema entering the endoneurial space. At both the peripheral nerve and nerve root, external pressures may lead to an obstruction of venous return with resultant oedema (Sunderland 1976). Oedema may then increase compression of the nerve, with subsequent deleterious effects of increased intrafascicular pressure, in addition to maintaining an acidic nerve environment which may enhance peripheral nerve sensitivity (Steen et al. 1996). Reducing oedema would therefore be particularly beneficial to patients with peripheral neuropathic pain.

It has been postulated that both slider and tensioner techniques (see description of these in detail below) could disperse oedema due to a milking or pumping effect caused by oscillatory techniques (Coppieters & Butler 2008). Intraneurally injected dye has been demonstrated to disperse along the nerve after nerve mobilization techniques in both the peripheral nerve (Brown et al. 2011) and the nerve root (Gilbert et al. 2007) in cadavers. Whilst the limitations of cadaveric research limit to an extent the extrapolation to clinical practice, another study has demonstrated reduced oedema post nerve mobilization proximal to the carpal tunnel in patients with carpal tunnel syndrome (Schmid et al. 2012). Whilst this was not significantly different to a group of participants who only wore resting night splints, the study suggests that both management strategies to control compression by preventing wrist flexion or techniques which move the nerve are beneficial to reducing oedema. It may be more favourable to use movement-based techniques due to additional neurophysiological and biomechanical effects of movement.

Immune Cell Changes

Oedema is one of the cardinal signs of inflammation, and it has been well established that inflammation is a feature in some entrapment neuropathies (Kobayashi et al. 2004; Rothman & Winkelstein 2007; Hubbard & Winkelstein 2008; Schmid et al. 2013). Inflammatory mediators can lower the threshold for firing and may therefore result in spontaneous pain. Such lowered firing of afferent nerves would warrant caution when applying movement-based treatment approaches, especially techniques such as tensioners where elongation of the nerve may provoke further discharge (Dilley et al. 2005). Glial cells become activated in neuropathic pain conditions, and these cells synthesize proinflammatory cytokines, glutamate and nitrous oxide (DeLeo & Yezierski 2001) as well as increased production of nerve growth factor. Hence an elevation of glial cells may result in heightened nerve sensitivity (Herzberg et al. 1997; DeLeo & Yezierski 2001).

Normalization of both glial cell activity and the presence of nerve growth factor have been demonstrated in rats with experimentally induced neuritis after neural mobilizations (Martins et al. 2011; Santos et al. 2012). These changes suggest that neural mobilization may lead to a downplay in the immune response after peripheral nerve injury. These changes were associated with a decrease in mechanical (Martins et al. 2011; Santos et al. 2012) and thermal hyperalgesia (Santos et al. 2012).

Descending Inhibitory Pain Pathways

Supraspinal pain-inhibitory mechanisms have been suggested as one of the ways in which neurodynamic mobilization may be beneficial. Animal studies have demonstrated improvements in pain-related behaviour after nerve mobilizations in rats with nerve injury (Bertolini et al. 2009; Martins et al. 2011: Santos et al. 2012). Interestingly, in two of these studies (Bertolini et al. 2009; Santos et al. 2012), the positive changes to pain were found after a tensioner mobilization, suggesting that, in these animals, improvements in pain (and indeed, immune cell changes) can be found even after mobilizations which have been suggested to be more aggressive forms of treatment (Nee & Butler 2006). In patients, the careful monitoring of symptoms would be essential to ensure that no aggravation of the condition occurs in a more irritable situation.

More compelling evidence of descending inhibitory pain mechanisms after neurodynamic mobilizations has been demonstrated by Santos et al. (2014). After chronic constriction injury of the sciatic nerve in rats, a decrease in opioid receptor levels in the periaqueductal grey matter was shown which normalized after 10 sessions of neurodynamic tensioner treatment undertaken every other day. Taken together with the pain behaviour changes, this suggests that one of the mechanisms responsible for beneficial changes after nerve mobilizations is an endogenous pain-inhibitory mechanism.

Blood Flow and Axonal Transport Systems

Improvements in blood flow and axonal transport systems after mobilizations are one of the theories proposed for many tissues around the body. Improvements in these systems would be of potential benefit to enhance normal healing processes, and provide the nerve with essential nutrients and an oxygen supply which may be restricted due to the deleterious effects of compression (Rydevik & Lundborg 1977; Rydevik et al. 1981; Ogata & Naito 1986). Limited research exists which demonstrates changes to these systems, particularly the changes to axonal transport systems possibly due to the complexities of the methodology required to do so. Compression of nerves can cause impairment of axonal transport systems; pressure as small as 20 mmHg (much lower than those demonstrated to occur in patients with compression neuropathies) have been shown to affect transport systems detrimentally in animal studies (Dahlin et al. 1986) and therefore if such techniques could improve these transport systems, substantial benefits may be associated with such changes.

With respect to blood flow, Driscoll et al. (2002) found that stretching rabbits' sciatic nerve beyond 8% of their resting length for an hour resulted in a decrease in blood flow, but on release an increase of around 151% of baseline occurred. Whilst the amount of strain may be similar during nerve mobilization techniques (Coppieters et al. 2006; Boyd et al. 2013), the duration of the stretch is clearly well outside those given during those techniques, and therefore it is not clear how well this applies to clinical practice. It does suggest, however, that circulation can be affected by applying a technique which lengthens and then releases the nerve and its accompanying circulatory system.

BIOMECHANICAL EFFECTS OF NERVE TREATMENT

As mentioned previously, oedema is a common finding in neuropathic pain presentations, and if it is not dispersed it can lead to intra- and extraneural fibrosis

(Sunderland 1989; Mackinnon 2002), which may result in a restriction in the nerve's ability to glide through the interfacing structures as well as the connective tissue layers gliding alongside each other. Such restrictions could result in pain as the nerve is moved through the interfaces, and may be one situation where the concept of influencing the connective tissue properties of the nerve via creep and hysteresis (see Chapter 3) is an attractive proposition. One caution to such potential mechanisms is that it is not well established if nervous tissue becomes restricted after injury. Some studies have shown no differences in the amount of nerve excursion in individuals with and without painful neuropathies (Erel et al. 2003; Dilley et al. 2008; Ridehalgh et al. 2015), although two studies did show differences (Hough et al. 2007; Korstanje et al. 2012). Such inconsistencies in results may be accounted for by differences in methodology. It is also conceivable that the restriction of the connective tissue layers within the nerve, which cannot be measured accurately with ultrasound imaging, may contribute to pain, and therefore techniques which aim to lengthen the connective tissue, such as tensioners, may still alter the nerve biomechanically in a positive way.

Tensioners and sliders have been proposed to influence the nervous tissue differently, due to the biomechanical changes that occur during the two techniques. Tensioners can be described as a combination of a series of joint movements with the aim of lengthening the targeted nerve. Sliders on the other hand consist of a combination of joint movements which aim to lengthen the nerve bed at one length whilst simultaneously releasing it at the other end. The result of this is a larger overall excursion of the targeted nerve, whilst limiting the amount of nerve strain.

Despite their advocation, it is only within the last 10 years that the biomechanical and clinical efficacy of sliding techniques has been scrutinized. Two in vitro biomechanical studies appear to provide evidence that sliding techniques do indeed produce large nerve excursion without significant increases in nerve strain (Coppieters & Alshami 2007; Coppieters & Butler 2008). In the most recent of these studies, longitudinal excursion and strain of the medial and ulnar nerves during tensioning and sliding movements were examined in two embalmed cadavers (Coppieters & Butler 2008). The median nerve was tensioned by extending the elbow and wrist, whilst the sliding manoeuvre consisted of elbow extension with wrist flexion and vice versa (Fig. 7.6). The ulnar nerve was tensioned by extending the wrist, flexing the elbow and abducting the shoulder, whilst the sliding manoeuvre consisted of elbow extension with shoulder abduction and vice versa. Although there was no statistical confirmation of the trends identified, the sliding techniques produced more excursion than the tensioning techniques whilst producing less strain. For example, the median nerve sliding technique produced 12.6 mm of excursion and a 0.8% increase in strain at the wrist, compared with the tensioning technique, which produced 6.1 mm of excursion and a 6.8% increase in strain at the wrist. Along with the small sample size and lack of statistical confirmation, a major limitation of these cadaveric studies is that it is not clear whether these findings would accurately reflect nerve excursion and strain in vivo.

More recently, studies using ultrasound imaging have further supported the biomechanical events during the two techniques (Coppieters et al. 2009, 2015; Ellis et al. 2012). Whilst this technology has not yet been able to give accurate estimates of strain, measurements of excursion have been shown to be reliable (Ellis et al. 2008; Ridehalgh et al. 2012) and valid (Dilley et al. 2001; Ridehalgh 2014). Coppieters et al. (2009) found 3.6 mm of median nerve excursion measured proximal to the elbow during the tensioner manoeuvre and 10.2 mm in the slider manoeuvre. Whilst Ellis et al. (2012) found sciatic nerve excursion in the posterior thigh of 2.6 mm during the slump tensioner manoeuvre and 3.2 mm during the slider manoeuvre, and this difference was statistically significant, such small differences could be attributed to measurement error, which was in the region of 0.5 mm (smallest detectable difference). Larger differences were found during a modified SLR (Coppieters et al. 2015) (Fig. 7.7); sciatic nerve excursion in the posterior thigh during the tensioner manoeuvre was in the region of 3.2 mm and the slider was 17 mm.

Taken together, the ranges of motion in themselves are probably not important, but the significance of the findings is that with a slider technique larger amounts of overall nerve excursion occur whilst smaller amounts of strain (or stretch) of the nerve occur. As mentioned previously, this may suggest that, where the patient has severe and irritable symptoms, movements which impose

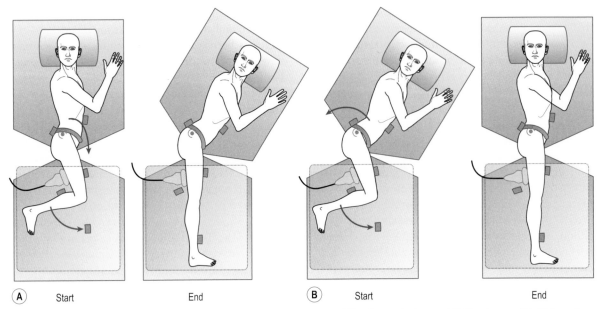

FIG. 7.7 ■ Modified slider and tensioner straight-leg raise (SLR) mobilization techniques. (A) Tensioner. (B) Slider. *(From Coppieters et al. 2015.)*

less strain on the nerve may be warranted. However, where symptoms are not severe and irritable, the evidence presented in the section above may suggest that tensioners might induce a number of positive neurophysiological effects. In addition, studies which have used tensioners in vivo in symptomatic populations have also found beneficial effects (see below). Ultimately it is the close monitoring and reassessment of treatment which will determine the effectiveness of the technique.

Nerve Interface Treatments

Nerve interface treatments refer to the treatment of specific locations (interfaces) along the course of a nerve where nerve function may be compromised as it winds its way around bone, or through muscle or fascia. Examples of possible nerve interfaces where function may be compromised include the median nerve passing beneath the flexor retinaculum of the wrist into the carpal tunnel, the common peroneal nerve passing around the superior tibiofibular joint and the tibial nerve passing through the tarsal tunnel into the foot. If a nerve becomes entrapped and loses its ability to move, slide and glide within the interface, the aim of treatment may often be to move the interface relative

to the nerve. For example, a patient may have signs of L5 nerve root compression, comprising pain in the lumbar spine with anterolateral calf pain, reduced sensation to fine touch over the anterolateral calf, together with weakness of the big-toe extensors. The SLR test position of hip flexion, knee extension and foot dorsiflexion may be limited to 45° hip flexion, reproducing the patient's pain, with the pain increased on cervical flexion, giving a positive SLR. In addition, there may be positive findings on passive accessory movements of the lumbar spine; for example, the patient's back and calf pain may be reproduced with a unilateral posteroanterior pressure on L5 with a caudad inclination, and S1 with a cephalad inclination. It could be speculated in this scenario that the pain may be emanating from the nerve root as it exits the intervertebral foramen at the L5–S1 level and so the accessory movement could be considered an interface treatment. In this example, it could be argued that treating the interface to offload the neural structures may be a priority to improve the nerve root environment (e.g. reduce inflammatory exudate, improve circulation, reduce compression and improve pain through descending inhibitory pain pathways). Following each intervention, the objective markers of altered sensation and strength and restricted SLR would need to be reassessed to establish the effectiveness of the technique.

Another example of an interface treatment may be treatment of a patient whose symptoms suggest a carpal tunnel syndrome. Treatment may be aimed at increasing the space within the carpal tunnel to reduce the compression on the median nerve. For example, joint accessory movements may be applied to the carpal bones (Tal-Akabi & Rushton 2000).

Soft-tissue techniques could also be applied as an appropriate interface technique. Examples of common soft-tissue interfaces include the supinator as it interfaces with the posterior interosseous nerve or piriformis muscle as it interfaces with the sciatic nerve.

If the condition is non-severe and non-irritable, the clinician may wish to replicate a nerve-provocative position corresponding to an aggravating factor, and apply the interface technique in this position. Where the symptoms are severe and/or irritable, the interface technique may be performed away from a position of pain, which may be with the limb/trunk in a neutral position. It is possible that there may be a greater effect on the nerve when positioned in the nerve-provocative position. Examples of this could be to perform a unilateral posteroanterior to the lumbar spine with the leg in an SLR position if the patient complained of pain on heel strike during gait, or in a slump position if the patient complained of pain in sitting or flexion.

It has been found that the point of symptomatic range of SLR coincides with the point of greatest restriction of the nerve root adjacent to lumbosacral disc herniation, which reduces after surgical disc removal (Kobayashi et al. 2003). It is plausible therefore that greater biomechanical effects might occur in the position of provocation of symptoms, which would potentially lead to positive neurophysiological effects. These may occur as a result of possible changes to the pressure on the nerve, potentially resulting in restoration of blood circulation and dispersal of inflammatory exudates in addition to descending inhibitory pathways. These are of course hypothetical consequences, but since compression of the nerve has many negative effects, as discussed in Chapter 6, altering pressure or improving circulation would produce a likely positive response.

Treatment Dose: Considerations in Relation to Nerve Treatment (Table 7.2)

Time and Repetitions

In terms of treatment dose, time relates to the amount of time spent performing the technique, be it a direct nerve treatment or an interface technique. It is often confusing to establish the best treatment times and

TABLE 7.2

Examples of Treatment Dose Utilized in Some Studies on Effectiveness of Neurodynamic Treatment

Authors	Neurodynamic Treatment	Dose
Adel (2011)	SLR tensioner	5 sets sustained for 30 seconds
Allison et al. (2002)	Lateral glide Cx spine and single joint movements to Cx spine and shoulder	Lateral glide not specified Single joint movements, up to 10 repetitions 1–3 times daily
Bialosky et al. 2009	ULNT1 tensioner	5 sets of 10 repetitions for sessions 1–3 then 7 sets of 10 repetitions for sessions 4–6
Cleland et al. (2006)	Slump tensioner	5 sets sustained for 30 seconds
Heebner & Roddey 2008	ULNT1 tensioner	10 repetitions each held for 5 seconds 3–5 times daily
Nagrale et al. (2012)	Slump tensioner	5 sets sustained for 30 seconds. HER 2 X 30 seconds hold
Nee et al. (2012)	ULNT1 slider and tensioner	10–15, 3 times daily as HER
Oskouei et al. (2014)	ULNT1	
Ridehalgh et al. (2016)	SLR tensioner	3 sets of oscillations for 60 seconds
Schäfer et al. (2011)	Side-lying SLR slider	5 sets of oscillations for 30 seconds
Schmid et al. (2012)	ULNT1 slider	10 repetitions
Tal-Akabi & Rushton (2000)	ULNT1 mobilization	Dose not specified

Cx, cervical; HER, home exercise regime; SLR, straight-leg raise; ULNT, upper-limb neurodynamic test.

repetitions to administer from the literature as many studies have used a variety of treatment doses (see Table 7.2 for an example of some of these). Spinal joint mobilizations have been shown to have a more influential effect on pain after four sets, but no difference was found between 30 and 60 seconds (Pentelka et al. 2012). However it must be noted that the participants for this study were asymptomatic, and it is not clear if the same trend would be the same in symptomatic participants. More research is needed on symptomatic participants to see if the same trend follows.

Whether these times or repetitions would have similar effects for neurodynamic treatment is not currently clear. The clinician is guided by the patient's symptoms and rigorous evaluation of reassessment asterisks as a guide to the optimal treatment time for the individual patient. It is worth noting that the choice of time and repetition that has been demonstrated to be beneficial in the treatment room should be maintained for any home exercises prescribed.

Grades of Movement

The reader is referred back to Chapter 3 for a comprehensive discussion of the grades of movement. There is no specific guide for neurodynamic treatment, although it may be wise in the early stages of treatment to consider the use of grade III over grade IV where nerve circulation could be impaired, and sustained stretches into resistance have the potential to reduce circulation (Boyd et al. 2005), even for short transitions of time. Of course, functional activities normally involve some degree of sustained positions, where the nerve is in a more lengthened state, and it is therefore essential that at some stage the patient is able to tolerate such tensile loads. This may mean that grade IV and even sustained neurodynamic positions are required prior to discharge.

Symptom Response

The clinician decides which symptom, and to what extent, is to be provoked during treatment. Choices include:

- no provocation
- provocation to the point of onset, or increase in resting symptoms
- partial reproduction
- total reproduction.

The decision as to what extent symptoms are provoked during treatment depends on the severity and irritability of the symptom(s) and the nature of the condition. If the symptoms are severe, the clinician would choose not to provoke them. The clinician may also choose not to provoke symptoms if they are irritable. If, however, the symptoms are not severe and not irritable, then the clinician is able to reproduce the patient's symptoms during treatment; the extent to which symptoms are reproduced will depend on the patient's tolerance. The nature of the condition may also limit the extent to which symptoms are produced, such as a recent traumatic injury, or where neuropathic symptoms such as pins and needles and numbness are being reproduced, it may be wise to treat to P1. Such symptoms may suggest that intraneural circulation is being compromised (Schmid 2015).

It is suggested that inexperienced clinicians alter only one aspect of treatment dose at an attendance so that they fully understand the value of the alteration; in this way they will quickly develop valuable clinical experience and clinical mileage, which will contribute to growth in their clinical learning skills. The immediate and more long-term effect of the alteration can then be evaluated by reassessment of the subjective and physical asterisks.

Active Movement by the Patient

The factors defining the treatment dose when patients apply their own treatment are exactly the same as the clinician applying a passive technique (Table 7.3). The only difference is that, in this instance, the patient is in total control of the movement and relies on his or her own perception of stretch and symptom production to determine the way the movement is carried out. The patient needs to be fully informed as to how to carry out the movement; that is, how forceful to be and to what extent to reproduce the symptoms. The clinician in this case takes on a more educational and advisory role.

ADDRESSING THE BIOPSYCHOSOCIAL ASPECTS OF SYMPTOMS

Pain is a complex scenario which has multiple manifestations and associated pain behaviours. There is some suggestion that high levels of psychosocial factors are

	TABLE 7.3	
	Treatment Dose for Passive Mobilization by the Clinician and Active Movement by the Patient	
Factors	Passive Mobilization by the Clinician	Active Movement by the Patient
Patient's position	E.g. supine	E.g. sitting, standing with heel on a stool with knee extended
Direction of movement	E.g. hip flexion	E.g. active knee extension
Magnitude of force applied	Related to therapist's perception of resistance: grades I–V	Related to patient's perception of stretch
Amplitude of oscillation	Static or small or large	Static or small or large
Speed	Slow or fast	Slow or fast (if fast, may be referred to as ballistic)
Rhythm	Smooth or staccato	Smooth or staccato
Time	Of repetitions and number of repetitions	Of repetitions and number of repetitions
Symptom response	Short of symptom production Point of onset or increase in resting symptom Partial reproduction of symptom Full reproduction of symptom	Short of symptom production Point of onset or increase in resting symptom Partial reproduction of symptom Full reproduction of symptom

more prevalent in neuropathic pain conditions (Walsh & Hall 2009), although other studies have not shown differences between those with neuropathic pain and others with mechanical nociceptive disorders of similar regions (Jensen et al. 2010; Ridehalgh et al. 2016). Regardless, individuals with high levels of psychosocial factors may respond more poorly to interventions than those with lower levels (Jensen et al. 2010; Haugen et al. 2012). The exploration of such factors and management of people with these factors are critical, and may be the main focus of treatment. This is no easy task, and to do it well requires a high level of skill in active listening. Active listening involves putting our own thoughts, beliefs and feelings to one side and choosing instead to hear what the patient has to say. It involves trying to understand patients and their world, through their eyes, and trying to avoid the all-too-easy error of reinterpreting through our eyes. It requires the clinician to listen with compassion and patience, and without judgement. It involves the clinician using words carefully and meaningfully, and using open-ended questions, to search for information, until understanding is reached. It involves sensitive verbal and non-verbal communication, thus encouraging safe and open communication. This is a tall order, but the benefits of truly being able to come alongside the patient will far outweigh the effort of developing these skills. These concepts are explored more fully in Chapters 8 and 9.

MODIFICATION, PROGRESSION AND REGRESSION OF TREATMENT

The continuous monitoring of the patient's subjective and physical asterisks guides the entire treatment and management programme of the patient. The clinician judges the degree of change with treatment and relates this to the expected rate of change from the prognosis, and then decides whether or not a treatment needs to be altered in some way. The nature of this alteration can be to modify the technique in some way, to progress the treatment or regress the treatment. Regardless of which alteration is made, the clinician makes every effort to determine what effect this alteration has on the patient's subjective and physical asterisks. In order to do this, the clinician alters one aspect of treatment at a time and reassesses immediately to determine the value of the alteration.

The clinician may modify the treatment given to a patient by altering an existing treatment, adding a new treatment or stopping a treatment. At all times the treatment should have the functional goals of the patient in mind. Altering an existing treatment involves altering some aspect of the treatment dose, as discussed earlier. The immediate and more long-term effect of the alteration is then evaluated by reassessment of the subjective and physical asterisks. The clinician then decides whether, overall, the patient is better, the same or worse, relating this to the prognosis. For instance, if a quick improvement was expected, but only some improvement occurred, the clinician may progress treatment. If the patient is worse after treatment, the dose may be regressed in some way, and if the treatment made no difference at all, then a more substantial modification may be made. Before discarding a treatment it is worth making sure that it has been fully utilized, as it may be that a much stronger or much weaker treatment dose may be effective.

EFFECTIVENESS OF NERVE TREATMENT

There has been a steady stream of studies examining the effectiveness of nerve treatments over the past 15 years. In general these studies tend to support nerve treatment (Cleland et al. 2006; Adel 2011; Nagrale et al. 2012; Nee et al. 2012), but many have methodological limitations, and some show no difference compared to standard care alone (Scrimshaw & Maher 2001; Akalin et al. 2002; Heebner & Roddey 2008; Bardak et al. 2009), or when nerve treatment alone was compared to different subgroups (Ridehalgh et al. 2016). Tensioner treatments in addition to standard care have been found to be superior to standard care alone in patients with spinally referred leg pain (Cleland et al. 2006; Adel 2011; Nagrale et al. 2012), but there are limitations associated with these study designs. Such limitations include the use of multiple T tests (Cleland et al. 2006; Adel 2011) which could lead to a type 1 error (risk of falsely accepting the alternative hypothesis) and the disparity of time/attention that the participants in the standard care plus nerve treatment group received, which could account in part for the more favourable findings in this group. Schäfer et al. (2011) and Ridehalgh et al. (2016) investigated whether the effectiveness of nerve treatment differed dependent on the subgroup that participants with spinally referred leg pain were allocated to. Schäfer et al. (2011) found that the group with nerve mechanosensitivity (without neurological loss) showed significant improvements in a number of outcomes (including Global Perceived Change Scale and functional disability) over other subgroups; however, the small number of participants in this group ($n = 9$) makes the extrapolation of these results less convincing. Ridehalgh et al. (2016) looked at the immediate changes to treatment

after a single session of an SLR tensioner and found no significant differences in outcomes between subgroups or indeed after treatment. However the short treatment duration (3×1 minute) may not be sufficient to show changes to pain, and measurement only immediately after treatment may have missed any longer-term effects. Indeed, De-la-Llave-Rincon et al. (2012) found significant changes to pressure pain thresholds 1 week after nerve treatment, but no immediate changes.

Studies investigating treatment for carpal tunnel syndrome have produced some equivocal results. Whilst nerve treatments have been found to produce significant benefits compared to baseline scores, frequently no additional benefit has been found to the addition of nerve treatment to standard care (Akalin et al. 2002; Heebner & Roddey 2008; Bardak et al. 2009). However, in contrast, Oskouei et al. (2014) found a significantly greater improvement in functional scales and symptoms in the standard care plus nerve treatment. Studies differed in methodology, and one of the limitations of the studies of Akalin et al. (2002) and Bardak et al. (2009) was that nerve gliding exercises, rather than neurodynamic mobilization, were performed. Whilst the aim of such treatments is to focus the nerve mobilization to the median nerve locally within the hand and wrist, it is possible that greater effects could be ascertained with a more global mobilization of the nerve, such as that utilized by Oskouei et al. (2014). Heebner and Roddey (2008) utilized a home exercise regime of tensioner-type stretches, but the exercises were in a full ULNT 1 with the hand fixed into extension against the wall, which could have been inappropriate for those with more severe symptoms. In addition patients were diagnosed by electroconductive testing which may be suggestive of those with a greater functional loss and therefore more severe symptoms, since these tests are commonly negative in patients with carpal tunnel syndrome (Finsen & Russwurm 2001; Atroshi et al. 2003).

Cervical radicular pain has been investigated with some positive midterm findings (Deepti et al. 2008; Nee et al. 2012). Nee et al. (2012) found that the numbers-needed-to-treat analysis favoured neurodynamic treatment using sliders and tensioners in addition to cervical spine mobilizations compared to a control group on a number of measures, including pain, Global

Rating of Change Scale and disability. Deepti et al. (2008) found significant improvements in pain and disability in a neurodynamic tensioner group compared to participants who had a cervical lateral glide treatment.

Despite some assertions of potentially harmful effects of neurodynamic treatment, there is little literature published which supports such a notion. Ridehalgh et al. (2016) found no statistical differences in vibration thresholds after an SLR tensioner in participants with and without identifiable neurological loss of function, suggesting that nerve function is not detrimentally affected even in those with a reduction in function. Nee et al. (2012) found that patients with cervical radicular pain who reported adverse symptoms after neurodynamic treatment recovered quickly and did no worse than those who did not report adverse effects.

Philosophical Considerations

Most papers in this field have followed a positivist approach with a linear look at cause and effect. Whilst many are considered to be high on the hierarchy of evidence (Oxford Centre for Evidence-Based Medicine 2011), the approach has been considered by some to be reductionist, and limits a true understanding of the complexities of treating people with pain and illness (Miles & Asbridge 2013). In essence, the individualized nature of musculoskeletal practice where the patient (person) is at the centre of the interaction is undermined by the strict control of variables and an assumption that individuals will behave mostly like the average (mean) of a particular group. It is, of course, no surprise that human beings do not all behave in a very linear way, but outcome is influenced by much more than the application of a neural mobilization. The very essence of practice should be centred on the person and his or her unique set of circumstances which places the patient in front of the clinician.

More pragmatic research which incorporates the individual needs of patients, and enables the therapist to utilize high-level clinical reasoning processes and joint decision making with the patient is needed. In addition, the acceptance of other methodological designs such as case studies and qualitative methodologies which explore the patient's and clinician's experience and perspective is required from an array of clinicians, academics, journal editors and, importantly, policy makers.

CLINICAL EXAMPLE

Assessment

A 45-year-old accountant presented with a 4-week history of pain and tingling in the median nerve distribution of his left hand. He could not recall a specific mechanism of injury but his symptoms started at the end of the financial year, which was his busiest time. Typing was the principal aggravating factor but he also developed pain with sustained wrist flexion and the pain and tingling woke him at night regularly. He could not continue to type once the pain started, and often he found that, even if he stopped typing before pain, some time later he would notice his pain even if he was relaxing. Systemically he was fit and well. He had previously enjoyed swimming twice a week, but had stopped due to his wrist.

On examination he had full painfree range of movement of the cervical spine. Combined movements of the cervical spine and palpation from the occiput to the mid-thoracic spine were painfree. There was no atrophy to the thenar muscles of the left hand. Wrist flexion reproduced his pain at 45°, Tinel's sign was positive and he had reduction in pinprick sensation in the median nerve distribution (all other neurological integrity test findings were normal). An anteroposterior (AP) glide to the radiocarpal joint (RCJ) on the left reproduced discomfort and tingling in the median nerve distribution at mid third resistance. His ULNT1 was as follows:

Cx neutral √/ Sh depression √/ sh abduction √/ sh external rotation√/sup√/ EE√//WE immed pain and P + N/Cx ipsilateral LF ↓pain

Treatment Session 1

As the condition was deemed irritable, a sliding technique was chosen as an initial treatment in a supine position. With shoulder depression, abduction and external rotation, supination and the wrist maintained in 10° of wrist flexion, elbow extension was coupled with ipsilateral cervical side flexion for 4 × 30 seconds (Fig. 7.1). Reassessment revealed reduced wrist discomfort and increased wrist flexion to 50° before pain and wrist extension in the ULNT1 position had improved to 20° before symptoms were reproduced. As the response to treatment was favourable, the patient was asked to replicate the sliding technique as a home exercise in supine with the same treatment dose of 4 × 30 seconds. He was advised to wear a resting splint at night to prevent wrist flexion. The patient's perceptions of what might be causing his problem were discussed and any worries he had about the future and the prognosis were addressed by adopting an open and patient-centred approach.

Treatment Session 2

The patient's subjective markers had improved and he reported that he could now sustain a flexed wrist position and could continue typing once his symptoms had begun. He was waking less at night. He was only complaining of intermittent paraesthesia in the median nerve distribution, mainly at night. Physical examination revealed the improved wrist flexion had been maintained with discomfort at 50°. Neurological examination was unremarkable. ULNT1 again revealed discomfort with the addition of wrist extension. As the clinician deemed the condition to be no longer irritable, the sliding technique was progressed to a slider with the wrist extended to the onset of symptoms. Reassessment revealed reduced discomfort but no change in wrist flexion at 50°. ULNT had improved with wrist extension reproducing mild pain and minimal pins and needles at the end of range.

As the clinician was confident of the patient's response to treatment, 4 × 30 seconds of a grade III AP RCJ mobilization in 50° of wrist flexion was employed as a hypothesized interface treatment. Reassessment revealed an increase in wrist range to 60°. The patient was asked to progress the sliding technique as a home exercise in supine, as described above. The same treatment dose of 4 × 30 seconds was to be used in the home exercise. The contributing factors of posture and prolonged computer work were discussed with the patient. He was advised to take regular breaks every half-hour for a few minutes and to use a gel or memory foam wrist rest when typing.

Treatment Session 3

The patient's subjective markers had once again improved. He was sleeping through the night without pain or paraesthesia. He only noticed discomfort at the wrist after an hour of typing. Physical examination revealed mild discomfort at 60° of wrist flexion, unremarkable neurology and only mild discomfort at end-of-range wrist extension during ULNT1 with

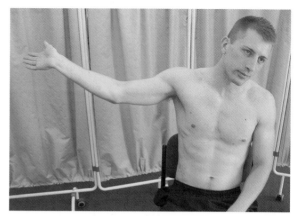

FIG. 7.8 ■ Upper-limb neurodynamic test 1 (ULNT1) tensioner in sitting.

contralateral side flexion. The slider technique was progressed into a tensioner in contralateral side flexion using the wrist extension, grade III+ in sitting to replicate the patient's principal aggravating factor more closely (Fig. 7.8). On reassessment ULNT was full and painfree, wrist flexion was ISQ. Wrist mobilizations were progressed to a grade IV AP RCJ for 4 × 30 seconds. Reassessment revealed a maintained full ULNT1 and full painfree wrist flexion. The patient was asked to perform the home tensioning exercise in sitting. It was recommended that aerobic exercise involving upper-limb movement such as swimming might help to maintain nerve, as well as general health benefits. The patient was advised to try sleeping without the splint, given an open appointment and advised to continue his home exercise programme until his symptoms had completely resolved.

REFERENCES

Adel, S.M., 2011. Efficacy of neural mobilization in treatment of low back pain dysfunctions. J. Am. Sci. 7, 566–573.

Akalin, E., El, O., Peker, O., et al., 2002. Treatment of carpal tunnel syndrome with nerve and tendon gliding exercises. Am. J. Phys. Med. Rehabil. 81, 108–113.

Allison, G., Nagy, B., Hall, T., 2002. A randomized clinical trial of manual therapy for cervico-brachial pain syndrome: a pilot study. Man. Ther. 7, 95–102.

Atroshi, I., Gummesson, C., Johnsson, R., et al., 2003. Diagnostic properties of nerve conduction tests in population-based carpal tunnel syndrome. BMC Musculoskelet. Disord. 7, 4–9.

Bardak, A.N., Alp, M., Erhan, B., et al., 2009. Evaluation of the clinical efficacy of conservative treatment in the management of carpal tunnel syndrome. Adv. Ther. 26, 107–116.

Bertolini, G.T.F., Silva, T.S., Trindade, D.L., et al., 2009. Neural mobilization and static stretching in an experimental sciatica model – an experimental study. Braz. J. Phys. Ther. 13, 493–498.

Bialosky, J.E., Bishop, M.D., Price, D.D., et al., 2009. A randomised sham-controlled trial of a neurodynamic technique in the treatment of carpal tunnel syndrome. J. Orthop. Sports Phys. Ther. 39, 709–723.

Boyd, B.S., Puttlitz, C., Jerylin, G., et al., 2005. Strain and excursion in the rat sciatic nerve during a modified straight leg raise are altered after traumatic nerve injury. J. Orthop. Res. 23, 764–770.

Boyd, B.S., Topp, K.S., Coppieters, M.W., 2013. Impact of movement sequencing on sciatic and tibial nerve strain and excursion during the straight leg raise test in embalmed cadavers. Journal of Orthopaedic and Sports Physical Therapy 43, 398–403.

Brown, C.L., Gilbert, K.K., Brismee, J.-M., et al., 2011. The effects of neurodynamic mobilization on fluid dispersion within the tibial nerve at the ankle: an unembalmed cadaveric study. J. Man. Manip. Ther. 19, 26–34.

Butler, D.S., 1991. Mobilisation of the nervous system. Churchill Livingstone, Melbourne.

Cleland, J.A., Childs, J.D., Palmer, J.A., et al., 2006. Slump stretching in the management of non-radicular low back pain: a pilot clinical trial. Man. Ther. 11, 279–286.

Coppieters, M.W., Alshami, A.M., 2007. Longitudinal excursion and strain in the median nerve during novel nerve gliding exercises for carpal tunnel syndrome. J. Orthop. Res. 25, 972–980.

Coppieters, M.W., Butler, D.S., 2008. Do 'sliders' slide and 'tensioners' tension? An analysis of neurodynamic techniques and considerations regarding their application. Man. Ther. 13, 213–221.

Coppieters, M.W., Alshami, A.M., Babri, A.S., et al., 2006. Strain and excursion of the sciatic, tibial, and plantar nerves during a modified straight leg raising test. J. Orthop. Res. 24, 1883–1889.

Coppieters, M.W., Hough, A.D., Dilley, A., 2009. Different nerve gliding exercises induce different magnitudes of median nerve longitudinal excursion: an in vivo study using dynamic ultrasound imaging. Journal of Orthopaedic and Sports Physical Therapy 39, 164–171.

Coppieters, M.W., Andersen, L.S., Johansen, R., et al., 2015. Excursion of the sciatic nerve during nerve mobilization exercises: an in vivo cross-sectional study using dynamic ultrasound imaging. Journal of Orthopaedic and Sports Physical Therapy 45, 731–737.

Dahlin, L., Danielsen, N., Ehira, T., et al., 1986. Mechanical effects of compression of peripheral nerves. J. Biomech. Eng. 108, 120–122.

Deepti, C., Kavitha, R., Ganesh, B., et al., 2008. Effectiveness of neural tissue mobilization over cervical lateral glide in cervico-brachial pain syndrome – a randomized clinical trial. Indian J. Physiother. Occup. Ther. 2, 47–52.

De-La-Llave-Rincon, A.I., Ortega-Santiago, R., Ambite-Quesada, S., et al., 2012. Response of pain intensity to soft tissue mobilization and neurodynamic technique: a series of 18 patients with chronic carpal tunnel syndrome. J. Manipulative Physiol. Ther. 35, 420–427.

DeLeo, J.A., Yezierski, R.P., 2001. The role of neuroinflammation and neuroimmune activation in persistent pain. Pain 90, 1–6.

Dilley, A., Greening, J., Lynn, B., et al., 2001. The use of cross-correlation analysis between high-frequency ultrasound images to measure longitudinal median nerve movement. Ultrasound Med. Biol. 27, 1211–1218.

Dilley, A., Lynn, B., Pang, S., 2005. Pressure and stretch mechano-sensitivity of peripheral nerve fibres following local inflammation of the nerve trunk. Pain 117, 462–472.

Dilley, A., Odeyinde, S., Greening, J., et al., 2008. Longitudinal sliding of the median nerve in patients with non-specific arm pain. Man. Ther. 13, 536–543.

Driscoll, P.J., Glasby, M.A., Lawson, G.M., 2002. An in vivo study of peripheral nerves in continuity: biomechanical and physiological responses to elongation. J. Orthop. Res. 20, 370–375.

Ellis, R., Hing, W., Dilley, A., et al., 2008. Reliability of measuring sciatic and tibial nerve movement with diagnostic ultrasound during a neural mobilisation technique. Ultrasound Med. Biol. 34, 1209–1216.

Ellis, R., Hing, W., McNair, P., 2012. Comparison of longitudinal sciatic nerve movement with different mobilization exercises: an in vivo study utilizing ultrasound imaging. Journal of Orthopaedic and Sports Physical Therapy 42, 667–675.

Erel, E., Dilley, A., Greening, J., et al., 2003. Longitudinal sliding of the median nerve in patients with carpal tunnel syndrome. J. Hand Surg. Br. 28B, 439–443.

Finsen, V., Russwurm, H., 2001. Neurophysiology not required before surgery for typical carpal tunnel syndrome. J. Hand Surg. Am. 26, 61–64.

Gilbert, K.K., Brismee, J.-M., Collins, D.L., et al., 2007. Lumbosacral nerve root displacement and strain: part 2: straight leg raise conditions in unembalmed cadavers. Spine 32, 1521–1525.

Haugen, A.J., Brox, J.I., Grovle, L., et al., 2012. Prognostic factors for non-success in patients with sciatica and disc herniation. BMC Musculoskelet. Disord. 13, 183.

Heebner, M.L., Roddey, T.S., 2008. The effects of neural mobilization in addition to standard care in persons with carpal tunnel syndrome from a community hospital. J. Hand Ther. 21, 229–241.

Herzberg, U., Eliav, E., Dorsey, J.M., et al., 1997. NGF involvement in pain induced by chronic constriction injury of the rat sciatic nerve. Neuroreport 8, 1613–1618.

Hough, A.D., Moore, A.P., Jones, M.P., 2007. Reduced longitudinal excursion of the median nerve in carpal tunnel syndrome. Arch. Phys. Med. Rehabil. 88, 569–576.

Hubbard, R.D., Winkelstein, B.A., 2008. Dorsal root compression produces myelinated axonal degeneration near the biomechanical thresholds for mechanical behavioural hypersensitivity. Exp. Neurol. 212, 482–489.

Jensen, O.K., Nielsen, C.V., Stengaard-Pedersen, K., 2010. Low back pain may be caused by disturbed pain regulation: a cross-sectional study in low back pain patients using tender point examination. Eur. J. Pain 14, 514–522.

Kobayashi, S., Shizu, N., Suzuki, Y., et al., 2003. Changes in nerve root motion and intraradicular blood flow during an intraoperative straight leg raise test. Spine 28, 1427–1434.

Kobayashi, S., Yoshino, N., Yamada, S., 2004. Pathology of lumbar nerve root compression. Part 1: intraradicular inflammatory changes induced by mechanical compression. J. Orthop. Res. 22, 170–179.

Korstanje, J.-W.H., Scheltens-de boer, M., Blok, J.H., et al., 2012. Ultrasonographic assessment of longitudinal median nerve and hand flexor tendon dynamics in carpal tunnel syndrome. Muscle Nerve 45, 721–729.

Lundborg, G., 2004. Nerve injury and repair: regeneration, reconstruction, and cortical remodelling, 2nd ed. Elsevier, Churchill Livingstone, Philadelphia.

Lundborg, G., Rydevik, B., 1973. Effects of stretching the tibial nerve of the rabbit: a preliminary study of the intraneural circulation and the barrier function of the perineurium. J. Bone Joint Surg. Br. 55B, 390–401.

Mackinnon, S.E., 2002. Pathophysiology of nerve compression. Hand Clin. 18, 231–241.

Martins, D.F., Mazzardo-Martins, L., Gadotti, V.M., et al., 2011. Ankle joint mobilization reduces axonotmesis-induced neuropathic pain and glial activation in the spinal cord and enhances nerve regeneration in rats. Pain 152, 2653–2661.

Miles, A., Asbridge, J.E., 2013. Contextualizing science in the aftermath of the evidence-based medicine era: on the need for person-centered healthcare. Eur. J. Pers. Cent. Healthc. 1, 285–289.

Nagrale, A.V., Patil, S.P., Ghandi, R.A., et al., 2012. Effect of slump stretching versus lumbar mobilization with exercises in subjects with non-radicular low back pain: a randomized clinical trial. J. Man. Manip. Ther. 20, 35–42.

Nee, B.J., Butler, D., 2006. Management of peripheral neuropathic pain: integrating neurobiology, neurodynamics, and clinical evidence. Phys. Ther. Sport 7, 36–49.

Nee, R.J., Vincenzino, B., Jull, G.A., et al., 2012. Neural tissue management provides immediate clinically relevant benefits without harmful effects for patients with nerve-related neck and arm pain: a randomised trial. J. Physiother. 58, 23–31.

Ogata, K., Naito, M., 1986. Blood flow of peripheral nerves effects of dissection, stretching and compression. J. Hand Surg. Am. 11B, 10–14.

Oskouei, A.E., Talebi, G.A., Shakouri, S.K., et al., 2014. Effects of neuromobilization maneuver on clinical and electrophysiological measures of patients with carpal tunnel syndrome. J. Phys. Ther. Sci. 26, 1017–1022.

Oxford Centre for Evidence-Based Medicine. Available online at: http://www.cebm.net/index.aspx?o=5653.

Pentelka, L., Hebron, C., Shapleski, R., et al., 2012. The effect of increasing sets (within one treatment session) and different set durations (between treatment sessions) of lumbar spine posteroanterior mobilisations on pressure pain thresholds. Man. Ther. 17, 526–530.

Petty, N.J., Ryder, D., 2017. Musculoskeletal examination and assessment: a handbook for therapists, 5th ed. Churchill Livingstone, Edinburgh.

Ridehalgh, C. 2014 Straight leg raise treatment for individuals with spinally referred leg pain: exploring characteristics that influence outcome. Doctoral thesis. University of Brighton. Available online at: http://eprints.brighton.ac.uk/12511/.

Ridehalgh, C., Moore, A., Hough, A., 2012. Repeatability of measuring sciatic nerve excursion during a modified passive straight leg raise test with ultrasound imaging. Man. Ther. 17, 572–576.

Ridehalgh, C., Moore, A., Hough, A., 2015. Sciatic nerve excursion during a modified passive straight leg raise test in asymptomatic participants and participants with spinally referred leg pain. Man. Ther. 20, 564–569.

Ridehalgh, C., Moore, A., Hough, A., 2016. The short term effects of straight leg raise neurodynamic treatment on pressure pain and vibration thresholds in individuals with spinally referred leg pain. Man. Ther. 23, 40–47.

Rothman, S.M., Winkelstein, B.A., 2007. Chemical and mechanical nerve root insults induce differential behavioural sensitivity and glial activation that are enhanced in combination. Brain Res. 1181, 30–43.

Rydevik, B., Lundborg, G., 1977. Permeability of intraneural microvessels and perineurium following acute graded experimental nerve compression. Scand. J. Plast. Reconstr. Surg. 11, 179–187.

Rydevik, B., Lundborg, G., Bagge, U., 1981. Effects of graded compression on intraneural blood flow: an in vivo study on rabbit tibial nerve. J. Hand Surg. Am. 6, 3–12.

Santos, F.M., Silva, J.T., Giardini, A.C., et al., 2012. Neural mobilization reverses behavioral and cellular changes that characterize neuropathic pain in rats. Mol. Pain 8, 57.

Santos, F.M., Grecco, L.H., Pereira, M.G., 2014. The neural mobilization technique modulates the expression of endogenous opioids in the periaqueductal gray and improves muscle strength and mobility in rats with neuropathic pain. Behav. Brain Funct. 10, 19.

Schäfer, A., Hall, T., Müller, G., et al., 2011. Outcomes differ between subgroups of patients with low back and leg pain following neural manual therapy: a prospective cohort study. Eur. Spine J. 20, 482–490.

Schmid, A., 2015. The peripheral nervous system and its compromise in entrapment neuropathies. In: Jull, G., Moore, A., Falla, D., et al. (Eds.), Grieve's modern musculoskeletal physiotherapy. Elsevier, Edinburgh, pp. 78–92.

Schmid, A., Elliott, J.M., Strudwick, M.W., et al., 2012. Effect of splinting and exercise on intraneural edema of the median nerve in carpal tunnel syndrome – an MRI study to reveal therapeutic mechanisms. J. Orthop. Res. 1343–1350.

Schmid, A., Coppieters, M.W., Ruitenberg, M.J., et al., 2013. Local and remote imuune-mediated inflammation after mild peripheral nerve compression in rats. J. Neuropathol. Exp. Neurol. 72, 662–680.

Scrimshaw, S.V., Maher, C.G., 2001. Randomized controlled trial of neural mobilization after spinal surgery. Spine 26, 2647–2652.

Shacklock, M.O., 2005. Clinical neurodynamics: a new system of musculoskeletal treatment. Elsevier/Butterworth Heinemann, Edinburgh.

Steen, K.H., Steen, A.E., Kreysel, H.W., et al., 1996. Inflammatory mediators potentiate pain induced by experimental tissue acidosis. Pain 66, 163–170.

Sunderland, S., 1976. The nerve lesions in the carpal tunnel syndrome. J. Neurol. Neurosurg. Psychiatry 39, 615–626.

Sunderland, S. 1989 Features of nerves that protect them during normal daily activities. Paper presented at: Manipulative Therapy Association Australia (Adelaide).

Tal-Akabi, A., Rushton, A., 2000. An investigation to compare the effectiveness of carpal bone mobilisation and neurodynamic mobilisation as methods of treatment for carpal tunnel syndrome. Man. Ther. 5, 214–222.

Walsh, J., Hall, T., 2009. Classification of low back-related leg pain: do subgroups differ in disability and psychosocial factors? Journal of Manual and Manipulative Therapy 17, 118–123.

Section 2

PRINCIPLES OF PATIENT MANAGEMENT

8

UNDERSTANDING AND MANAGING PERSISTENT PAIN

HUBERT VAN GRIENSVEN

CHAPTER CONTENTS

INTRODUCTION

The assessment, examination and management of a range of painful musculoskeletal conditions are discussed in preceding chapters and in Petty and Ryder (2017). They have a bias towards physical structures and dysfunctions as the source of pain. The assumption is that, if a physical source of pain can be identified correctly, treatment aimed at that source can be expected to lead to the resolution of pain. This way of thinking is referred to as the tissue pathology model. Neurophysiologists may call it an end-organ model, because it focuses on the tissues rather than the function of the nervous system innervating those tissues.

In musculoskeletal examination and treatment, the tissue pathology model is applied much of the time. Information about the inciting event and the way the pain behaves helps the clinician to form a hypothesis about the tissues that may have been damaged. This hypothesis can then be refined by testing whether the application of pressure or stretch to different tissues increases or decreases the patient's pain. Over time the

same tests are repeated to evaluate treatment efficacy and recovery.

In patients whose pain has become persistent, the tissue pathology model may no longer be meaningful. For example, pain may be present in absence of any evidence of tissue damage. If there was an inciting injury, the pain may have persisted beyond the healing time. The level of pain may be out of proportion with the original injury. Sometimes persistent pain leads to disability, which can be a greater obstacle to the patient's recovery than the physical pathology itself. These and other aspects of persistent pain are the consequence of changes in the way the sensory nervous system works, behaviour and psychology.

This chapter first provides an understanding of physiological, behavioural, psychological and social aspects associated with persistent pain. Although these are discussed in separate sections for didactic purposes, it is important to remember that several of these can be present in an individual patient. Next an overall approach to the assessment of patients with persistent pain will be discussed, which complements the information provided in Ryder and van Griensven (2017) and van Griensven and Ryder (2017). The final section provides strategies for managing persistent pain.

UNDERSTANDING PERSISTENT PAIN

Acute, Subacute and Persistent Pain

Pain is the body's warning system in the tissue pathology model. As such it can be referred to as adaptive, i.e. it helps us to change our behaviour in order to deal with injury. Pain makes us avoid circumstances, postures and activities that are likely to aggravate or maintain our injury. It can also make us take positive action, for instance, applying compression or seeking help. As the injury resolves, the pain associated with it settles down. Our protective behaviour reduces and we gradually return to normal function, although some local pain and functional limitation may remain if healing was incomplete or inadequate.

Pain associated with injury or recovery from injury is classed as acute or subacute, respectively (Loeser & Melzack 1999). It is the result of the stimulation of nociceptive neurons, types C and Aδ. They have a high stimulation threshold, so they are normally activated only when a stimulus is intense. The stimulation threshold may be lowered by sensitizing chemicals such as bradykinin or prostaglandin, which are released as part of the inflammatory process and tissue injury. When this happens, stimuli which are normally too weak to reach the stimulation threshold become capable of activating nociceptive neurons. For example, a fresh bruise may not hurt spontaneously but gentle pressure can make it sore because the local nociceptors are sensitized. This is mechanical allodynia, i.e. pain in response to mechanical stimulation which is not normally painful.

It is important to distinguish between nociception and pain. Nociception is sensation as a consequence of stimulation of nociceptive neurons, while pain is a subjective experience. While the two often coincide, it is possible to stimulate nociceptive neurons in a non-noxious manner (Gardner & Johnson 2013) or to experience pain in the absence of nociceptive stimulation (Fisher et al. 1995). The full definition of pain is: 'an unpleasant sensory and emotional experience associated with actual or potential tissue damage, or described in terms of such damage' (www.iasp-pain.org). According to this definition, pain may or may not be a consequence of nociceptive stimulation. It is worth taking time to consider its elements and the implications for the understanding of pain.

Tissue damage and its associated pain are expected to resolve within a few months. Pain which has been present for more than 3–6 months can be called chronic or persistent arbitrarily (Loeser & Melzack 1999). Some authors instead base their definition of persistent pain on the inability of the body to restore its normal homeostasis (Loeser & Melzack 1999), or to respond to curative treatment or pain control (Merskey et al. 1994). In this sense, pain may be called persistent once the expected time for recovery has passed and there has been a lack of response to treatment.

The relationship between persistent pain and tissue damage is often unclear. As a consequence, persistent pain can be unreliable as an indicator of what is happening in the body. This makes it a poor guide to pain-related behaviour, so the pain can no longer be said to have a protective function. It is therefore called maladaptive. Reasons for the maladaptive nature of persistent pain can be found in changes in neurophysiology, psychology, behaviour and social circumstances. Physiologically, the patient's sensory nervous system may become hypersensitive and create an inaccurate and exaggerated experience of physical sensations. Persistent pain is likely to influence a patient's emotions and behaviour, together with the patient's pain-related thoughts and beliefs. Socially, relationships, work and leisure activities can be affected. The remainder of this chapter explains the role that these aspects of pain can play for patients.

Physiological Aspects of Persistent Pain

Sensory Transmission in the Dorsal Horn

Fig. 8.1 shows how primary nociceptive neurons, type C and Aδ, terminate in the dorsal horn of the spinal cord and synapse with secondary neurons (Galea 2013). Aβ fibres carrying non-noxious mechanoreceptor signals do not end at the spinal cord level, but continue up the dorsal column to the medulla. They do however have collateral fibres which influence secondary neurons and inhibitory interneurons (Galea 2013). Secondary neurons in the dorsal horn which receive input from nociceptive fibres only are classed as nociceptive specific neurons, while those receiving stimulation from both

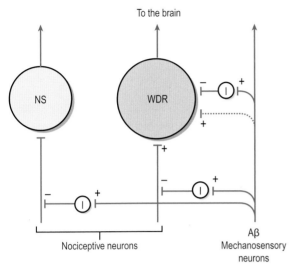

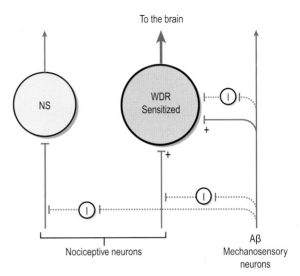

FIG. 8.1 ■ Simplified diagram of sensory transmission in the dorsal horn. Nociceptive neurons terminate at the dorsal horn and synapse either with nociceptive-specific (*NS*) neurons or wide dynamic range (*WDR*) neurons. Aβ mechanosensory neurons do not terminate at dorsal horn level, but stimulate local inhibitory interneurons (*I*). They also have a low-level excitatory influence on the WDR (dotted line). The interneurons play a role in controlling nociceptive transmission, either presynaptically or postsynaptically. Neurons can exert either an excitatory (+) or inhibitory (–) influence.

FIG. 8.2 ■ Simplified diagram of central sensitization in the dorsal horn. When wide dynamic range (*WDR*) neurons become sensitized (dark green on diagram), input from nociceptive neurons and Aβ neurons is amplified. This leads to hyperalgesia and tactile allodynia, respectively. Part of the central sensitization process is a reduction in inhibitory influence (dotted lines). As a consequence, control of nociceptive input is reduced and the WDR is more easily excited. Neurons can exert either an excitatory (+) or inhibitory (–) influence. *I*, interneurons; *NS*, nociceptive-specific.

nociceptive and Aβ fibres are called wide dynamic range cells (Basbaum & Jessell 2013). A complex system of interneurons keeps transmission of nociceptive information under control (Sandkühler 2013; Todd & Koerber 2013).

Central Sensitization

A persistent influx of nociceptive stimulation can lead to a heightened responsiveness of secondary neurons in the dorsal horn (Fig. 8.2). When this happens, nociceptive signals are subjected to facilitated transmission. This state of the dorsal horn neurons is referred to as central sensitization (www.iasp-pain.org), or long-term potentiation (Ruscheweyh et al. 2011). Central sensitization means that secondary neurons in the spinal cord develop a heightened responsiveness to sensory input. This manifests as hyperaesthesia (increased response to normal sensory stimulation) and hyperalgesia (increased response to a normally painful stimulus) (www.iasp-pain.org). The secondary neurons can also develop a new responsiveness to signals which are normally below the

stimulation threshold (allodynia) and to signals from a wider area (Woolf 2011). Finally, activation of secondary neurons can outlast the duration of the initiating stimulus (Woolf 2011). Similar changes may take place in pain pathways in the brain (Zhuo 2015). Central sensitization has been shown to play a role in patients with fibromyalgia syndrome and arthritic conditions (Lee et al. 2011; Meeus et al. 2012).

Clinical manifestations of central sensitization are listed in Box 8.1. It is important to be aware that signs and symptoms inconsistent with a purely musculoskeletal diagnosis may indicate changes in central sensory processing. When present, these changes may warrant further investigation.

Descending Inhibition and Facilitation

Sensory processing in the dorsal horn is influenced not only by nociceptive input, but also by the brain. This influence can be either positive (descending facilitation) or negative (descending inhibition). In other words, the brain selects the sensory input it requires by

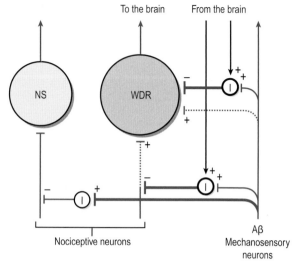

FIG. 8.3 ■ Simplified diagram of descending inhibition. Inhibitory neurons descending from the brain (wide arrows) stimulate inhibitory interneurons at the level of the dorsal horn. This enhances presynaptic inhibition of primary nociceptive input and postsynaptic inhibition of the wide dynamic range (WDR) (dark green on diagram), thus controlling both the input and transmission of nociceptive signals. Neurons can exert either an excitatory (+) or inhibitory (–) influence. I, interneurons; NS, nociceptive-specific.

enhancing or suppressing incoming information as soon as it enters the dorsal horn.

A non-specific pain-suppressing system is called the diffuse noxious inhibitory system (LeBars et al. 1979a, b). When a painful stimulus is given, neurons in the caudal medulla start to regulate activity in various centres in the central nervous system, which are important for the transmission of nociceptive information (Villanueva & Fields 2004). These centres include the dorsal horn and the thalamus (Villanueva & Fields 2004). The diffuse noxious inhibitory system can be activated from anywhere in the body and may therefore underpin counterirritation, i.e. inhibition of one pain by another.

Nociceptive transmission is controlled by cerebral networks in the periaquaductal grey, the rostroventro-medial medulla and the locus ceruleus (Basbaum & Jessell 2013; Heinricher & Fields 2013). Activation of these centres can generate a local release of endogenous opioids, which are the neurotransmitters that activate descending inhibitory neurons. These neurons terminate in the dorsal horn, releasing noradrenaline (norepinephrine) or serotonin, which stimulates the local inhibitory systems. This mechanism is known as descending inhibition (Fig. 8.3). It is important to note that there are similar pathways for descending facilitation. Through these systems the brain can be said to select its own input.

Pain-inhibitory systems can be activated in life-threatening situations in which pain may prevent one

from escaping to safety. This is known as stress-induced analgesia (Butler & Finn 2009). They can also be activated when there is expectation of pain relief (Benedetti et al. 1999). This is part of the placebo response, which also includes a wider range of hormone releases and immune responses (Benedetti 2009). Conversely, expectation of worsening of pain can lead to hyperalgesia through the activation of pain-facilitatory systems (Benedetti 2009). This is referred to as the nocebo response. It is likely that a patient's concerns and uncertainties about the origin and nature of the pain can also drive descending facilitation, i.e. descending facilitation can be viewed as the physiological correlate of pain-related vigilance. Finally, inhibitory systems can be activated by attention, for instance, by focusing on something else (Bushnell et al. 2004; Price & Bushnell 2004). This can be utilized therapeutically (Bushnell et al. 2004; Price & Bushnell 2004).

Behavioural Aspects of Persistent Pain

Because acute and subacute pain are largely adaptive, changing one's behaviour in response is likely to reduce

> **BOX 8.2**
> ## ACUTE AND SUBACUTE PAIN BEHAVIOURS
>
> Adaptive avoidance behaviour may consist of:
> - Reducing or avoiding painful activities
> - Not weight bearing on an affected leg
> - Taking time off work
> - Suspending social activities
>
> Adaptive actions may include:
> - Taking medications
> - Seeking information and advice
> - Using aids such as walking aids or supportive bandages
> - Applying ice, compression or massage
> - Seeking treatment

the risk of further harm and enhance recovery. In the early stages of an injury, a patient may avoid activities associated with harm or pain, while developing behaviours which are likely to promote healing (Box 8.2).

These changes in activity are known as pain behaviours (Waddell 2004). They can be adaptive ways of dealing with a recent injury, but they can become maladaptive when pain persists. In the longer term, pain behaviours are likely to have a negative impact on the individual as a whole, whether they are helpful in avoiding pain or not. Using the examples provided above, potential downsides of long-term pain behaviour include the following.

Actions Avoided

- Reducing or avoiding painful activities can reduce one's fitness, flexibility and strength over time. Not only does this increase the chance of ongoing pain and further injury, it can also interfere with one's ability to work, take part in social activities and relationships.
- The same applies to not bearing weight on an affected leg.
- Patients may think that giving up work will help their pain, but this is often not the case. Work can be a distraction from pain and a powerful motivator to overcome pain and injury. A lack of financial independence can also have a negative effect on the individual.
- Suspending social activities can lead to isolation.

Actions Taken

- Common long-term side-effects of analgesic medication include drowsiness, lack of concentration and gastrointestinal disturbance (Waller & Sampson 2015). Analgesics may be regarded as adaptive if they help a patient to cope, but maladaptive if the side-effects interfere with overall function.
- Patients may continue to seek information and advice from multiple practitioners if the pain continues. While it is possible that an answer is eventually found, there is also a risk that:
  - The patient's focus on finding the right opinion prevents her from looking at her current situation and finding ways to manage the pain.
  - The patient receives conflicting opinions, which may be confusing. Even when referring to similar problems, different practitioners may use different terms (e.g. zygapophyseal joint dysfunction, facet joint arthritis or spondylitis).
- Reliance on aids may be necessary but also carries the risk of maintaining disability.
- Applying ice, compression or massage is unlikely to be of long-term benefit.
- Targeted treatment can be appropriate if there is a specific injury or dysfunction that can be treated. In the longer term, pain treatment may need to be either combined with or replaced by pain management.

An example of an unhelpful combination of avoidance and action is the overactivity–underactivity cycle: the patient rests for long periods, followed by a rush of activity once the pain subsides (Harding & Watson 2000). The excessive periods of rest are likely to lead to deconditioning, which in turn increases the risk of further pain and injury during activity. This tends to create an overall deterioration in pain and activity.

It is important for a clinician to interpret the patient's coping strategies in the context of overall function and well-being, in order to decide the extent to which they may be adaptive or maladaptive.

Social Aspects of Persistent Pain

The social environment has an influence on various aspects of persistent pain (Craig & Fashler 2013). For example, the patient's assessment and emotions related to pain are influenced by the opinions and behaviour of relatives, carers, friends and colleagues. Conversely, these aspects affect the way a patient expresses the pain to those around him. Thus, there is a complex interaction between the social environment and the patient which influences pain-related behaviour. Engaging with carers and relatives may therefore be important for the rehabilitation process. For example, if the patient is asked to tolerate some pain in order to make gains in function, the relatives have to understand that they should not take over whenever the patient expresses pain. They may also need to be included when the patient is given an explanation of the fact that pain is not always an indication of tissue damage.

Clinicians must be aware that their own behaviour also influences the patient's behaviour in relation to the pain. When clinicians have a biomedical orientation and think that painful activities must be avoided, their patients tend to adopt fear avoidance beliefs, i.e. they tend to avoid painful activities because they fear negative consequences (Darlow et al. 2013). These patients are also more likely to receive sick certification, increasing the risk of long-term disability (Darlow et al. 2013). Clinicians are advised to complete some of the questionnaires themselves, in order to assess their own fear avoidance (Houben et al. 2005; Pincus et al. 2006; Bishop et al. 2007). The results can be used to reflect on one's own pain-related beliefs and understanding and to guide training.

Clinicians must remain aware of the complexities of interaction in clinic. Patients may modify the way they present their pain depending on their impression of the clinician (Toye et al. 2013; Froud et al. 2014; van Griensven 2016). For example, if they sense that they are not believed or at risk of not receiving the care they feel they need, they may present their symptoms more forcefully (van Griensven 2016). Communication skills are therefore essential (Gask & Usherwood 2002). Patients with persistent pain tend to value an open attitude from their clinician, a clear explanation of tests and outcomes, realistic reassurance and a clear plan of action (May 2001; Cooper et al. 2008; Slade et al. 2009; Kidd et al. 2011).

Psychological Aspects of Persistent Pain

Psychological aspects of pain can be divided into cognitive and affective components, which are

> ### BOX 8.3
> ### PSYCHOLOGICAL FACTORS WHICH MAY PREDICT THE DEVELOPMENT OF PERSISTENT MUSCULOSKELETAL PAIN (LINTON 2000; PINCUS ET AL. 2002; MALLEN ET AL. 2007)
>
> - Anxiety and/or depression
> - Higher somatic perceptions
> - Higher psychological distress
> - Having poor coping strategies
> - Somatization, or the unconscious expression of psychological distress as physical symptoms
> - Pain cognitions such as catastrophizing
> - Fear avoidance beliefs

interrelated. Cognitive or evaluative aspects include thoughts, interpretations, beliefs, attitudes and expectations. Affective or emotional aspects may include joy, anxiety or anger. A patient's psychology is likely to be influenced by persistent pain. Conversely, psychological factors influence his experience of the pain and the impact it has.

In the management and treatment of pain, psychology may be important from several points of view. Psychological factors have been found to be statistical predictors of the transition from acute to chronic pain (Box 8.3). They also affect how a patient responds to or deals with the pain.

It is important to remember that these factors cannot be used as absolute predictors of persistent pain in an individual; they are based on statistical data of large groups of patients. The presence of psychological risk factors does not mean that persistent pain is irreversible or that therapy should not be undertaken. In fact, therapists who are sensitive to these issues are more likely to help the patient to recover and reduce or avoid disability. This has been referred to as psychologically informed practice (Main & George 2011).

Numerous psychological factors of pain have been, and continue to be, identified. Two well-researched factors associated with the development and maintenance of persistent pain are catastrophizing and fear avoidance. Catastrophizing is a set of exaggerated cognitions in relation to current or anticipated pain (Sullivan et al. 2001). It can be subdivided into rumination (an inability to keep pain out of the awareness), magnification (persistent focus on pain and what might happen) and helplessness (Haythornthwaite 2013). There is a strong link between catastrophizing and poor function in patients with persistent pain (Haythornthwaite 2013). It may be assessed using the Pain Catastrophizing Scale (Sullivan et al. 1995).

Fear avoidance is the tendency not to undertake activities associated with pain, because the pain is experienced as threatening (Vlaeyen & Linton 2000). High threat value of the pain is thought to be associated with catastrophizing, leading to pain-related fear (Haythornthwaite 2013). The fear avoidance model suggests that patients who are willing and able to confront and/or accept their pain have a better chance of actively engaging with their recovery, thus reducing their chance of pain-related disability (Vlaeyen & Linton 2000). A useful assessment tool is the shortened Tampa Scale for Kinesiophobia (Woby et al. 2005).

Patients' pain cognitions have consequences for the way they experience and respond to their pain (Linton & Shaw 2011). Therapists can deal with unhelpful cognitions and behaviours by giving patients a realistic explanation of their pain, addressing concerns about its cause and providing strategies to deal with it. They can also help their patients to engage with their rehabilitation programme and allow them to set their own pace, as well as helping them to set goals which are meaningful to them as an individual. These issues are expanded on in the next section.

It is important for therapists to deal with psychological aspects of persistent pain, while remaining aware of their professional boundaries. Preexisting psychological conditions, such as anxiety or depression which are not a consequence of the patient's physical condition or pain, are likely to be beyond the scope of musculoskeletal therapy practice. Therapists are not expected to diagnose or manage psychological states or traits, and should suggest professional help for psychological and psychiatric conditions as appropriate. In line with this, it is advisable not to use psychological diagnostic terms in notes and letters; terms such as 'low mood' or 'feeling anxious' are preferable to 'depression' or 'anxiety disorder'.

ASSESSING PERSISTENT PAIN – GENERAL APPROACH

Musculoskeletal assessment is detailed in Petty and Ryder (2017), so this section provides only a brief overview of the assessment of a patient with persistent pain. From the preceding section it will be clear that persistent pain presents the clinician with diagnostic challenges because:

- It does not correlate well with a lesion or injury.
- It may involve multiple body regions.
- It may not respond to tests in a predictable fashion.
- It may be associated with general dysfunction, as well as psychological and social changes.

These issues can have the following consequences for the assessment:

- Musculoskeletal findings may be misleading.
- Musculoskeletal problems may be less relevant for the patient's overall progress than, for example, overall function, work status and social life.
- The clinician needs to decide what to prioritize in the assessment.

The clinician is advised to consider by the end of the subjective examination whether the patient's history of present complaint, symptom behaviour and other factors point to a specific musculoskeletal problem. One of the issues to look out for is consistency: a musculoskeletal problem may be multifactorial, but history and presentation tend to suggest specific mechanisms and tissues. Examples of issues that may not fit a musculoskeletal model well are:

- A patient feels that using a crutch helps his pain, but he is using it on the wrong side, i.e. he does not take pressure off the affected area and may even load it more.
- A patient diagnosed with fibromyalgia syndrome experiences pain in varying places in the body at different times.
- A patient has pain and hyperaesthesia in the whole of the right leg, which developed over years following a back injury years ago.
- A patient has given up work, is finding it increasingly difficult to leave the house and has become stiff, weak and unfit. The patient has become socially isolated and finds it difficult to go out because of pain.

For patients with a persistent pain presentation, the assessment has to be adapted to accommodate aspects beyond the strictly musculoskeletal. As mentioned in Chapter 3 of Petty and Ryder (2017), the traditional musculoskeletal therapy examination consists of ruling in conditions which are involved. For example, if a patient has back pain radiating to the hip area, the clinician will test various structures of the lumbar region, pelvis and hips. All the tissues which yield a positive test tend to be ruled in and the clinician will clinically reason how the findings can be combined to form a consistent diagnostic hypothesis.

This examination approach is not appropriate when symptoms are widespread, non-specific or, to a large extent, of a non-musculoskeletal nature. In this case, focusing on local structures carries a risk of missing the barriers to the patient's recovery and therapeutic targets. The clinician is therefore advised primarily to direct attention to general issues such as overall posture and movement, behavioural response to pain and general sensitivity to gentle stimuli. Where a specific musculoskeletal condition is tested, the clinician adopts an approach where tissues are ruled out: the examination is used to decide whether there is consistent evidence of a specific condition such as a ligament sprain. This is similar to the examination of a patient with a stroke: the overall physical and mental function forms the main target of the examination, but within that approach the clinician may check whether a frozen shoulder can be ruled out as an aspect of the patient's overall presentation.

The use of objective examination markers is recommended, as discussed in Ryder and van Griensven (2017). These can take the form of functional outcome measures, pain scores and questionnaires. This provides a means of evaluating the patient's progress. In patients with persistent pain this is particularly important, because they may not be aware that they are making functional gains if their pain does not change.

A word of caution: even when a patient has widespread persistent pain that does not seem to fit a specific musculoskeletal pattern, it is not sufficient to call this a pain syndrome and not to examine the patient. Even a patient with long-term pain can have a knee injury, for example.

At the end of the examination, the patient must be given an explanation of the findings. This ought to include what has been ruled out and address all concerns voiced by the patient. If the patient has been given conflicting information by others, the clinician must try to explain what this information may mean in the light of the examination findings. The clinician should also explain what she can and cannot do for the patient, and agree with the patient how to proceed (Main et al. 2008).

MANAGING PERSISTENT PAIN

Overview

By necessity, musculoskeletal therapy training tends to have a biomedical focus. Communication skills and understanding of psychological and social management of persistent pain have become more prominent over the years, but may still lag behind (Synnott et al. 2015). Therapists need to have an understanding of strategies to deal with wider aspects of persistent pain, because they are often first-line or second-line practitioners. Elements of a physiotherapy approach to persistent pain are listed in Box 8.4.

BOX 8.4
ELEMENTS OF MUSCULOSKELETAL THERAPY FOR PERSISTENT PAIN

Depending on the issues that the patient presents with, musculoskeletal therapy for persistent pain may include the following:

- Providing the patient with a helpful understanding of the pain and its consequences. This can also help to reduce the patient's fear
- Maximizing factors that are likely to enhance the patient's pain inhibition systems, such as:
  - Education about pain
  - Empowering the patient
  - Suggesting exercises and changes that are within the patient's control
  - Giving positive and realistic feedback
- Helping patients to identify what is important to them as an individual, setting goals accordingly, and developing an approach to rehabilitation that works towards those goals
- Adopting an active approach to rehabilitation, in a way that demonstrates to the patient that activity can be improved without making the pain worse. This can also help to reduce fear
- Relaxation techniques and sleep management
- Mindfulness-based approaches

Pain Education

Patient education is important for two main reasons. First, patients who understand their condition are likely to manage their pain more appropriately. If their situation changes, they have a better chance to adapt well. Second, the subjective threat represented by pain is likely to affect how it is perceived and whether pain-inhibitory systems are activated (Moseley & Butler 2015). A reduction of a patient's uncertainty and vigilance may therefore aid the activation of active pain inhibition, so that the perception of pain reduces even if the source of nociception remains the same (Moseley & Butler 2015).

For education and reassurance to be effective, it is essential that it addresses all of the patient's concerns; a blanket explanation is unlikely to reassure (Dowrick et al. 2004). The therapist therefore has to find out first what these concerns are and what the patient's assessment of the situation is. This can be done by asking questions such as, 'What do you think is happening?', 'What is the best explanation you have had for your pain?' or 'How do you see your future?' The clinician is advised to be open and listen to the patient's own answer, resisting the temptation to prompt (Gask & Usherwood 2002; Laerum et al. 2006). This leads to a better understanding of the patient's subjective experience, aids interaction and ensures that the clinician's educational strategy addresses the patient's concerns (Harding & Watson 2000).

If the clinician deems the patient's interpretation of the pain to be maladaptive and/or if there are indications of central sensitization, it may be advisable to educate the patient regarding pain physiology (Nijs et al. 2012). Understanding can be verified when the patient returns, either by asking a few questions or with the aid of a pain neurophysiology questionnaire (Moseley 2003b). Research has demonstrated that patients are capable of understanding pain physiology better than clinicians may anticipate (Moseley 2003b). The patient's new understanding of pain and central sensitization can be used to develop self-management strategies that are likely to enhance descending inhibition.

Family members and carers may need to be involved in pain rehabilitation. It can be difficult for relatives to see a loved one in pain, so they may feel obliged to take over tasks. This is sometimes necessary but can also reinforce unhelpful pain behaviour. It is important that relatives understand when the patient should engage with activities, even if these are associated with some pain. Patients can be given permission to refuse help when it is not in accordance with their rehabilitation programme, but to ask for help when they need it.

Active Pain Rehabilitation

Patients with persistent pain often lose function, with consequences for their work, leisure activities and other aspects of their social life. Patients are more likely to engage with rehabilitation if they can see how it will contribute to their overall recovery. It is therefore advisable to help patients to set personal goals that are meaningful to them.

Patient goals can be used to formulate a rehabilitation strategy, which may include stretches, strengthening exercises and increases in fitness and general activity (Harding & Williams 1995). A structured programme with clearly identified outcomes can provide patients with a view of how and when they are likely to achieve their goals. This can aid their motivation but also helps to shift their focus from pain (and pain reduction) to activity and life goals.

One of the strategies used to increase activity levels while avoiding lasting aggravation of pain is called activity pacing (Gil et al. 1988; Harding & Williams 1995). Patients start with exercises and functional activities at a level that feels safe to them and is unlikely to exacerbate the pain. The activity is then increased over time by very small amounts. Patients are asked to apply these activities in daily life. For example, if patients have increased their walking time to 5 minutes and have to undertake a 15-minute walk, they are advised to divide their walk into three sections and have a short rest in between. From a neurophysiological perspective this means that they are less likely to feed into central sensitization, while the achievement of relevant activities can enhance pain inhibition.

Patients are usually asked to apply objective markers to their activity pacing, such as the time that they stand, sit or walk, walking distance or the number of steps when using the stairs. Some patients can be taught to recognize when they are approaching their safe activity limit instead. This may be a more appropriate way for patients to learn to manage their activities, but it is essential that they recognize that they are approaching their safe limit before the pain forces them to stop.

Before embarking on a pain rehabilitation programme, patients need to be clear that their pain may or may not reduce, certainly in the first instance. The initial aim is to overcome deconditioning and to restore function, in order to help patients to return to (or maintain) activities that are important to them. This may or may not lead to the reduction of pain in the future, unless it is possible for the therapist to apply pain-reducing treatments alongside the programme. It is important that the patient understands and accepts that specific treatments are undertaken to support the overall rehabilitation programme.

Activity pacing can be useful for patients who persist in being active, albeit not in the most helpful way. On the other hand, other patients become so fearful of activities associated with pain that they end up doing very little. For these patients with so-called fear avoidance, a programme of graded exposure may be more appropriate (Meeus et al. 2016). Fear of movement can be further reduced by breaking the movements down into smaller, less threatening components, or by asking the patient to imagine performing the movement in a painfree manner (Moseley 2003a). As mentioned above, the clinician's own attitude may be equally important.

Apart from pain management approaches, patients may be helped by advice on posture, ergonomics such as the set-up of a workstation or other equipment, and manual handling. If necessary, a graded approach can help patients to increase their tolerance to postures and activities required for work (Main et al. 2008). Success of the application of what is gained may rely on involvement of family members and liaison with employer and general practitioner.

Relaxation and Mindfulness

Our discussion so far has focused on active approaches to pain rehabilitation, but it is equally important for patients to be able to relax. Relaxation techniques can help the patient to learn to relax both body and mind. It can also help in the treatment of negative pain-related emotions such as fear, distress or low moods (Linton & Shaw 2011). There are many books with relaxation techniques on the market. Patients who prefer to be guided

through the relaxation exercise can buy a CD. The CD by pain psychologist Neil Berry (www.paincd.org.uk) has tracks to teach relaxation, as well as provide education, advice and exercise. Another resource is the relaxation CD in the self-help book *The Pain Management Plan* (www.pain-management-plan.co.uk) (Lewin & Bryson 2010). A note of caution may be appropriate: while many patients benefit from relaxation techniques, some find a quiet environment without activity extremely uncomfortable.

Finally, pain management approaches based on mindfulness meditation have come to prominence in recent years. It is not possible to provide a full introduction to the field in this context, so the clinician is advised to access the resources below or others. Mindfulness has its roots in Buddhist meditation, but can be practised outside that context. At its core is learning to pay attention to what can be perceived in the present moment. Thoughts and feelings associated with past and future, including regrets, hopes and fears, are acknowledged but not adhered to or acted on. In pain management, mindfulness has the potential to allow patients to become aware of the difference between what is happening and what they are worried may happen, for example. It can help them to let go of the mind's drive constantly to think of ways to escape the pain, which can be problematic when this pain cannot be avoided. An important aspect of mindfulness is acceptance, which is not a passive 'giving up' but an acknowledgement of where one is at the present moment without judgement.

There is a growing body of literature about the efficacy of mindfulness in the management of persistent pain (Kabat-Zinn 1982; Chiesa & Serretti 2011; Theadom et al. 2015). A pioneer in the application of mindfulness in the treatment of stress and pain is John Kabat-Zinn, whose book *Full Catastrophe Living* (1990) continues to be one of the most thorough and accessible explorations of the topic. One of the most progressive yet traditionally rooted approaches in the UK has been developed by Breathworks (www.breathworks-mindfulness.org.uk), which provides training for patients and professionals, as well as books and CDs. It must, however, be stressed that, although many more resources are available, the only way to appreciate mindfulness fully and learn how to help others with it is to practise it.

CONCLUSION

This chapter has described how persistent pain may vary from acute and subacute pain in terms of neurophysiology, psychology, behaviour and social circumstances. It has provided a general strategy to assessing patients with persistent pain and discussed psychologically informed physiotherapy techniques that can be used to manage or treat them. When applied appropriately, physiotherapy has an important role to play in the management and treatment of persistent pain.

REFERENCES

Basbaum, A., Jessell, T., 2013. Pain. In: Kandel, E., Schwartz, J.H. (Eds.), Principles of neural science, fifth ed. McGraw-Hill, New York, pp. 530–555.

Benedetti, F., 2009. Placebo effects. Understanding the mechanisms in health and disease. Oxford University Press, Oxford.

Benedetti, F., Arduino, C., Amanzio, M., 1999. Somatotopic activation of opioid systems by target-directed expectations of analgesia. J. Neurosci. 19, 3639–3648.

Bishop, A., Thomas, E., Foster, N., 2007. Health care practitioners' attitudes and beliefs about low back pain: a systematic search and critical review of available measurement tools. Pain 132, 91–101.

Bushnell, M., Villemure, C., Duncan, G., 2004. Psychophysical and neurophysiological studies of pain modulation by attention. In: Price, D., Bushnell, M. (Eds.), Psychological methods of pain control: basic science and clinical perspectives. IASP Press, Seattle, pp. 99–116.

Butler, R., Finn, D., 2009. Stress-induced analgesia. Prog. Neurobiol. 88, 184–202.

Chiesa, A., Serretti, A., 2011. Mindfulness-based interventions for chronic pain: a systematic review of the evidence. J. Altern. Complement. Med. 17, 83–93.

Cooper, K., Smith, B., Hancock, E., 2008. Patient-centredness in physiotherapy from the perspective of the chronic low back pain patient. Physiotherapy 94, 244–252.

Craig, K., Fashler, S., 2013. Social determinants of pain. In: van Griensven, H., Strong, J., Unruh, A. (Eds.), Pain. A textbook for health professionals, second ed. Churchill Livingstone, Edinburgh, pp. 21–34.

Darlow, B., Dowell, A., Baxter, G., et al., 2013. The enduring impact of what clinicians say to people with low back pain. Ann. Fam. Med. 11, 527–534.

Dowrick, C., Ring, A., Humphris, G., et al., 2004. Normalisation of unexplained symptoms by general practitioners: a functional typology. Br. J. Gen. Pract. 54, 165–170.

Fisher, J., Hassan, D., O'Connor, N., 1995. Minerva. Br. Med. J. 310, 70.

Froud, R., Patterson, S., Eldridge, S., et al., 2014. A systematic review and meta-synthesis of the impact of low back pain on people's lives. BMC Musculoskelet. Disord. 15, 50.

Galea, M., 2013. Neuroanatomy of the nociceptive system. In: van Griensven, H., Strong, J., Unruh, A. (Eds.), Pain. A textbook for healthcare practitioners, second ed. Churchill Livingstone, Edinburgh, pp. 49–76.

Gardner, E., Johnson, K., 2013. The somatosensory system: receptors and central pathways. In: Kandel, E., Schwartz, J.H. (Eds.), Principles of neural science, fifth ed. McGraw-Hill, New York, pp. 475–479.

Gask, L., Usherwood, T., 2002. ABC of psychological medicine. The consultation. Br. Med. J. 324, 1567–1569.

Gil, K., Ross, S., Keefe, F., 1988. Behavioural treatment of chronic pain: four pain management protocols. In: Chronic pain. American Psychiatric Press, Washington, pp. 317–413.

Harding, V., Watson, P., 2000. Increasing acitivity and improving function in chronic pain management. Physiotherapy 86, 619–630.

Harding, V., Williams, A.C.d.C., 1995. Extending physiotherapy skills using a psychological approach: cognitive-behavioural management of chronic pain. Physiotherapy 81, 681–688.

Haythornthwaite, J., 2013. Assessment of pain beliefs, coping, and function. In: McMahon, S.B., Koltzenburg, M. (Eds.), Wall & Melzack's textbook of pain, sixth ed. Saunders, Philadelphia, pp. 328–338.

Heinricher, M., Fields, H., 2013. Central nervous system mechanisms of pain modulation. In: McMahon, S.B., Koltzenburg, M. (Eds.), Wall & Melzack's textbook of pain, sixth ed. Saunders, Philadelphia, pp. 129–142.

Houben, R., Gijsen, A., Peterson, J., et al., 2005. Do health care providers' attitudes towards back pain predict their treatment recommendations? Differential predictive validity of implicit and explicit attitude measures. Pain 114, 491–498.

Kabat-Zinn, J., 1982. An outpatient program in behavioural medicine for chronic pain patients based on the practice of mindfulness meditation: theoretical considerations and preliminary results. Gen. Hosp. Psychiatry 4, 33–47.

Kabat-Zinn, J., 1990. Full catastrophe living. How to cope with stress, pain and illness using mindfulness meditation. Piatkus, London.

Kidd, M., Bond, C., Bell, M., 2011. Patients' perspectives of patient-centredness as important musculoskeletal physiotherapy interactions: a qualitative study. Physiotherapy 97, 154–162.

Laerum, E., Indahl, A., Skouen, J., 2006. What is 'the good back-consultation'? A combined qualitative and quantitative study of chronic low back pain patients' interaction with and perceptions of consultations with specialitsts. J. Rehabil. Med. 38, 255–262.

LeBars, D., Dickenson, A., Besson, J.-M., 1979a. Diffuse noxious inhibitory controls (DNIC). 1. Effects on dorsal horn convergent neurones in the rat. Pain 6, 283–304.

LeBars, D., Dickenson, A., Besson, J.-M., 1979b. Diffuse noxious inhibitory controls (DNIC). 2. Lack of effect on non-convergent neurones, supraspinal involvement and theoretical implications. Pain 6, 305–327.

Lee, Y., Nassikas, N., Clauw, D., 2011. The role of the central nervous system in the generation and maintenance of chronic pain in rheumatoid arthritis, osteoarthritis and fibromyalgia. Arthritis Res. Ther. 13, 211.

Lewin, R., Bryson, M., 2010. The pain management plan: how people living with pain found a better life. Npowered, York.

Linton, S., 2000. A review of psychological risk factors in back and neck pain. Spine 25, 1148–1156.

Linton, S., Shaw, W., 2011. Impact of psychological factors in the experience of pain. Phys. Ther. 91, 700–711.

Loeser, J., Melzack, R., 1999. Pain: an overview. Lancet 353, 1607–1609.

Main, C., George, S., 2011. Psychologically informed practice for management of low back pain: future directions in practice and research. Phys. Ther. 91, 820–824.

Main, C., Sullivan, M., Watson, P., 2008. Pain management. Practical applications of the biopsychosocial perspective in clinical and occupational settings, second ed. Churchill Livingstone, Edinburgh.

Mallen, C., Peat, G., Thomas, E., et al., 2007. Prognostic factors for musculoskeletal pain in primary care: a systematic review. Br. J. Gen. Pract. 57, 655–661.

May, S., 2001. Patient satisfaction with management of back pain. Part 1: What is satisfaction? Review of satisfaction with medical management. Physiotherapy 87, 4–20.

Meeus, M., Nijs, J., Van Wilgen, P., et al., 2016. Moving on to movement in patients with chronic joint pain. Pain – Clinical Updates XXIV: 1–8.

Meeus, M., Vervisch, S., De Clerck, L., et al., 2012. Central sensitisation in patients with rheumatoid arthritis: a systematic literature review. Semin. Arthritis Rheum. 41, 556–567.

Merskey, H., Lindblom, U., Mumford, J., et al., 1994. Pain terms, a current list with definitions and notes on usage. In: Merskey, H., Bogduk, N. (Eds.), Classification of chronic pain. IASP Press, Seattle, pp. 207–214.

Moseley, G., 2003a. A pain neuromatrix approach to patients with chronic pain. Man. Ther. 8, 130–140.

Moseley, G., 2003b. Unraveling the barriers to reconceptualization of the problem in chronic pain: the actual and perceived ability of patients and health professionals to understand the neurophysiology. J. Pain 4, 184–189.

Moseley, G., Butler, D., 2015. Fifteen years of explaining pain: the past, present, and future. J. Pain 16, 807–813.

Nijs, J., van Wilgen, C., Van Oosterwijck, J., et al., 2012. How to explain central sensitisation to patients with 'unexplained' chronic musculoskeletal pain: practice guidelines. Man. Ther. 16, 413–418.

Petty, N., Ryder, D., 2017. Musculoskeletal examination and assessment: a handbook for therapists, fourth ed. Churchill Livingstone, Edinburgh.

Pincus, T., Burton, A., Vogel, S., et al., 2002. A systematic review of psychological factors as predictors of chronicity/disability in prospective cohorts of low back pain. Spine 27, E109–E120.

Pincus, T., Vogel, S., Santos, R., et al., 2006. The Attitudes to Back Pain Scale in musculoskeletal practitioners (ABS-mp). The development and testing of a new questionnaire. Clin. J. Pain 22, 378–386.

Price, D., Bushnell, M., 2004. Overview of pain dimensions and their psychological modulation. In: Price, D., Bushnell, M. (Eds.), Psychological methods of pain control: basic science and clinical perspectives. IASP Press, Seattle, pp. 3–17.

Ruscheweyh, R., Wilder-Smith, O., Drdla, R., et al., 2011. Long-term potentiation in spinal nociceptive pathways as a novel target for pain therapy. Mol. Pain 7, 20.

Ryder, D., van Griensven, H., 2017. Physical examination. In: Petty, N.J., Ryder, D. (Eds.), Musculoskeletal examination and assessment: a handbook for therapists. Churchill Livingstone, Edinburgh.

Sandkühler, J., 2013. Spinal cord plasticity and pain. In: McMahon, S.B., Koltzenburg, M. (Eds.), Wall & Melzack's textbook of pain, sixth ed. Saunders, Philadelphia, pp. 94–110.

Slade, S., Molloy, E., Keating, J., 2009. 'Listen to me, tell me': a qualitative study of partnership in care for people with non-specific chronic low back pain. Clin. Rehabil. 23, 270–280.

Sullivan, M., Bishop, S., Pivik, J., 1995. The pain catastrophizing scale: development and validation. Psychol. Assess. 7, 524–532.

Sullivan, M., Thorn, B., Haythornthwaite, J., et al., 2001. Theoretical perspectives on the relation between catastrophizing and pain. Clin. J. Pain 17, 52–64.

Synnott, A., O'Keeffe, M., Bunzli, S., et al., 2015. Physiotherapists may stigmatise or feel unprepared to treat people with low back pain and psychosocial factors that influence recovery: a systematic review. J. Physiother. 61, 68–76.

Theadom, A., Cropley, M., Smith, H., et al., 2015. Mind and body therapy for fibromyalgia. Cochrane Database Syst. Rev. (4), CD001980.

Todd, A., Koerber, H., 2013. Neuroanatomical substrates of spinal nociception. In: McMahon, S.B., Koltzenburg, M. (Eds.), Wall & Melzack's textbook of pain, sixth ed. Saunders, Philadelphia, pp. 77–93.

Toye, F., Seers, K., Allcock, N., et al., 2013. Patients' experiences of chronic non-malignant musculoskeletal pain: a qualitative systematic review. Br. J. Gen. Pract. e829–e841.

van Griensven, H., 2016. Patients' experiences of living with persistent back pain. Int. J. Osteopath. Med. 19, 44–49.

van Griensven, H., Ryder, D., 2017. Subjective examination. In: Petty, N.J., Ryder, D. (Eds.), Musculoskeletal examination and assessment: a handbook for therapists. Churchill Livingstone, Edinburgh.

Villanueva, L., Fields, H., 2004. Endogenous central mechanisms of pain modulation. In: Villanueva, L., Dickenson, A., Ollat, H. (Eds.), The pain system in normal and pathological states: a primer for clinicians. IASP Press, Seattle, pp. 223–243.

Vlaeyen, J., Linton, S., 2000. Fear-avoidance and its consequences in chronic musculoskeletal pain: a state of the art. Pain 85, 317–332.

Waddell, G., 2004. The back pain revolution, second ed. Churchill Livingstone, Edinburgh.

Waller, D., Sampson, A., 2015. Medical pharmacology and therapeutics, fourth ed. Saunders, Edinburgh.

Woby, S., Roach, N., Urmston, M., et al., 2005. Psychometric properties of the TSK-11: a shortened version of the Tampa Scale for Kinesiophobia. Pain 117, 137–144.

Woolf, C., 2011. Central sensitisation: implications for the diagnosis and treatment of pain. Pain 152, S2–S15.

Zhuo, M., 2015. Central sensitisation, synaptic potentiation, and microglia. In: Wilder-Smith, et al. (Eds.), Postoperative pain. Science and clinical practice. IASP Press, Washington DC, pp. 79–94.

9

PRINCIPLES OF COMMUNICATION AND ITS APPLICATION TO CLINICAL REASONING

LISA ROBERTS ■ NEIL LANGRIDGE

CHAPTER CONTENTS

The aim of this chapter is to develop your communication skills further to enhance your clinical practice and treatment outcomes.

THE POWER OF COMMUNICATION

Communication has been described as the most important aspect of practice that health professionals have to master (Wetherall et al. 1998). It impacts upon every clinical encounter and so must be one of the most highly developed skills in a therapist's toolkit. Furthermore, this high level of skill must be maintained throughout the patient's whole journey, from their first contact, right through to the time when they leave the service.

Whilst there are some core components to the communication skill set, these need to be finely tuned and tailored for every patient, as it is not the case that one size fits all. It is worth remembering too that, although it may not always be possible to achieve an excellent clinical outcome in every care episode, it should always be possible to ensure the patient has a positive experience.

Within healthcare, patient experience (or 'satisfaction') is increasingly used as an indicator of quality (Mazur et al. 2015) and is equally important across public and private health sectors. When patients go unheard, the result is 'careless communication, insincere apologies and unclear explanations' (Parliamentary and Health Service Ombudsman 2012). Furthermore, poor communication has been cited as one of the top three reasons for hospital complaints investigated by the Ombudsman Service, alongside errors in diagnosis and poor treatment (Parliamentary and Health Service Ombudsman 2014).

For such a key skill, it is interesting how little time therapists spend, once qualified, further developing communication skills, compared with clinical skills. Reading this, you might consider: how much time, in the last 12 months, have I dedicated specifically to improving my communication skills?

PREPARATIONS

Initial Contact

The first contact between a patient and the therapy service is an important marker for what is to follow. The patient may have initiated the contact, for example, through self-referral to the service, or it may be that the clinic has made contact by post, telephone, email or text, following receipt of a referral. It is important to give thought to both the appearance and content of this communication, as it shapes those all-important first impressions of the service. Asking patients for feedback about this part of the process when they have got to know the service can be illuminating and provide key insights for future service improvement.

For many patients, seeking healthcare is a considerable undertaking. They may have had to make complex plans to take time off from their usual activities, juggle roles as a carer, and encounter expense and hassle travelling to the clinic. They may be uncertain what therapy is and what an initial consultation might involve and have had considerable anxieties about this, ahead of their appointment.

It has been reported that many patients fail to get the best from their interactions with health professionals because they arrive 'unprepared and unequipped with the "right" questions' (Meredith et al. 1995). Providing clear information ahead of the consultation can help to minimize non-attendance, patients going to the wrong location, wearing inappropriate clothing, being unable to recall their current medication or not bringing reading glasses, for example.

Care must be taken to make any advice or instructions as patient-friendly as possible. During the course of our research, we encountered a patient with significant back pain who struggled into clinic carrying a huge bag of clothes, all because her appointment letter stated, 'please bring some shorts' and she didn't have any and so 'brought everything else in case', as she was so troubled by this single request and had lain awake thinking about it.

It is worth considering that communication skills are also an integral part of a raft of factors collectively known as 'non-specific treatment effects' that have the potential to impact significantly upon the outcome of a care episode. These include factors such as the Hawthorne effect (positive changes in behaviour that occur in individuals when interest is taken in them), touch, professionalism, the environment and the placebo effect. These cannot, and indeed should not, be ignored and it is important for clinicians to optimize these, to give their clinical skills the best chance of success.

Preparing Yourself

An important non-specific treatment effect that impacts greatly upon patients is the physical appearance of the clinician they are seeing. Does the clinician look neat and professional? Is the clinician's clothing clean and well ironed? These factors can readily be optimized, for example, by good personal hygiene, avoiding strong-smelling foods at mealtimes before working in clinic, avoiding strongly scented toiletries when in close proximity to the patient. As part of this close proximity, it is particularly important to think about the influence of touch in clinical practice, whether it be for empathic, facilitatory or therapeutic purposes. Good handling skills are a trademark of musculoskeletal practice and so extra care is needed to ensure nails are short and clean and any rough skin is well moisturized.

In addition to physical preparations, it is essential for clinicians to be aware of their own thought processes if they have received a referral letter ahead of the initial consultation:

Does it impact upon your thinking if you read any socioeconomic details like the patient:

- is currently off sick?
- has recurrent symptoms?
- is a single parent with a young family?
- has sustained a sporting injury?
- works as a health professional?
- has had multiple previous appointments in the service?
- has had previous therapy which the patient found to be unhelpful?
- is involved in litigation?

It is really important to be aware of these assumptions and to think about how they impact upon the communication style and content in the interaction that follows.

Preparing the Environment

Before inviting a patient into the clinical area, it is necessary to take a minute to check that the area is tidy, that there is clean paper on the couch and the furniture is arranged appropriately. This is all part of making the patient feel expected, welcome and valued (Fig. 9.1). As a parallel, think of a time when you have been staying somewhere unfamiliar, for example, on holiday, and that all-important moment when you first open the door to your accommodation. How would you feel if the furniture was strewn untidily and the bed unmade? Would you consider this to be acceptable?

Having a clinic room with solid walls rather than curtains can influence the communication that takes place, as patients may be more guarded if they perceive they can be overheard. Simple measures like having a radio or music playing could be an option, but in order to avoid copyright infringement in the UK, it is important to check whether the premises has a Performing Right Society (PRS) for Music licence for playing a radio or background music in public and also a Phonographic Performance Ltd (PPL) licence, which collects and distributes money for using recorded music on behalf of record companies and performers.

HISTORY TAKING

Meeting and Greeting

Taking time to smile and welcome patients can go a long way to making them feel at ease and it should not be underestimated how highly this is valued by patients. Indeed, for some, a smile has been deemed even more important than clinical competence. One patient in our research remarked: 'As long as there's a big smiley face I'm quite happy … a smiley face is more important than clinical skills!'

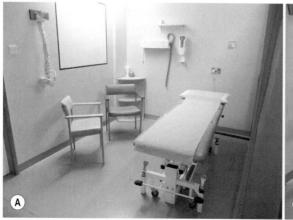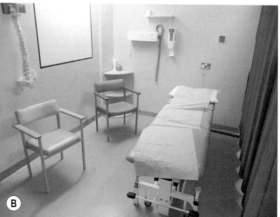

FIG. 9.1 (A, B) ■ You only have one chance to make a positive first impression – or not?

Do you introduce yourself with both first name and surname? Do you also give an indication of your level of experience, such as your job title? In undertaking a needs analysis with patients to develop a leaflet for our department, it was interesting that patients most wanted to know not only the name of their therapist, but also his or her level of experience (Roberts 2006), or as one patient put it, 'Are they any good?'

If the patient is attending with someone else, it is important to greet that person too, check that s/he has come with the patient and that the patient is happy for that individual to be present in the consultation, rather than waiting outside. It may sound simple, but we are aware of an instance when a parent and her son somehow managed to sit through an entire consultation for a totally unconnected patient. The situation occurred when the clinician called a patient's name and both adults and the child entered the clinic room, giving the appearance of being together. Neither party said anything about the other throughout the whole 45-minute lower-limb assessment. It was only at the end when the therapist gave the patient a slip to book in his next appointment and the woman stayed behind that the physiotherapist became aware they were not connected in any way!

Additional Clinicians

It may be that the clinician wishes an additional person to be present during a consultation, for example, a student, another colleague doing a peer observation, someone on work experience. It is essential that the clinician explains who this person is and why the individual wishes to be present. Where possible, it is preferable for patients to be asked in advance if they are willing for this, so that it is not sprung upon them as they arrive, or in the waiting room, without much time to think. Patients should be asked their opinion in a way that tries to reduce coercion as far as possible – i.e. in private, and away from the additional person, as the power differential in a clinician–patient relationship already makes it difficult for a patient to decline, and it is essential that the patient's autonomy be respected.

The Importance of First Impressions

As in any interaction, the clinician only has one chance to make a favourable first impression. Therefore it is essential that the therapist considers communication skills right from the outset, as it is reported to take only 39 ms for a first impression to be made (Bar et al. 2006) and 'many encounters' to change it (Tongue 2007).

Careful thought needs to be given to the use of small talk and social pleasantries. In our research, a therapist accompanied a patient from the waiting room into the clinic and, following an initial introduction, said to a patient 'How are you?' Later the patient confided to the researcher: 'It didn't start off well…when people say to me, "How are you?" I hate it, because that is like saying, I don't really care how you are actually, but I'm going to ask out of politeness.' Sincerity is key.

Having greeted the patient and entered the clinic room, according to Lipkin et al. (1995), there are three main purposes of a clinical consultation:

1. to gather information
2. to develop and maintain a therapeutic relationship
3. to communicate information.

The most important determinants of a 'good' consultation have been described in the literature as: (1) the patient's perception of being taken seriously; (2) giving an understandable explanation of the pain; (3) applying patient-centred care; (4) reassurance; and (5) being told what can be done (Lærum et al. 2006). Communication transcends all five of these.

The situation is further complicated by needing to consider not only what is said during a clinical encounter, but how the spoken word is conveyed, since communication traditionally incorporates verbal and non-verbal behaviours. The effectiveness of any verbal message passed on to another person relies on that person's ability to listen, hear and assimilate the message appropriately (Williams 1997). Meanwhile non-verbal communication describes all behaviours that convey messages without the use of verbal language (Oliver & Redfern 1991). There have been attempts in the literature to quantify the relative importance of these behaviours, with estimates of the non-verbal component comprising 55–97% (Caris-Verhallen et al. 1999), 90% (Hall & Lloyd 1990) and 93% of the message (Mehrabian 1971) and, although the figures vary, the non-verbal aspects of communication are consistently thought to be more influential than the verbal. Therefore, as Waddell says (2004), when the non-verbal message conflicts with the verbal message, we will probably not believe what is said.

Building Rapport

Along with compassion and empathy, rapport has been described as a cornerstone of a positive clinical encounter (Raja et al. 2015). During the initial phase, it begins to develop and history taking, if done well, resembles a conversation that tends to be paced and directed by both participants (McAllister et al. 2004), rather than an interview or, worse still, an interrogation.

Rapport is not only built by verbal communication skills, but is also affected by non-verbal gestures such as offering a handshake on introduction, making eye contact without prolonged staring or maintaining an open, non-threatening body posture (Casella 2015). Therefore, it is important for clinicians to think about how they sit during a consultation to show they are attentive and interested. Sitting back or slouching may give an impression of disengagement; meanwhile, a very forward-leaning posture can be intimidating, particularly if the clinician is positioned relatively close to the patient.

WHAT COMMUNICATION HAPPENS DURING A MUSCULOSKELETAL CONSULTATION?

The early stages of the clinical encounter are when patients present their problems to the clinician. Heritage and Robinson (2006) introduced the term 'problem presentation' to describe the stage at which patients disclose information about their symptoms to the clinician. This important component is reported to be the only time in a healthcare encounter when patients are given the opportunity to describe their condition in their own words and address their own personal agenda (Heritage & Robinson 2006).

Research has highlighted that clinicians' communication, and in particular, how they phrase their questions about the problem presentation can affect patient 'satisfaction' (Heritage & Robinson 2006; Robinson & Heritage 2006) as well as adherence to treatment (Zolnierek & Dimatteo 2009). Therefore, the clinician's skill in questioning is vital in establishing a good interpersonal relationship and setting the scene for the rest of the consultation.

Opening Questions

Communication within therapy is still underexplored, and little attention has been given to how 'best' to open clinical encounters. To study this phenomenon, our team audio-recorded 42 initial consultations and 17 first follow-up encounters between qualified physiotherapists and patients with back pain in an adult musculoskeletal, primary care outpatient setting (Chester et al. 2014). We identified 11 different opening questions in the initial consultations (Table 9.1) and seven in the follow-up visits (Table 9.2), which we then used to determine clinicians' preferences in a national survey, posted on the four most relevant professional networks (sports medicine, orthopaedics, massage and soft-tissue

TABLE 9.1
Results From the National Survey Showing the Preferred Phrasing of the Key Clinical Question in Initial Consultations Between Physiotherapists and Patients With Low-Back Pain (Chester et al. 2014)

Preferences	Score	Phrase
1st	83	Do you want to just tell me a little bit about [problem presentation, e.g. knee, back] first of all?
2nd	77	I've had this referral through. Tell me what's happened
3rd	71	The referral says you've got [problem presentation]; is this correct?
4th	65	How can I help you today?
5th	57	What we'll do today is just have a bit of a chat about [problem presentation], I believe it is. All right?
6th	45	It's your [problem presentation] that you're here for, is it?
7th	35	What problem are you having at the moment?
8th	30	Do you want to tell me your story?
9th	29	Do you want to start off by telling me whereabouts you're getting your pain at the moment?
10th	28	I know a little bit from the GP; when did this start?
11th	17	How long have you had [problem presentation] for?

TABLE 9.2

Results From the National Survey Showing the Preferred Phrasing of the Key Clinical Question in a Follow-Up Clinical Encounter Between Physiotherapists and Patients With Low-Back Pain (Chester et al. 2014)

Preferences	Score	Phrase
1st	158	How have you been since I last saw you?
2nd	131	How did you get on with the [treatment, e.g. exercises, hydro, injection, massage]?
3rd	82	How have you been feeling from a [problem presentation, e.g. knee, back] point of view?
4th	71	How are you getting on?
5th	54	How have you been?
6th	18	Are the [problem presentation] symptoms ongoing?
7th	12	What was the take-home message that you got from me last time?

therapy, and pain management) of the national, interactive Chartered Society of Physiotherapy (iCSP) website, to canvass opinion more widely.

The preferred 'key clinical question' for an initial encounter among the 43 physiotherapists who responded was: 'Do you want to just tell me a little bit about [your problem presentation] first of all?' and, for follow-up encounters: 'How have you been since I last saw you?' Although the survey response in this study was small, this paper has generated much debate among clinicians on their preferences for opening patient encounters and optimizing non-specific treatment effects.

Questioning Styles

Developing skills in questioning is key to gaining information in a clinical encounter and enhancing the therapeutic relationship. It is important to keep questions short and simple, ensuring that they only address one issue at a time. Asking closed questions, for example, 'Have you got another appointment booked?' is likely to result in a short, focused answer to this yes/no interrogative. Meanwhile, open questions such as, 'How is your knee pain affecting you?' will invite patients to

give a fuller account and can be particularly helpful in establishing the history and impact of the patient's symptoms.

'TED' questions can provide a rich source of data, and these are questions that involve: 'tell', 'explain' or 'describe' stems. For example: 'Can you tell me how your neck pain started?'; 'Can you explain how these symptoms are affecting your life at the moment?'; 'Can you describe the feeling in your leg?' These can really encourage patients to share their experiences with the clinician and provide useful insights when it comes to mutually identifying possible treatment goals.

Sensitive Questioning

It is worth considering your own personal values when asking certain questions, as the reason to ask the question should ultimately be to inform clinical reasoning. Care must be taken to ensure questions do not come across as judgemental or bias the patient to give a socially desirable answer, especially when, in practice, clinicians often want to ask about levels of activity, working status and current personal relationships. The clinician wishes to know this to allow links to be made in the narrative story, and insight to be gained into the psychological and social aspects of the presentation (Nicholas et al. 2011). The nature of the question may drive an emotional reaction from patients, such as asking about social activities, as possibly patients have not been able to engage in sports/leisure pursuits for some time due to their pain and this may lead to them finding the question upsetting to consider. Therefore, although this question helps in the reasoning process, it may have a negative consequence on how patients perceive themselves, and therefore on the patient–clinician relationship. You might consider asking the question in a less direct way, to take away the personal value of the question:

> Clinician: 'In many cases like this the patient tends to find certain activities challenging to get back to.'
> Patient: 'Yes, I can imagine.'
> Clinician: 'Are you in a similar position?'
> Patient: 'Yes, I am.'
> Clinician: 'Can you tell me about that?'

This leaves the question open, is less threatening and allows the narrative reasoning to be explored and perhaps even narrowed down once the patient has begun the process. It is also important to offer a non-judgemental style towards patients who have life choices that do not concur with your own values. For example, healthcare professionals who themselves have higher fear avoidance beliefs towards their own healthcare are more likely to advise rest rather than activity (Ostelo et al. 2003), and so, when communicating behavioural change, it is just as important to consider your own motivations before applying these to patient care. Therefore, whilst needing to know about habits, health values and life choices to aid in understanding patients as well as their condition, applying communication skills sensitively offers the opportunity to explore with depth as rapport builds and the patient–clinician relationship moves forward.

Handing Over Control

As well as giving patients opportunities to address their agenda through careful opening questions and judicious use of silence, it can be really helpful to ask questions during history taking that are phrased in a way specifically to hand over control. For example, 'You know your body better than anyone; what do you think is happening in your [problem presentation, e.g. neck]?' This shifts the balance of power to the patient, as the clinician is not presupposing a specific angle or problem, or displaying prior knowledge of the patient's problem, in what Heritage (2012) calls a less knowledgeable (K–) epistemic status. This can reveal some interesting and important beliefs; for example, if a patient has concerns that the label of 'degeneration' in their spine means they think their spine is crumbling, this will be a useful starting point to discuss their beliefs, in readiness for any decisions about possible treatment options. It is useful to explore these beliefs and what or who has influenced them, especially as many patients now search the internet before seeking healthcare.

Another particularly revealing question to ask at the end of history taking can be, 'Before we go on to have a look at your [problem presentation, e.g. back], is there anything else that we haven't talked about that you think is important and want to raise?' Again, this provides an opportunity for patients to address their agenda, add further detail to what has already been mentioned and lessen the chance of new problems being identified in the closing minutes of the consultation.

ACTIVE LISTENING

Sacks et al. (1974) maintain that people take turns to talk by following a set of conventional rules that assign speaker time and direction, and any deviation could indicate a person's attempt to display power, status or influence. Practical guides to clinical communication skills concur with Sacks' model and the two most important skills have been identified as: the ability to allow the patient to speak without interruption; and the ability truly to hear what the patient is trying to say (Jackson 2006).

In developing patient-centred care, clinicians are advised to attend not only to the disease, but to patients' experience of symptoms, the impact of the condition and what really matters for them (Pollock 2001; Walseth et al. 2011).

Silence Is Golden

As well as knowing what to say, a key skill for the clinician to master is to know when to be silent and, as in the title of the book by Cathy Jackson, to *Shut up and Listen!* (Jackson 2006). Even short pauses can be very empowering for patients and provide them with an opportunity to bring up an issue that is really important to them.

Audio-recording consultations, with patients' permission, can be a really useful learning tool to help clinicians see whether there are any periods of silence in their consultations and, if so, what follows from the patient: is it a question; a more affective account of their symptoms and how they are impacting upon the patient's life; or an expression of a deeper worry or concern?

Empathy

Empathy is difficult to define and is considered in medicine to be an understanding and communication of a patient's experience (Pedersen 2008). Cox et al. (2012) define empathy as the 'ability to understand and identify with the feelings or emotional states of others… comprising both affective and cognitive aspects', which Misch and Peloquin (2005) describe as 'having empathy' and 'showing empathy', respectively.

It is not clear when or how some clinicians successfully acquire a high level of empathic skills. When Millie Allen, in our group, conducted three focus groups with different grades of physiotherapists about empathy, the majority of clinicians considered it to be an innate characteristic. For example, one senior clinician said: 'It's not something that you can just go on a course and learn, accept that it is something that will probably get better and better over time … accept that it is there as something to be developed as part of your practice.' This much-coveted, holy grail of communication is both highly valued and worthy of future research.

The Content of Musculoskeletal Consultations

In comparison with medicine, there has been little work identifying communication practices within physiotherapy and even less examining the associations between communication practice and outcomes (Parry 2008). We undertook a cross-sectional, observational study to measure the verbal communication taking place between clinicians and 25 patients with back pain in a UK primary care setting (Roberts et al. 2013). The mean duration of the initial consultations was 38 minutes and 59 seconds (range 26 minutes 21 seconds–53 minutes 16 seconds). The content of the audio recordings was categorized using the Medical Communications Behavior System (Wolraich et al. 1982), which categorizes 13 clinician behaviours and seven patient behaviours and has three miscellaneous categories (as shown in Table 9.3, with added examples from our research).

Our results showed that the physiotherapists spoke more than the patients (49.5% vs. 33.1%, respectively), with the most prevalent categories of speech being 'history/background probes' and 'content remarks', respectively, as clinicians asked questions about patients' symptoms and patients discussed how these affected their lives. Both groups spent little time overtly discussing emotions (1.4% and 0.9%, respectively). Analysis further highlighted the prominence of 'advice' given in the initial consultation, constituting 12.5% of the total time, establishing it as a key player in the physiotherapist's treatment repertoire, which should not be underestimated (Roberts et al. 2013).

Interruptions

In this work mapping the verbal content of physiotherapy consultations, we noted that concurrent talk was more prevalent among experienced clinicians compared with less experienced practitioners (7.6% vs. 2.6%, respectively) and interruptions were common (Roberts et al. 2013). A further analysis of 42 audio-recorded initial consultations demonstrated that physiotherapists interrupted patients answering the key opening question about their back pain in 60% of cases. This is not unique to physiotherapy: Marvel et al. (1999) found, in a sample of 264 consultations with primary care family physicians in the USA, that 45.5% of patients were interrupted (or 'redirected') while giving their 'statement of concerns' and this was associated with fewer concerns mentioned by patients, late-arising concerns and missed opportunities to gather important patient data. On average, patients were given 23.1 seconds to itemize their concerns before interruption from the physician (Marvel et al. 1999).

Langewitz et al. (2002) reported that patients will take, on average, 92 seconds to explain their problem in an outpatient setting if they are not interrupted. Studies have shown, however, that 25–76% of patients are interrupted by physicians before they finish talking, and the mean talking time is reduced to only 12–23 seconds (Beckman & Frankel 1984; Marvel et al. 1999; Rhodes et al. 2001). Interruptions are not restricted to the problem presentation stage; they can occur at any time during the clinical encounter and be by either the patient or clinician (Beckman & Frankel 1984). Such interruptions may lead to delays in patients expressing their concerns (Irish & Hall 1995) and the clinician missing opportunities to gather relevant information (Beckman & Frankel 1984; Marvel et al. 1999).

Two different types of 'interruptions' have been identified: 'overlaps' and 'interruptions'. Kitzinger (2008) has described an interruption as a start-up at a point in a speaker's talk where it cannot possibly be completed, and an overlap as an error in projecting where a speaker is planning to end his or her turn. At present these definitions are not universal and, in practice, the two terms are often applied interchangeably (Drummond 1989; Kitzinger 2008).

It is important for clinicians to be aware of the extent to which they interrupt patients and the impact this has on an interaction.

THE 'THREATENED STATE' AND COMMUNICATION

In a clinical environment, patients may be presenting with increased social and emotional stresses placed upon them and these 'yellow flags' are well documented in

TABLE 9.3			
Examples of the Categories in the Medical Communications Behavior System (MCBS) **(Wolraich et al. 1982)**			
	Category	**Includes**	**Example From Research**[a]
Physiotherapist	Content behaviours	History/background probes	'And did you have the back discomfort at the time or was it purely just the leg pain?' (patient 5: line 33)
		Checks for understanding information	'When you were told about you having the sort of wear and tear and the arthritis … was it explained to you exactly what is going on?' (patient 1: line 412)
		Advice/suggestion	'If you bring your leg up towards your chest for me and just hug the knee, can you feel that sort of stretching out the back here?' (patient 5: line 781)
		Restatement	'Just to go back to when it started, you said it started to get worse about a year ago?' (patient 7: line 54)
		Clarification	(Following a patient's description of her recurring symptoms): 'So it [the back pain] was sort of episodic?' (patient 4: line 37)
	Affective behaviours	Emotional probes	'How would you feel about … me referring you to one of the community rehabilitation teams, who can come out and see you in your home … and see if there's anything that we can do to help you?' (patient 9: line 385)
		Reassurance/ support	'So the fact that you can control it [the back pain] quite well – not to worry at the moment' (patient 1: line 477)
		Reflection of feelings	Patient: 'I'm just concerned it might be arthritis going into my back …' Therapist: 'Right. That's what you, how you're thinking?' (patient 1: line 776)
		Encourages/ acknowledges	'I know what you mean' (patient 1: line 547)
	Negative behaviours	Disapproval	'Tsk. OK. OK. So, I'm still trying to ascertain when the right hip pain came on' (patient 20: line 116)
		Disruptions	(Knock at the door) 'Oh sorry, do you mind if I just quickly answer that?' (patient 2: line 1011)
		Jargon	'I'm going to teach you an exercise … which is to work on your transversus abdominis, which is a deep, core stabilizing muscle, OK?' (patient 4: line 605)
Patient	Content behaviours	Content questions	(Responding to an answer on a health questionnaire to the question 'Do you have diabetes?'): 'Did I tick that by mistake?' (patient 10: line 81)
		Content remarks	'Oh well, I crouched down to get the bag from under my bed and you know, something went' (patient 3: line 39)
		Checks for understanding	'What I'm gathering is, I have to re-strengthen the muscles that have become … like an elastic band. They've gone really thin? Huh?' (patient 2: line 1306)
	Affective behaviours	Encourages	'I would say that was spot on' (patient 14: line 90)
		Emotional expressions	'I think it's the old situation of, I've hurt myself, I'm a bit scared and I don't really want to do anything again, yeah' (patient 2: line 585)
	Negative behaviours	Disapproval	Therapist: 'It's too hot outside?' Patient: 'Well, it is when you've got to walk round in circles in this hospital' (patient 7: line 5)
		Disruptions	e.g. Knock on the door from another clinician enquiring whether the room contains a particular piece of equipment
	Miscellaneous categories	Social amenities	'Come on in and have a seat. Right. Did you catch my name?' (patient 6: line 4)
		Silence	
		Unclassifiable	e.g. When the physiotherapist and patient talk over each other

[a]Research of Roberts et al. (2013).

the literature. Melzack (1999) details many of the factors that can precipitate persistent pain after injury and suggests that cortisol, as well as autoimmune chemicals, can have a negative effect on the psychological status associated with stress, which can, if not addressed, subsequently lead to hypersensitivity and poor tissue health. A stressor can be defined as any stimulus that threatens normal homeostatic mechanisms (Melzack 2001) and can include events such as sudden changes in body temperature or blood pressure, prolonged reduction in food intake, illness, infection and pain (Dickerson et al. 2009), in addition to fear, worry, bereavement or unemployment.

The body's first defence against homeostatic challenge is the sympathetic nervous system response of fight or flight. This response is felt to be addressed by the hypothalamic–pituitary–adrenocortical (HPA) axis that regulates the release of cortisol, an important hormone associated with psychological, physiological and physical health functioning (Dickerson & Kemeny 2004). Fig. 9.2 outlines the relationship between the hormones and ongoing action between the axis; the negative feedback relates to the release of cortisol and suppressing further action.

However, as well as providing the energy substrates that support the sympathetic responses, the HPA stress axis is responsible for both the cognitive assessment of the stressful situation as well as the behavioural and endocrine adaptation to stress (Melzack 2001). Therefore, the clinician needs to understand the 'threatened state' in patients presenting with ongoing pain to enable the clinical encounter to be as successful as possible. In acknowledging this physiological state, clinicians should

be aware of their own words and actions that could result in further stressing the patient and leading to additional negative emotional, behavioural and physiological responses that in essence are revealed as negative responses to treatment. Good communication skills here are vital, as the patient will likely attend with worry, anxiety and concern as to the nature of the presentation and outcome of the care episode.

Key components in addressing the 'threatened state' include good observation of the patient's initial communicative behaviours, facial expression, body positions, sounds and actions associated with movement, which all may display some catastrophizing traits. When placed in the context of a clinical examination, these behaviours may become magnified as patients try to communicate to the clinician the levels of pain and distress that they are experiencing (Vlaeyen et al. 2009). It is worth remembering that reported pain and associated reduction in facial expression can occur during times of perceived social threat, as demonstrated by Peeters and Vlaeyen (2011), who noted, in patients with high levels of catastrophizing, that when a perceived painful stimulus is applied with an associated rise in pain, facial expression is reduced.

When asking about certain activities and social interactions, it is worth noting the patient's facial expression, whether the patient's body position is open, or any associated behaviours indicating anxiety, such as nail biting or hand clasping, which may communicate to the clinician a level of associated stress. As the clinician, you may wish to explore these at the time of interview. This may put patients in a less anxious state if they are reassured that they will not be asked to perform anything that they are uncomfortable with. It will be worth asking and exploring what the barriers and concerns may be in attempting certain physical movements, such as bending, or picking an object up. This method of communicative inquiry will enable the clinician to start to understand the barriers to recovery, and the behavioural changes needed that will enhance recovery. Posing the question about certain tasks can be as simple as: 'You look worried about that, is anything in particular concerning you?' And it can easily be followed up with the social context, as in the example of bending. The way to reinforce positive messages about bending would be to communicate it is safe, that it won't cause damage, that it may be uncomfortable but

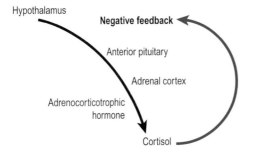

FIG. 9.2 ■ The hypothalamic–pituitary–adrenocortical (HPA) axis.

this is the body's way of overprotecting itself, and that together you will work through this; whilst acknowledging the patient's pain, you will explain that the exercises will be gentle and manageable. This communication is valuable and even in the early phases of the clinical assessment it can powerfully aid in reducing anxiety, encourage confidence and therefore improve the pain experience.

Challenging Conversations

Sometimes it can be difficult to discuss social and emotional issues with patients. Indeed, it has been reported that doctors have been loath to inquire about the social and emotional impact of patients' problems for fear it will increase the patients' distress, take up too much time and threaten their own emotional survival. Consequently, they respond to emotional cues with strategies to block further disclosure: offering advice and reassurance before the main problems have been identified, explaining away distress as normal, attending to physical aspects only, switching topic or 'jollying' patients along (Maguire & Pitceathly 2002). It is important for therapists to be aware of times when they are tempted to, or indeed do, use such strategies and the consequences.

Another source of challenging conversation can be when a patient becomes upset during a clinical encounter. It is essential to have a box of tissues to hand that the patient can readily access, should the need arise. Sharing such moments can be a powerful component in a therapeutic relationship, as the patient conveys emotional distress and, although the clinician may be feeling quite helpless and not know what to say, sometimes words are not necessary and just being there and listening is a source of comfort.

If given time and space to cry, patients will stop at their own pace. Ensuring privacy is important and it might help to use phrases like, 'I'm so sorry this is so difficult for you', or 'please take your time', which gives them some space, whilst acknowledging they are really struggling. However difficult the situation, it is important to resist any urges to ask the patient to stop crying, or for clinicians to display their own embarrassment or awkwardness. This is a time when it can be really helpful to relinquish control and let the patient lead. It can be an opportunity to find out more about the patient's coping skills and what has helped in the past – knowledge

that can be useful to help the patient think about facing the difficulties that lie ahead.

Even the most experienced clinicians can feel really challenged when patients become angry or distressed and it is important to seek support and debrief with colleagues to help process the experience and further develop your healthy coping skills for the future.

When feeding back to colleagues about experiences, it is essential to avoid labelling patients as 'yellow flaggy', 'heart sink', displaying 'psychological overlay' or 'supratentorial'. This has damaging consequences for the patient, for your credibility and for the profession. An example of explaining findings in a professional, non-judgemental way might be: 'The patient presented with causal beliefs that his pain was the direct result of the lifting incident at work, with subsequent loss of personal control, negative treatment beliefs and significant consequences, including loss of earnings, potential job security and inability to return to his twice-weekly football.' Feeding back to referring medical colleagues about the care episode provides an opportunity to demonstrate the professional, sensitive and thorough communication skills that therapists can deliver.

THE PHYSICAL EXAMINATION

When the clinician has completed the clinical interview, it is of value to summarize the findings and explain the possible diagnoses that are being considered as this again will inform the patient whilst giving the context to the physical examination.

Having completed the history-taking aspect of the consultation, the next stage is usually to undertake a physical examination. It is important for therapists not to lose sight of anxieties patients may feel at having to get undressed. Simple measures, like leaving the cubicle while the patient undresses and providing a towel/ blanket nearby to preserve the patient's dignity can all help in this respect. The therapist's communication skills can go a long way to smoothing what might be a potentially difficult situation here. For example, explaining to patients why it is necessary to ask them to remove an item of clothing is only courteous. It is important to think about the wording of such a question and avoid potentially patronizing phrases such as, 'Please could you take off your shirt for me'. Are you asking them to remove an item of clothing or instructing them?

Do they have any choice in the matter? What verb have you used – need, want, invite, encourage? Are you being culturally sensitive?

It is vital during initial observations that the therapist explains what s/he is looking for, so that s/he does not appear just to be staring at the patient in a state of undress, which patients can find degrading and humiliating. For example, in our research about expectations, when we asked patients about what they were hoping would happen at their first appointment, one patient (who had previously attended physiotherapy) replied, 'not asking you to do things that make you look absolutely ridiculous like take too many clothes off and stand/walk around like it'.

The therapist can help allay some concerns when observing the patient's posture by simply explaining that s/he is looking at the shape of the person's spine, comparing the muscle formations on the right and left side and looking for any signs of swelling or spasm. Not only is this showing respect for the patient, it can also lessen the chance of dissatisfaction with the consultation, as examples exist where patients have formally complained about clinicians 'making' them get undressed and staring at them, which they found 'humiliating'.

A physical test can be significantly influenced by the patient's state of fear, concern and anxiety and this will ultimately affect the outcome. By reducing this threatened state the clinician is more able to find reproducible outcomes that will make clinical sense – a patient who is experiencing high sensitivity, when examined with poor communication but great handling, will ultimately give false positives. So, set the scene: 'I would like to place my hands here and lift your leg, and the reason to do this is to test…'; follow that with 'the responses that may occur might be…could you inform me if you feel these or anything else?', and lastly, 'you are in charge; if you would like me to stop please tell me'. This will help gain a clearer understanding and will fully inform the patient of what is expected whilst enabling a reasoning cycle to be informed by the clinical data.

THE POWER OF TOUCH AND ITS ROLE IN COMMUNICATION

With the patient suitably undressed and the physical examination under way, it is important for clinicians specifically to think about their touch, which is considered a core element of therapeutic practice in many health disciplines. Touch can be communicating a form of emotion or delivering elements of clinical enquiry as part of the reasoning process. It can be considered a non-verbal form of expression that links directly to the verbal components of communication, and so when delivered in harmony, these two components can be very powerful. It also has a number of different roles for the clinician: it may be something you use when you meet a patient, to help with building rapport, such as greeting the patient with a handshake; it can help pinpoint areas of pain or discomfort and/or may have featured as an affective behaviour demonstrated by the clinician during history taking, to help express empathy. For the therapist, it also forms a key therapeutic skill; for example, when delivering treatment, it can be used to demonstrate an exercise and provide feedback to the patient when s/he attempts to follow this advice, as well as in a therapeutic manner, for example, to deliver treatment (such as manual therapy). Nathan (1999) describes communicating through manual therapy as a complex mixture of non-invasive, non-threatening assessments and treatments that are patient-centred and caring in nature. Considering the nature, manner and context of touch can also be regarded as a powerful therapeutic mediator, engaging psychological and physiological responses.

When working through a clinical interview, a patient may have anxieties and concerns that may be expressed to the clinician when discussing the clinical details. Whilst wanting to explore these concerns, it can be helpful, when displaying empathy and sincerity, to communicate this through affective touch, such as placing a hand on the patient's arm or hand. Importantly, this would not linger and would be context-appropriate, yet by doing so the clinician is able to reinforce the care and attention being shown. In a qualitative study exploring the role of touch in physiotherapy (Hiller et al. 2015), the research highlighted themes including the demonstration of care, empathy and reassurance. When the clinicians were interviewed they surprisingly reported rarely using touch as a method of communication, as opposed to the patients, who felt it reproduced a sense of genuine care. Patients therefore in this study expected and welcomed appropriate communicative touch as part of the clinical experience. This was also supported in primary care in a qualitative study, where general practitioners felt touch was an 'instinctive' element of the clinical interaction, and subsequently improves a patient's well-being (Cocksedge et al. 2013).

Touch can also help identify areas of discomfort and pain as part of the palpatory exploration. This can demonstrate to the patient that the clinician has knowledge, is responsive and confirms a level of skill, and so by doing so this can reduce the 'threatened state' of the patient and allow the context of the pain to be established. 'Finding' or reproducing pain with touch and palpation is an important communicative medium of assessment, and helps with confirming a diagnosis or source of pain. It may highlight the sensitivity of the patient's tissues, or lead the clinician to understand better the pain mechanism, such as neuropathic pain/sensitivity and sensory change. This can be particularly helpful in supporting or refuting a clinical hypothesis. Once again, it is vital to explain the nature of touch and the importance of the communication from the patient whilst s/he experiences the palpation.

Communicating what is a normal response and understanding what might be abnormal, painful or natural discomfort is imperative for clinical accuracy. For example, palpating tissues firmly without communicating what the clinician is doing, why s/he is doing it, and what information is needed from the patient is likely to be threatening, confusing and uncomfortable. Clearly explaining what you are doing and how this helps in developing a clinical diagnosis is important.

Clinician: 'I would like to put my hands on you to see how your muscles feel. Is that OK?'
Patient: 'Yes, that is fine'.
Clinician: 'Some of my pressure may be a bit uncomfortable. I won't be doing anything that could damage you. Is that OK?'
Patient: 'Yes, that's fine'.
Clinician: 'I'm really interested to know if my pressure causes discomfort and perhaps it may be the familiar pain you have been experiencing. It would be really helpful to know if that happens'.
Patient: 'OK, I'll tell you'.
Clinician: 'If I perhaps first press an area that is not normally painful so you can understand the pressure and the normal response, that will then help you to help me work out where you might be feeling your symptoms, OK?'

Patients attending a clinical assessment may expect that an element of touch will occur and may also feel it is a vital component of being examined and understood. If effective hands-on assessment and treatment are not given or offered, it is vital that it is effectively communicated to the patient as this will be therapeutically unhelpful if poorly explained. Expectation is well documented to have a significant role in non-specific treatment effects, which can enhance recovery; therefore the role of touch or not touching must be explained.

When providing treatment that involves touch, the clinician has to set the scene by clearly explaining what to expect and the language that accompanies treatment can be very powerful. For example, McCabe et al. (2008) demonstrated that the application of cream was enhanced when the cream was described as 'rich moisturizing' versus 'basic'. In this study of 12 healthy volunteers one single lotion was used; however, the labelling was different in its description. The experimenter was blinded to the labels and the subjects reported ratings of pleasantness and richness. Functional magnetic resonance imaging testing, that enables a picture of brain activation, demonstrated activation with the 'rich moisturizing' expectation was more widespread and correlated to an improved subjective experience. In a study involving 11 male and 11 female healthy volunteers, the team examined the physiological response to touch massage to the hands and feet; the authors observed a decrease in heart rate (within 5 minutes and sustained for 65 minutes) and a reduction in cortisol levels, indicating a reduction in stress/threat (Lindgren et al. 2010). The mechanical elements of this treatment would be minimal; however, the non-verbal communication of touch delivered via therapeutic treatment was physiologically and psychologically likely to be beneficial.

A manual therapist with good handling techniques will not be successful if that mechanical expertise is not accompanied by expert communication. An example of this interaction is set out below.

Clinician: 'I would like to apply some hands-on treatment now. It may begin with being a little sore; is that OK?'

Patient: 'Yes, that is fine'.
Clinician: 'If it becomes too sore, please let me know'.
Patient: 'Yes, I will'.
Clinician: 'I would expect as you get used to the treatment that the initial soreness subsides. Would you also let me know if this is the case?'

Conversely, patients expecting treatment to be painful and inclusive of their symptoms need to be informed that perhaps a certain treatment will not be painful, and the reasons why this is the case. It is also appropriate practice to explain the rationale, expected benefits, expected side-effects and the science behind what you are doing (see Gaining consent, below).

ARTICULATING THE ASSESSMENT FINDINGS

Perceptions of Diagnosis

One of the most challenging aspects of a clinical consultation is to explain to the patient the findings from the assessment, in readiness for discussions about further investigations or potential treatment options. When the going gets tough, it is common for clinicians to regress to using jargon and to make assumptions about the patient's level of knowledge. The only way to be clear about patients' understanding of their symptoms is to ask them, which is why questions like, 'You know your body better than anyone; what do you think is happening?' are an excellent place to start.

Patients essentially want to know what is causing the problem, what can be done about it and how quickly/will it resolve? They want a simple strapline of what is wrong so that when a family member, friend or work colleague asks how they got on at their appointment, they can legitimize their symptoms and give a short account of what is at fault.

Unfortunately, clinicians do not help the situation when using words like 'chronic', to mean the symptoms have prevailed for more than 3 months, as one use of 'chronic' in everyday language, often used by teenagers, is more akin to dire. Then there is the notion of 'degeneration': we don't talk about the skin or hair degenerating with age and a 'degenerative spine' conjures up all sorts of horrors for patients. A less fearful option to use is 'age-related changes'. Likewise, 'wear and tear' can induce fear, as patients are left wondering what is

actually tearing? It is little wonder, then, if a clinician tries to minimize concerns by saying, 'Your chronic back pain is caused by mild degeneration and a small amount of wear and tear to the spine', the patient becomes fearful, as s/he may be hearing the situation is dire, the spine is crumbling and physically weakening by structures that are tearing. Ouch!

CLINICAL REASONING AND ITS INFLUENCE ON COMMUNICATION

The clinical reasoning process is a complex interaction of knowledge, clinical data, experience and patient understanding. As clinicians, we are asking questions of our patients, ourselves and the literature to help construct a clinical diagnosis and formulate a treatment plan. The challenge is to do this all at the same time whilst building and maintaining rapport, which is not easy. This demanding environment is a symbiotic relationship, underpinned by relationship building and knowledge, and is one that is considerably enhanced by good communication skills. Alongside the flexibility in communication style, it is imperative to have flexibility in reasoning style, as they are interdependent, and together enable patient-centred care.

Clinical reasoning is about assimilating all the available evidence, gleaning information about the patient prior to the consultation, such as the referral letter (if one is available) or reviewing any previous notes, followed by a clinical interview that helps the clinician formulate hypotheses, that are then tested in the physical examination. Throughout a clinical encounter, the clinician is using evidence from both verbal and non-verbal skills to gain an understanding of the clinical presentation, its impact and the rehabilitation goals and also ensuring safety, such as interpreting questions regarding cauda equina syndrome or cervical arterial symptoms.

The structure and order of the questions can be vital in gaining this information and therefore constructing hypotheses, in collaboration with the patient, using knowledge gleaned from observation, interpretation and communication, will ultimately allow this process to seem a comfortable experience for both parties. It may also be helpful to explain why certain questions are being asked, as this will help patients understand the context and encourage them to speak freely. In an

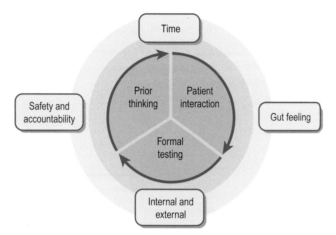

FIG. 9.3 ■ A model to demonstrate the clinical reasoning processes of physiotherapists assessing patients with low-back pain. *(From Langridge et al. 2015, with permission.)*

observational study of 10 physiotherapists discussing their clinical reasoning processes following an assessment of a patient with low-back pain in primary care, clinicians were asked to discuss their reasoning and how they came to understand the patient presentation (Langridge et al. 2015). The clinicians discussed elements of communication and how they interpreted this as well as their interaction with the patients. From the data, the key features of this process were identified (Fig. 9.3).

Within this model, the internal features of patient interaction, prior thinking and formal testing are all integral to the clinical assessment and require good communication skills to elicit data, used to inform the clinician. There are also other themes noted, such as being safe, which require communication/interpretation skills, leading to a contextual understanding of important information, such as changes in bladder/bowel function in cauda equina syndrome. Fig. 9.4 highlights a hypothetico-deductive model, underpinned by knowledge, data collection and synthesis. This further demonstrates that, although this reasoning approach is a cognitive process, reasoning is collaborative and therefore, without effective communication, constructive clinical reasoning is not possible. Planning and conducting the clinical interview will involve multiple models of reasoning and this chapter is not designed to explore every one of those, but shows how communication skills link to commonly cited models of reasoning and makes suggestions on how best to enhance these skills.

When planning a physical examination, clinical reasoning should underpin every question that is asked, and every test that is completed. A clinical question should help support a possible presentation, pathology or syndrome that the clinician may be considering as the cause of the symptoms; however, some questions may also mean that the hypothesis is less likely, allowing the clinician to build a picture of the diagnosis and potential treatment plan. Being adaptive in styles of questioning will help support the clinician in understanding different elements of the presentation. For example, a more narrative approach allows a clinical story to unfold (Mattingly 1991), allowing the patient to speak without interruption which may feel as if you, as the clinician, are unable to get the information that you feel is needed; however, it is likely that, if allowed to, the patient will give many of the answers that are required.

The hypothetico-deductive method of reasoning is a more focused approach and, as its name suggests, is a way of being specific from a general position in a logical way (Edwards et al. 2004). Patients will expect specific questions and it is generally advisable to start with the open approach and, once a basic understanding of the possible problems has been gained, the clinician can then begin to ask specific questions that narrow the possibilities down. These questions need to be clear, and it is also important not to repeat questions later in the interview, as this will suggest to the patient that

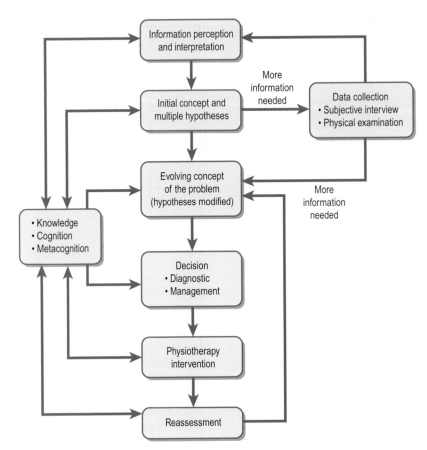

FIG. 9.4 ▪ Clinical reasoning model for physical therapists. *(From Jones 1992.)*

the clinician is not actively listening to the responses. It is however good practice to clarify the responses and this will offer patients reassurance that they have been listened to and heard.

There may be occasions in the reasoning process when the clinician feels confident of the clinical diagnosis and is able quickly to link the data to previous experience and knowledge. This form of reasoning is described as 'pattern recognition' (Noll et al. 2001) and is a proposed 'faster' method of considering the clinical data and variables by being able to see a familiar pattern of symptoms that fit a standard clinical picture. This reasoning process, if not appropriately supported in good communication, may feel to the patient that the clinician has not listened or appears uninterested, but equally a sense of confidence from the clinician may raise the levels of reassurance for the patient. A poor

experience of this type of reasoning is easily negated by good follow-up comments such as, 'yes, this is not uncommon' or perhaps, 'I have seen this before', which will foster a decrease in threat and a feeling of confidence in the clinician.

EXPLORING YOUR OWN BELIEFS AND BIAS

When reasoning through a patient presentation and trying to make sense of the information, a clinician will use past experiences to support the diagnosis. Sometimes clinicians can be at fault for making assumptions about a presentation and also trying to make the presentation 'fit' their own model of what might be wrong. Commonly, the reason for doing this is so the clinician can then apply a standard mode of treatment that fits the proposed diagnosis. Clinicians may use leading questions and in some cases encourage a certain answer that then corroborates their own beliefs and justifies the diagnosis. This has been described as 'confirmation bias' (Nickerson 1998) and can lead to methods of communication that fail to help in understanding patients from their perspective. This can continue into the physical examination, where further testing is designed to support the clinical hypothesis and so leading communication such as, 'that hurts, doesn't it?' or 'that feels easier, right?' means that ineffective communication based on a flawed reasoning process that is driven by bias is underpinning the clinician–patient interaction.

CLINICIAN EMOTION, COMMUNICATION AND REASONING

When communicating with patients whilst clinically reasoning through their presentation, it is worthwhile considering your own emotion at the time of the clinical encounter. As clinicians we are aware of the need to understand patients' possible 'yellow flags', psychosocial elements that may be playing a part in patients' ongoing symptoms and inhibiting recovery. However, it is important to recognize our own anxieties when dealing with trying to reason a condition and how this may affect the interaction.

Consider a worrying presentation: you may feel your heart rate increase, your breathing rate change and a sensation deep in your stomach. This could also occur in a challenging scenario where a patient is distressed or even angry. The interaction at this point is vital; how the clinician deals with these feelings will ultimately affect the patient experience. It is recognized that this process of decision making at a cognitive level can be assisted by emotion-related signals, known as emotional/somatic markers (Velasquez 1998). Emotional/somatic markers can be described as homeostatic changes that occur in different levels of the brain and body in given situations, and link the body to the emotional response (Bechara & Damasio 2005). When making decisions, an emotional reaction to an option is generated and this is suggested to create what is known as an emotional/somatic marker that includes sensations from the viscera, skeletal and smooth muscles. These would be the physical

and emotional feelings associated with a decision and they are suggested to serve as an indicator of the importance of what is about to be decided upon (Langridge et al. 2016). Therefore, as a clinician you will feel physical and emotional reactions to the patient data and this will possibly alert you to a concern or generate a position of empathy from you that is genuine, as your emotional centres react to the emotion of the patient. These functions help the clinician provide a sense of safety which has been described in the medical literature as a 'gut feeling' (Langridge et al. 2013), or it can help in the emotional understanding of the patient's perspective, which has also been described as intuitive practice (Buckingham & Adams 2000).

Realizing these mechanisms can be helpful in 'tailoring' the communication style at the right time. For example, in the case of a 'gut feeling,' the sensation that there is something that does not fit will lead the clinician to question carefully, using closed-style questions to be very specific and exact. Meanwhile, sensing emotion and being intuitive to the language, body position and non-verbal cues may lead the clinician to a more narrative approach, using open questions, delivered with a relaxed body position that aims to encourage dialogue from the patient.

These features and interactions will be affected by how clinicians are feeling themselves. Perhaps they have had a particularly challenging week, or stress levels are higher than normal. This could lead to a different communication style with some patients, and so recognizing this can be very helpful when reflecting on practice and planning a communication style for patients. It is good practice to evaluate yourself in terms of your emotional status, before attempting to understand those elements in your patients and significant others.

Shared Decision Making

Having reached a clinical diagnosis, it is important to think about how the findings are communicated and the process of collaboratively negotiating the various treatment options. Shared decision making is described as both a philosophy and a process whereby clinicians engage patients as partners, to make choices about care based on clinical evidence and patients' informed preferences (Coulter & Collins 2011). At present, a universally agreed definition is lacking and a systematic

---

BOX 9.1

THE CORE COMPONENTS OF SHARED DECISION MAKING (ELWYN & CHARLES 2009)

Identifying and clarifying the issue
Identifying potential solutions
Discussing options and uncertainties
Providing information about the potential benefits, harms and uncertainties of each option
Checking that patients and professionals have a joint understanding
Gaining feedback and reactions
Agreeing a course of action
Implementing the chosen treatment
Arranging follow-up
Evaluating outcomes and assessing the next steps

---

review cited 161 definitions using 31 concepts (most commonly 'patient preferences' and 'options') (Makoul & Clayman 2006).

The principal components of shared decision making have been identified (Elwyn & Charles 2009) and are summarized in Box 9.1.

Observational studies have shown shared decision making is rarely implemented in practice and our team set about measuring the prevalence of shared decision making in 80 clinical encounters involving physiotherapists and patients with back pain (Jones et al. 2014), using the 12-item OPTION scale (Elwyn & Charles 2009). Although initially devised to rate general practice consultations, the scale contains generic phasing 'applicable to any clinical setting' (Elwyn & Charles 2009). It measures the overall shared decision making, scoring the clinician-initiated behaviour from an observer's perspective.

The tool rates 12 behavioural concepts on an ordinal scale, ranging from 0 – 'the behaviour is not observed', to 4 – 'the behaviour is observed and executed to a high standard'. Scores are summated and scaled to give an overall percentage and, the higher the score, the greater the shared decision-making competency attained, with 60% generally accepted to correlate with the lowest meaningful competency level (Elwyn & Charles 2009). The reliability of the OPTION tool has been demonstrated, with the interrater intraclass correlation coefficient (0.62), kappa scores for interrater agreement (0.71), Cronbach's alpha (0.79) and intrarater test–retest reliability (0.66) all above acceptable thresholds (Elwyn & Charles 2009).

In our study, there were 42 initial and 38 follow-up appointments (and care episodes ranged from one to six appointments per patient), giving a total of 80 consultations. Initial consultations were allocated 45 minutes and follow-up consultations were allocated 30 minutes. The overall mean OPTION score was 24% (range 10.4–43.8%), with 23.6% and 24.5% for the initial and follow-up consultations, respectively. Table 9.4 shows mean score for the individual scale items, including minimum and maximum ranges and score distributions. The modal score for 10 out of 12 items in the OPTION scale was 1 out of a possible 4, which indicates the clinicians consistently demonstrated only a 'minimal' attempt to perform these behaviours. The exceptions were: 'exploring the patient's concerns', which was consistently 'not observed' and therefore scored 0, and 'expressing the need to review the decision', which scored 2, indicating clinicians regularly achieved the 'baseline skill level'. No shared decision-making behaviour was consistently performed to a 'good' or 'high' standard (Jones et al. 2014).

Providing patients with a list of options was the only behaviour that was exhibited by every clinician across all observed encounters ($n = 80$), but in nearly three-quarters (73.8%) of consultations, this was only done to a 'perfunctory' level. In only 1.3% of consultations the option to defer treatment ($n = 2$) or take no action ($n = 1$) was provided – evidence that physiotherapists rarely considered doing nothing a viable option in this cohort of patients reporting back pain.

These findings concur with other clinical contexts and healthcare professions. In the only other physiotherapy study using the OPTION scale, Dierckx et al. (2013) analysed 210 Flemish encounters from 13 self-employed clinicians and reported a mean score of 5.2% (range 0–31%), considerably lower than the mean of 24% identified in this UK study. More broadly, Couët et al. (2015) conducted a systematic review of 2489 consultations across 29 international studies, involving general practitioners, cardiologists, psychiatrists, oncologists, dieticians and nurses, treating a variety of medical conditions (most frequently cancer, diabetes and depression) and identified a mean OPTION score of 23% (9–37%).

TABLE 9.4

Shared Decision Making in Consultations Between Physiotherapists and Patients With Low-Back Pain (Jones et al. 2014)

Item	Shared Decision-Making Behaviour	Mean Score (Min – Max)	0 (%)	1 (%)	2 (%)	3 (%)	4 (%)
1	The clinician draws attention to an identified problem as one that requires a decision-making process	0.7 (0–3)	48.8	33.8	16.3	1.3	0.0
2	The clinician states that there is more than one way to deal with the identified problem	0.8 (0–3)	41.3	36.3	21.3	1.3	0.0
3	The clinician assesses the patient's preferred approach to receiving information to assist decision making	0.6 (0–3)	58.8	27.5	10.0	3.8	0.0
4	The clinician lists 'options', which can include the choice of 'no action'	1.4 (1–3)	0.0	73.8	25.0	1.3	3.8
5	The clinician explains the pros and cons of options to the patient	0.8 (0–3)	42.5	38.8	15.0	3.8	0.0
6	The clinician explores the patient's expectations (or ideas) about how the problem(s) are to be managed	1.0 (0–4)	41.3	27.5	22.5	6.3	2.5
7	The clinician explores the patient's concerns (fears) about how problem(s) are to be managed	0.3 (0–2)	77.5	17.5	5.0	0.0	0.0
8	The clinician checks that the patient has understood the information	1.3 (0–3)	17.5	36.3	43.8	2.5	0.0
9	The clinician offers the patient explicit opportunities to ask questions during the decision-making process	1.2 (0–2)	18.8	46.3	35.0	0.0	0.0
10	The clinician elicits the patient's preferred level of involvement in decision making	0.7 (0–3)	58.8	16.3	22.5	2.5	0.0
11	The clinician indicates the need for a decision-making (or deferring) stage	1.2 (0–3)	7.5	70.0	20.0	2.5	0.0
12	The clinician indicates the need to review the decision (or deferment)	1.7 (0–4)	5.0	42.5	31.3	18.8	2.5

Key (Elwyn & Charles 2009)
0 = The behaviour is not observed.
1 = A minimal attempt is made to exhibit the behaviour.
2 = The clinician asks the patient about his or her preferred way of receiving information to assist decision.
3 = The behaviour is exhibited to a good standard.
4 = The behaviour is observed and executed to a high standard.

In the current climate, it is vital that clinicians involve patients appropriately in decisions affecting their healthcare to maximize non-specific treatment effects, reduce the potential for complaints and litigation, and enhance patients' experiences. Our findings indicate that shared decision making was underdeveloped in this cohort of back pain consultations and this aspect of practice would be a good area for physiotherapists to invest time in, to enhance their skills further.

CHANGING BEHAVIOUR

Implementing evidence-based practice and public health agendas depends on successful behaviour change interventions (Michie et al. 2011), which are common to physiotherapy practice. A plethora of theories and frameworks exist, including the behaviour change wheel, which was developed from 19 frameworks, incorporating capability, opportunity, motivation and behaviour. It comprises:

- physical capability, which can be achieved through physical skill development or potentially through enabling interventions such as medication, surgery or prostheses
- psychological capability, which can be achieved through imparting knowledge or understanding, training emotional, cognitive and/or behavioural

skills or through enabling interventions such as medication

- reflective motivation, which can be achieved through increasing knowledge and understanding, eliciting positive (or negative) feelings about behavioural target
- automatic motivation, which can be achieved through associative learning that elicits positive (or negative) feelings and impulses and counter-impulses relating to the behavioural target, habit formation or direct influences on automatic motivational processes (e.g. via medication)
- physical and social opportunity, which can be achieved through environmental change (Michie et al. 2011).

The behaviour change wheel starts with the question: 'What conditions internal to individuals and in their social and physical environment need to be in place for a specified behavioural target to be achieved?' This comprehensive approach is highly pertinent to physiotherapy (Fig. 9.5).

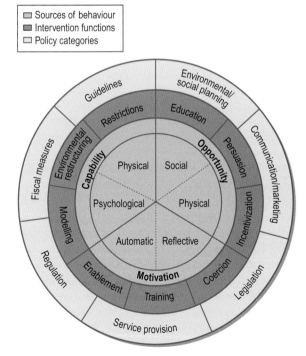

FIG. 9.5 ■ The behaviour change wheel. (From Michie et al. 2011, with permission.)

Motivational Interviewing

Motivational interviewing is a collaborative, goal-oriented style of communication with particular attention given to the language of change and has become popular within physiotherapy. It is designed to strengthen personal commitment to a specific goal by eliciting and exploring the patient's own reasons for change, within an atmosphere of acceptance and compassion (Miller & Rollnick 2013).

With this approach, the therapist uses active listening and communication skills to elicit the patient's own positive reasons for change, with the aim of avoiding confrontation or resistance to behaviour change, which can be particularly helpful when encouraging patients to make difficult lifestyle changes such as taking more exercise, or reducing their alcohol intake.

GAINING CONSENT

Appropriately and adequately gaining consent is vital in providing safe, patient-centred, collaborative care. There is a legal, ethical and clinical necessity to gain informed consent from the patient in front of you. Information regarding an intervention or treatment should be disclosed inclusive of the 'material' risks, benefits, alternatives and information regarding not accepting any treatment at all. In a landmark case in 2015 (Montgomery v. Lanarkshire Health Board), there was a move from the 'reasonable clinician' to the 'reasonable patient' and the test of materiality is:

> whether, in the circumstances of the particular case, a reasonable person in the patient's position would be likely to attach significance to the risk, or the doctor is or should reasonably be aware that the particular patient would be likely to attach significance to it.

In a therapeutic environment, there may be an assumption that, as patients have attended, they have consented to receive treatment; however, this is not the case. Therefore, after an assessment, it is the clinician's responsibility to communicate the diagnosis in a way that patients are able to understand clearly the nature of their condition and the options available. On understanding this, patients should still have the option of not receiving any treatment, including any benefits or potential risks/consequences, and this should always be made clear to them and accurately documented.

Best-practice models propose that the consent process is voluntary, patients consent freely and in a non-coercive environment and that patients have the capacity to make decisions whilst having the opportunity to ask questions (Goldfarb et al. 2012). For an excellent summary of the components of consent, see Sim (1996).

COMMUNICATING THE TREATMENT

When working with a patient in a rehabilitation environment, a positive patient–clinician relationship is imperative to a successful outcome. Treatment adherence, compliance and collaboration are enhanced and improved by effective communication, built on a basis of understanding and rapport. Kenny (2004) outlines a cycle of frustration that patients feel when they perceive not being listened to or have been stigmatized and so, to action behavioural change, such as movement or lifestyle, the author proposes that the clinician must build:

- trust
- collaboration
- empowerment
- respect.

In doing so, the patient gets a sense of engagement and so adherence to change is more likely. The belief in the treatment, sometimes referred to as non-specific treatment effects, which include placebo, is a physiological response to expectation and the above emotions. Non-specific positive treatment effects are generally attributable to the therapeutic encounter and are linked to the context, environment and the interpretation of the intervention itself. Clinical procedures are proposed to be associated with a complex psychosocial context that can influence the therapeutic outcome (Linde et al. 2011). Placebo has been described as the clinical psychosocial context that surrounds the patient and contributes to healing (Benedetti et al. 2003). The emotional, empathic, communicative style of the clinician can possibly enhance the action of neurobiological mechanisms, such as the release of endorphins, dopamine and cannabinoids, whilst also stimulating different areas of the brain (such as the amygdala, prefrontal cortex and anterior insula), all of which are also linked to similar mechanisms of pain relief medication (Finniss

et al. 2010). The clinician is best placed to use these effects by promoting reassurance, developing trust and providing encouragement. Sutterlin et al. (2015) support these features, but also make a case for non-personal elements of non-specific treatment effects, such as environmental factors, comfort, warmth, familiarity, and even the acoustics that can support endogenous outputs from clinical interactions. Fig. 9.6 demonstrates the relationship of belief/expectancy and the painful gate control. This mechanism is worth remembering when discussing with patients what they feel they need; always consider those discussions as a therapy in itself.

It is important to recognize that non-specific treatment effects are more than just different colours of pills but the effects of clinical interactions that can dramatically enhance the effects of medications (Kaptchuk & Miller 2015). Acknowledging the possible benefit of enhancing the treatment through expectation and interaction means that there is also the possibility of a poor experience causing an adverse response. This has been described as 'nocebo', which is likely driven by expectation of negative effects, or heightened vigilance towards or awareness of a painful condition that possibly has been driven by a distressing experience.

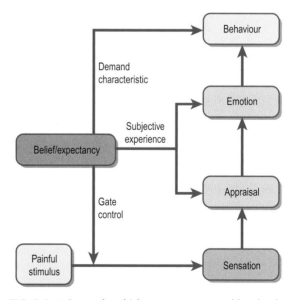

FIG. 9.6 ■ Routes by which expectancy, created by placebo treatments, may lead to changes in pain processing. (*Adapted from Wager 2005, with permission.*)

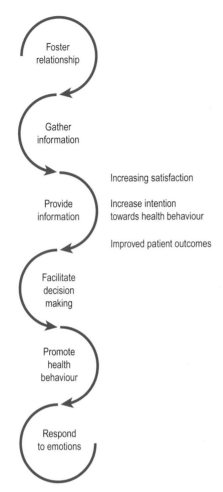

FIG. 9.7 ■ The role of healthcare professional and patient in enhancing communication during consultation. *(Adapted from de Haes and Bensing 2009, with permission.)*

Fig. 9.7 outlines the interlinkages of interaction that naturally lead to a better patient experience. Patient outcomes in persistent low-back pain have been shown to be enhanced by a mutual understanding of pretreatment expectation and also by setting individualized pain, impairment and disability goals (Hazard et al. 1994). Therefore, by using all these features effectively the clinician is best placed to support the therapeutic encounter.

NEGOTIATING AN EXIT

Leaving a positive final impression of the consultation is vitally important. Silverman et al. (1998) have proposed four main skills that contribute to a satisfactory ending of the consultation:

1. summarizing the session
2. contracting with the patient about what happens next
3. providing a safety net of what to do if the plan is not working, including when and how to seek help
4. final checks that the patient is comfortable with the plan and has the opportunity to ask questions or discuss any other items.

If all has gone to plan, patients should be leaving the consultation with a clear understanding of their clinical diagnosis and any further investigations or potential treatment options. Most importantly, they should have had a positive experience of physiotherapy. The clinician should also have experienced a positive interaction and optimized the non-specific treatment effects, to maximize the outcome of the care episode.

SUGGESTIONS TO ENHANCE YOUR COMMUNICATION SKILLS FURTHER

1. Think about a recent initial consultation that you have completed. Did it go well? Can you list any contributing factors as to why you think it went well, relating to: (a) the patient; (b) you; (c) the patient's problem presentation; (d) the environment; (e) anything else?
2. Think about a recent initial consultation that has not gone quite so well. Can you list any contributing factors as to why this might be, relating to: (a) the patient; (b) you; (c) the patient's problem presentation; (d) the environment; (e) anything else? What has given you the impression that this encounter could have gone better? At what point in the consultation did you get this impression? What can you learn from this?
3. In thinking about a recent consultation, what (if any) topics did you cover with the patient before you sat down at the start of the assessment (e.g. walking through to the clinic room)? What topics did you cover before asking about the patient's problem presentation? How did you phrase the specific opening question about the patient's problem presentation? Do you always use a similar form of words to this when taking a history?

4. With the patient's consent, try audio recording a clinical consultation. How frequently do you interrupt patients and what effect does this appear to have had?

5. Using the audio recording, how many of the 12 shared decision-making behaviours in the OPTION tool can you identify in your practice?

6. When planning supervision sessions and in-service training programmes, try to include topics on communication regularly to enhance your skills further.

Acknowledgements

Dr Lisa Roberts' research has been supported by an academic fellowship funded by Arthritis Research UK (17830) and a senior clinical lectureship from the National Institute for Health Research.

The authors wish to acknowledge the work of the research team, in particular: Chris Whittle, Lucy Jones, Emily Chester, Natalie Robinson, Faye Burrow, Millie Allen and the patients and staff in the UK who have generously given their time, shared their knowledge and made these studies possible.

REFERENCES

Bar, M., Neta, M., Linz, H., 2006. Very first impressions. Emotion 6, 269–278.

Bechara, A., Damasio, A.R., 2005. The somatic marker hypothesis: a new theory of economic decision. Games Econ. Behav. 52, 336–372.

Beckman, H.B., Frankel, R.M., 1984. The effect of physician behaviour on the collection of data. Ann. Intern. Med. 101, 692–696.

Benedetti, F., Pollo, A., Lopiano, L., et al., 2003. Conscious expectation and unconscious conditioning in analgesic, motor, and hormonal placebo/nocebo responses. J. Neurosci. 23, 4315–4323.

Buckingham, C.D., Adams, A., 2000. Classifying clinical decision making: interpreting nursing intuition, heuristics and medical diagnosis. J. Adv. Nurs. 32, 990–998.

Caris-Verhallen, W., Kerkstra, A., Bensing, J.M., 1999. Non-verbal behavior in nurse–elderly patient communication. J. Adv. Nurs. 29, 808–818.

Casella, S.M., 2015. Therapeutic rapport: the forgotten intervention. J. Emerg. Nurs. 41, 252–254.

Chester, E.C., Robinson, N.C., Roberts, L.C., 2014. Opening clinical encounters in an adult musculoskeletal setting. Man. Ther. 19, 306–310.

Cocksedge, S., George, B., Renwick, S., et al., 2013. Touch in primary care consultations: qualitative investigation of doctors' and patients' perceptions. Br. J. Gen. Pract. 63, e283–e290.

Couët, N., Desroches, S., Robitaille, H., et al., 2015. Assessments of the extent to which health-care providers involve patients in decision making: a systematic review of studies using the OPTION instrument. Health Expect. 18, 542–561.

Coulter, A., Collins, A., 2011. Making shared decision-making a reality. No decision about me, without me. The King's Fund. Available online at: http://www.kingsfund.org.uk/.

Cox, C., Uddin, L., Di Martino, A., et al., 2012. The balance between feeling and knowing: affective and cognitive empathy are reflected in the brain's intrinsic functional dynamics. Soc. Cogn. Affect. Neurosci. 7, 727–737.

De Haes, H., Bensing, J., 2009. Endpoints in medical communication research, proposing a framework of functions and outcomes. Patient Educ. Couns. 74, 287–294.

Dickerson, S.S., Gable, S.L., Irwin, M.R., et al., 2009. Social-evaluative threat and proinflammatory cytokine regulation: an experimental laboratory investigation. Psychol. Sci. 20, 1237–1244.

Dickerson, S.S., Kemeny, M.E., 2004. Acute stressors and cortisol responses: a theoretical integration and synthesis of laboratory research. Psychol. Bull. 130, 355–391.

Dierckx, K., Deveugele, M., Roosen, P., et al., 2013. Implementation of shared decision making in physical therapy: observed level of involvement and patient preference. Phys. Ther. 93, 1321–1330.

Drummond, K., 1989. A backward glance at interruptions. West. J. Speech Commun. 53, 150–166.

Edwards, I., Jones, M., Carr, J., et al., 2004. Clinical reasoning strategies in physical therapy. Phys. Ther. 84, 312–330.

Elwyn, G.M., Charles, C., 2009. Shared decision-making: the principles and the competencies. In: Edwards, A., Elwyn, G. (Eds.), Evidence-based patient choice. Oxford University Press, Oxford, pp. 118–143.

Finniss, D.G., Kaptchuk, T.J., Miller, F., et al., 2010. Biological, clinical, and ethical advances of placebo effects. Lancet 375, 686–695.

Goldfarb, E., Fromson, J.A., Gorrindo, T., et al., 2012. Enhancing informed consent best practices: gaining patient, family and provider perspectives using reverse simulation of medical ethics. J. Med. Ethics doi:10.1136/medethics-2011-100206.

Hall, T., Lloyd, C., 1990. Non-verbal communication in a health care setting. Br. J. Occup. Ther. 53, 383–387.

Hazard, R.G., Haugh, L.D., Green, P.A., et al., 1994. Chronic low back pain. The relationship between patient satisfaction and pain, impairment and disability outcomes. Spine 18, 881–887.

Heritage, J., 2012. Epistemics in action: action formation and territories of knowledge. Res. Lang. Soc. Interact. 45, 1–29.

Heritage, J., Robinson, J.D., 2006. The structure of patients' presenting concerns: physicians' opening questions. Health Commun. 19, 89–102.

Hiller, A., Delany, C., Guillemin, M., 2015. The communicative power of touch in the patient–physiotherapist interaction. WCPT Congress 2015/Physiotherapy 2015.101, Supplement eS427–eS632.

Irish, J.T., Hall, J.A., 1995. Interruptive patterns in medical visits: the effects of role, status and gender. Soc. Sci. Med. 41, 873–881.

Jackson, C., 2006. Shut up and listen! A brief guide to clinical communication skills. Dundee University Press, Dundee, p. 1.

Jones, M.A., 1992. Clinical reasoning in manual therapy. Phys. Ther. 72, 875–884.

Jones, L.E., Roberts, L.C., Little, P.S., et al., 2014. Shared decision-making in back pain consultations: an illusion or reality? Eur. Spine J. 23 (Suppl. 1), S13–S19.

Kaptchuk, T.J., Miller, F.G., 2015. Placebo effects in medicine. NEJM 373, 8–9.

Kenny, D.T., 2004. Constructions of chronic pain in doctor–patient relationships: bridging the communication chasm. Patient Educ. Couns. 52, 297–305.

Kitzinger, C., 2008. Conversation analysis: technical matters for gender research. In: Harrington, K., Litosseliti, L., Sauntson, H., et al. (Eds.), Gender and language research methodologies. Palgrave Macmillan, Hampshire, pp. 119–138.

Lærum, E., Indahl, A., Sture Skouen, J., 2006. What is 'the good back consultation'? A combined qualitative and quantitative study of chronic low back pain patients' interaction with and perceptions of consultations with specialists. J. Rehabil. Med. 38, 255–262.

Langewitz, W., Denz, M., Keller, A., et al., 2002. Spontaneous talking time at start of consultation in outpatient clinic: cohort study. Br. Med. J. 325, 682–683.

Langridge, N., Roberts, L., Pope, C., 2013. The place of 'gut feeling' in clinical reasoning. J. Bone Joint Surg. 95-B (Suppl.), 179.

Langridge, N., Roberts, L., Pope, C., 2015. The clinical reasoning processes of extended scope physiotherapists assessing patients with low back pain. Man. Ther. 20, 745–750.

Langridge, N., Roberts, L., Pope, C., 2016. The role of clinician emotion in clinical reasoning: balancing the analytical process. Man. Ther. 21, 277–281.

Linde, K., Fassler, M., Meissner, K., 2011. Placebo interventions, placebo effects and clinical practice. Philos. Trans. R. Soc. Lond. B Biol. Sci. 366, 1905–1912.

Lindgren, L., Rundgren, S., Winso, O., et al., 2010. Physiological responses to touch massage in healthy volunteers. Auton. Neurosci. 158, 105–110.

Lipkin, M., Putnam, S.M., Lazare, A., 1995. The medical interview: clinical care, education and research. Springer, New York.

Maguire, P., Pitceathly, C., 2002. Key communication skills and how to acquire them. Br. Med. J. 325, 697–700.

Makoul, G., Clayman, M.L., 2006. An integrative model of shared decision making in medical encounters. Patient Educ. Couns. 60, 301–312.

Marvel, M.K., Epstein, R.M., Flowers, K., et al., 1999. Soliciting the patient's agenda: have we improved? J. Am. Med. Assoc. 281, 283–287.

Mattingly, C., 1991. The narrative nature of clinical reasoning. Am. J. Occup. Ther. 45, 998–1005.

Mazur, M., McEvoy, S., Schmidt, M.H., et al., 2015. High self-assessment of disability and the surgeon's recommendation against surgical intervention may negatively impact satisfaction scores in patients with spinal disorders. J. Neurosurg. Spine 22, 666–671.

McAllister, M., Matarasso, B., Dixon, B., et al., 2004. Conversation starters: re-examining and reconstructing first encounters within the therapeutic relationship. J. Psychiatr. Ment. Health Nurs. 11, 575–582.

McCabe, C., Rolls, E.T., Bilderbeck, A., et al., 2008. Cognitive influences on the affective representation of touch and the sight of touch in the human brain. Soc. Cogn. Affect. Neurosci. 3, 97–108.

Mehrabian, A., 1971. Silent messages. Wadsworth, Belmont, CA.

Melzack, R., 1999. From the gate to the neuromatrix. Pain Suppl. 6, S121–S126.

Melzack, R., 2001. Pain and the neuromatrix in the brain. J. Dent. Educ. 65, 1378–1382.

Meredith, P., Emberton, M., Wood, C., 1995. New directions in information for patients. Br. Med. J. 311, 4–5.

Michie, S., van Stralen, M.M., West, R., 2011. The behaviour change wheel: a new method for characterising and designing behaviour change interventions. Implement. Sci. 6, 42.

Miller, W.R., Rollnick, S., 2013. Motivational interviewing. Helping people change, third ed. Guilford Press, New York.

Misch, D., Peloquin, S., 2005. Developing empathy through confluent education. J. Phys. Ther. Educ. 19, 41–51.

Montgomery (Appellant) v Lanarkshire Health Board (Respondent), 2015. UKSC 11, on appeal from [2013] CSIH 3; [2010] CSIH 104.

Nathan, B., 1999. Touch and emotion in manual therapy. Churchill Livingstone, New York, pp. 35–85.

Nicholas, M.K., Linton, S.J., Watson, P.J., et al., 2011. Early identification and management of psychological risk factors ('yellow flags') in patients with low back pain: a reappraisal. Phys. Ther. 91, 1–17.

Nickerson, R., 1998. Confirmation bias: a ubiquitous phenomenon in many guises. Rev. Gen. Psychol. 2, 175–220.

Noll, E., Key, A., Jensen, G., 2001. Clinical reasoning of an experienced physiotherapist: insight into clinician decision-making regarding low back pain. Physiother. Res. Int. 6, 40–51.

Oliver, S., Redfern, S., 1991. Interpersonal communication between nurses and elderly patients: refinement of an observational schedule. J. Adv. Nurs. 16, 30–38.

Ostelo, R., Stomp-van Den berg, S., Vlaeyan, J., et al., 2003. Health care providers' beliefs towards chronic low back pain: the development of a questionnaire. Man. Ther. 8, 214–222.

Parliamentary and Health Service Ombudsman, 2012. Listening and learning: the Ombudsman's review of complaint handling by the NHS in England 2011–12. London: The Stationery Office, p. 7.

Parliamentary and Health Service Ombudsman, 2014. Complaints about acute trusts, Q1 2013–14 and Q2 2014–15. London: The Stationery Office, p. 8.

Parry, R., 2008. Are interventions to enhance communication performance in allied health professionals effective, and how should they be delivered? Direct and indirect evidence. Patient Educ. Couns. 73, 186–195.

Pedersen, R., 2008. Empathy: a wolf in sheep's clothing? Med. Health Care Philos. 11, 325–335.

Peeters, P.A., Vlaeyen, J.W., 2011. Feeling more pain, yet showing less: the influence of social threat on pain. J. Pain 12, 1255–1261.

Pollock, K., 2001. 'I've not asked him, you see, and he's not said': understanding lay explanatory models of illness is a prerequisite for concordant consultation. Int. J. Pharm. Pract. 9, 105–117.

Raja, S., Hasnain, M., Vadakumchery, T., et al., 2015. Identifying elements of patient-centered care in underserved populations: a qualitative study of patient perspectives. PLoS ONE 10, e0126708.

Rhodes, D.R., McFarland, K.F., Finch, W.H., et al., 2001. Speaking and interruptions during primary care office visits. Fam. Med. 33, 528–532.

Roberts, L., 2006. First impressions: an information leaflet for patients attending a musculoskeletal out-patient department. Physiotherapy 92, 179–186.

Roberts, L., Whittle, C., Cleland, J., et al., 2013. Measuring verbal communication in initial physical therapy encounters. Phys. Ther. 93, 479–491.

Robinson, J.D., Heritage, J., 2006. Physicians' opening questions and patients' satisfaction. Patient Educ. Couns. 60, 279–285.

Sacks, H., Schegloff, E.A., Jefferson, G., 1974. A simplest systematics for the organization of turn-taking for conversation. Language 50, 696–735.

Silverman, J., Kurtz, S., Draper, J., 1998. Skills for communicating with patients. Radcliffe Medical Press, Oxford, p. 10.

Sim, J., 1996. Informed consent and manual therapy. Man. Ther. 1, 104–106.

Sutterlin, S., Egner, L.E., Lugo, R.G., et al., 2015. Beyond expectation: a case for non-personal contextual factors in a more comprehensive approach to the placebo effect and the contribution of environmental psychology. Psychol. Res. Behav. Manag. 8, 259–262.

Tongue, S., 2007. Every day brings a first impression. Nurs. Stand. 22, 62.

Velasquez, J.D., 1998. When robots weep. Emotional memories and decision-making. Presented at the 15th National Conference on Artificial Intelligence, Madison, WI.

Vlaeyen, J.W., Hanssen, M., Goubert, L., et al., 2009. Threat of pain influences social context effects on verbal pain report and facial expression. Behav. Res. Ther. 47, 774–782.

Waddell, G., 2004. The back pain revolution, second ed. Churchill Livingstone, Edinburgh, p. 243.

Wager, T.D., 2005. Expectations and anxiety as mediators of placebo effects in pain. Pain 115, 225–226.

Walseth, L.T., Abildsnes, E., Schei, E., 2011. Lifestyle, health and the ethics of good living: health behaviour counselling in general practice. Patient Educ. Couns. 83, 180–184.

Wetherall, D., Silverman, J., Kurtz, S., et al., 1998. Skills for communicating with patients. Radcliffe Medical Press, Oxford, p. vii.

Williams, D., 1997. Communication skills in practice, A practical guide for health professionals. Jessica Kinglsey, London, pp. 1–27.

Wolraich, M., Albanese, M., Reiter-Thayer, S., et al., 1982. Factors affecting physician communication and parent–physician dialogues. J. Med. Educ. 52, 621–625.

Zolnierek, K.B., Dimatteo, M.R., 2009. Physician communication and patient adherence to treatment: a meta-analysis. Med. Care 47, 832–834.

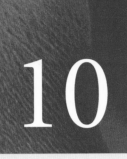

10 PRINCIPLES OF EXERCISE REHABILITATION

LEE HERRINGTON ■ SIMON SPENCER

INTRODUCTION

The goal when treating musculoskeletal injuries is restoration of function, to the greatest degree, in the shortest possible time. For all clinicians the overarching aim when rehabilitating a patient is to achieve a safe return of the individual to, or as close as possible to, preinjury levels of function. It becomes clear that, with this as the primary goal of the therapeutic intervention, to relieve the patient of symptoms solely, though significant, does not necessarily mean this primary goal has been attained. The tissues of the body are designed to function under and adapt to the loads applied to them; consequently, the absence of load has a negative impact on these tissues. The simplest means to relieve the primary symptom patients present with, that is pain, is to offload the irritated tissue. This takes away the cause of the pain, and symptoms can be resolved. This situation then presents the clinician with a dilemma: resting/offloading the tissues relieves pain and irritation, but it also weakens the tissue, making it more likely to reinjure and moving the patient further away from the goal of restoring full function. The primary aim of this chapter is to introduce concepts which will aid the clinician in the decision-making process regarding when, how and by how much to reload the tissues, in order to rebuild the patient's level of function through the use of targeted exercise intervention.

RELOADING IN REHABILITATION: A PHYSIOLOGICAL CONSTRUCT

This section will present the concept of tissue homeostasis and how this relates to the development of both acute and overuse injury and their rehabilitation. The section will also look at how loading of the tissues impacts on tissue homeostasis through the process of mechanotherapy.

Mechanotherapy and Tissue Homeostasis

Injuries occur when a tissue is stressed beyond its ability to cope with the load applied to it. In a biomechanics laboratory this is easy to visualize: the two ends of a muscle, tendon or ligament are pulled apart and eventually the forces applied are great enough that the structure tears. This is shown graphically in the load deformation curve (Fig. 10.1). Initially as a biological structure is loaded, the tissue deforms slowly (toe region), then more rapidly, until it reaches a point of microfailure. Prior to this point, if the load is removed the tissue returns to its previous form. Once the tissue has been loaded beyond the elastic region it is permanently changed. This model applies equally to all musculoskeletal tissues when loaded; the shape of the curve varies slightly and the loads required to bring about change might be different, but the overall processes are the same.

The model of loading presented above has significant implications for those working in the field of injury rehabilitation. If we wish to bring about changes in a tissue and make it more tolerant to load, for example, that is, shifting the microfailure zone to the right in Fig. 10.1, then we have to create some tissue damage in a controlled manner. This brings about a sequence of physiological events which create an anabolic environment causing positive adaptive changes in the tissues loaded. Mueller and Maluf (2002) describe this process within the Physical Stress Theory (PST).

The basic premise of the PST (Mueller & Maluf 2002) is that changes in the relative level of load cause a predictable adaptive response in all biological tissue. Tissues accommodate to physical stress by altering their structure and composition to meet the mechanical demands of routine loading best. Deviations from routine or steady-state loading provide a stimulus for tissue adaptation that allows tissues to meet the mechanical demands of the new loading environment. Response to loading is believed to occur along a continuum of threshold levels, defining the highest and lowest loads required to produce a specific tissue response. These thresholds can be viewed as boundaries for the effective dose–response to physical loading. There are five qualitative responses to physical stress depending on the level of load applied: decreased stress tolerance (e.g. atrophy); maintenance (tissue homeostasis); increased stress tolerance (e.g. hypertrophy); injury; and permanent damage.

Scott Dye (2005) has presented a tissue homeostasis model to describe the aetiology of patellofemoral pain. This model can be expanded potentially to describe what happens to any tissue and fits nicely with the PST model. The model of tissue homeostasis is shown in Fig. 10.2. Most uninjured biological structures can accept a broad range of loading (from less than one to nearly eight times body weight) and still maintain tissue homeostasis, a balance between cellular breakdown and growth. This range of load acceptance is called the zone of homeostatic loading, the outer limits of which are defined by the envelope of function. If an increased load is placed on a tissue, for example, repetitive low loading involved in distance running or the single high

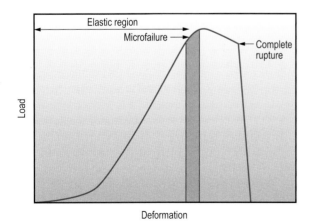

FIG. 10.1 ■ Load deformation curve.

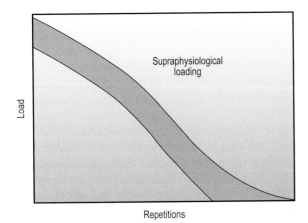

FIG. 10.2 ■ Tissue homeostasis model.

load of a rugby tackle, loss of soft- or hard-tissue homeostasis can result, characterized by low-level (cellular) damage to the tissue. This application of increased loading, insufficient to cause immediate overt structural damage, is termed to be within the zone of supraphysiological overload. At this point the tissue is weakened (losing its current homeostatic envelope) and, if subjected to repeated loads, is likely to deteriorate further (be less tolerant of load – its envelope of function shifting further to the left), eventually resulting in tissue failure. If sufficient recovery is allowed prior to application of a repeated loading, the tissues develop a tolerance to that load; they adapt and become stronger through reinforcement and orientation of tissue in direct response to the stress loading.

The PST model (Mueller & Maluf 2002) describes this process, whereby persistent loading levels below the maintenance level (homeostatic envelope of function) lead to tissue atrophy and decreased tolerance to load (in Fig. 10.1 the microfailure zone moves to the left, and in Fig. 10.2 the envelope of function moves to the left). If loading occurs within the maintenance range, there is no net change in load tolerance and homeostasis is maintained. Loading beyond this level results in tissue overload and increased load tolerance (the zones moving to the right in Figs 10.1 and 10.2), or, conversely, tissue breakdown, injury and cell death. A major consideration in determining which of these situations actually occurs is dependent on the nature of the applied load – a composite value, relating to magnitude, time, direction and recovery (repetition rate), with tissue breakdown

typically resulting from high-magnitude, short-duration or low-magnitude, long-duration loading.

Wolff's law of soft tissue states that tissue remodelling and the response to load (and so any exercise) are determined by the specific adaptation of the tissue to the imposed level of demand. Khan and Scott (2009) have described the overarching process as 'mechanotransduction', which is the processes whereby cells convert physiological mechanical stimuli into biochemical responses. They break down mechanotransduction into three steps: (1) mechanocoupling, (2) cell–cell communication and (3) the effector response. The mechanocoupling refers to physical load (often shear, tensile or compression) causing a physical perturbation to cells that make up a tissue. These forces elicit a deformation of the cell that can trigger a wide array of responses depending on the nature of loading. The forces need to perturb the cell directly or indirectly, which then acts as a trigger to a variety of chemical responses both within and between cells, the extent of which is dependent on the magnitude and duration of the load. The effector response following the transmission of chemical triggers from cell to cell is increased protein synthesis and, therefore, the addition of tissue in response to the stress loading. These physiological explanations lead logically to the development of 'mechanotherapy', where mechanotransduction is utilized therapeutically for the stimulation of tissue repair and remodelling.

It can be seen from the discussion above that movement and load appear to be critical in not only maintaining normal musculoskeletal tissue function, but in improving load tolerance (strengthening/hypertrophy of the tissue) to enhance function, sporting performance or recovery from injury. The tissue response to loading is likely to be a dynamic one, with a myriad of factors influencing how the tissue responds to loading, especially repetitive loading. A significant factor is likely to be the direction force that is applied. This is likely to be more specifically reflected in the alignment of the limb as it is loaded, as malalignment has the potential to cause the application of asymmetrical loads and concentration of those loads on specific tissues or even areas of tissues. An obvious example here is an increased Q angle increasing the load on the lateral facet of the patellofemoral joint. The components of movement and alignment which are very significant to maintaining optimal movement patterns are muscle performance (force development and capacity), motor control, posture and alignment, and physical activity, all of which will be discussed later.

A major emphasis within this chapter will be placed on the assessment and application of targeted progressive loading within the rehabilitation process.

FUNDAMENTALS OF MOBILITY AND MOTOR CONTROL TRAINING

Here the basic principles of motor control and skill learning will be covered, how they practically apply to injury rehabilitation and how rehabilitation exercise programmes can be progressed to reflect the chaotic environments individuals have to function in, to prepare patients best for return to their chosen activities.

Mobility and Stability Paradox

Mobility is defined as freedom of movement at articular segments, where a joint or series of joints demonstrates ease of motion through an appropriate anatomical range. In that sense, mobility forms the basis of motor control, where the performance of a skilled motor task is governed by an appropriate balance of mobility, passive stability (form closure), active stability and neuromuscular control (force closure). Vleeming et al. (2008) define functional stability as 'the effective accommodation of the joints to each specific load demand through an adequately tailored joint compression, as a function of gravity, coordinated muscle and ligament forces, to produce effective joint reaction forces under changing conditions'. Maintenance of joint integrity during skilled movement tasks is therefore dependent not only on muscular capacity, but also on the ability to process sensory input, interpret the status of stability and motion, and establish strategies to overcome predictable and unexpected movement challenges (Hodges & Moseley 2003).

Considerations When Rehabilitating to Regain Mobility

Deficits in movement are frequently identified in patients with a history of pain and pathology, where changes in mobility are a product of the interaction between soft tissue and articular dysfunction. Whilst aberrant connective tissue remodelling following injury may influence joint mobility, it is also plausible that abnormal movement patterns or repetitive directional loading could result in the consistent absence of mechanical tension, associated with connective tissue remodelling and eventual loss of muscle fibre length (Sahrmann 2002; Langevin & Sherman 2007). Loss of mobility could also represent an adaptive or maladaptive mechanism by which the body attempts to achieve active stability and maintain a level of function in the presence of pain, physical stress or failed motor control. Clinical assessment of joint range of motion (ROM) typically involves the use of goniometry or inclinometry as an accurate means of measuring and comparing joint displacement against normative reference angles in appropriate planes of motion and directions permitted at a specific joint. The development of affordable and portable movement analysis technologies (e.g. motion capture systems/software and inertial sensors) supports functional movement assessment outside of the traditional laboratory setting, with the caveat that measurement reliability and validity remain highly dependent on the technology, method of application and skill of the user.

A myriad of therapeutic interventions are employed to influence neurophysical mechanisms associated with loss of mobility (hypomobility), such as focal articular/tissue restriction, pain and altered muscular tone. Mechanical loading strategies attempt to influence the biomechanical properties of soft tissue and facilitate collagen reorganization, neural function and restoration of optimal movement kinematics. The nature of exercise prescription required to bring about an intended adaptation is highly individualized, as are the expectations of an intervention outcome. For example, consider a healthy, active individual presenting with an adaptive loss of mobility following an acute episode of low-back pain versus a sedentary patient presenting with a chronic loss of mobility 24 months post ankle surgery. Practitioners must therefore carefully consider how, in context, mechanical loading variables (e.g. direction, intensity, duration) could facilitate the desired physical effect. Increases in ROM following mobility (stretching) exercises are a product of the passive extensibility of the muscle–tendon unit (MTU), where joint ROM is unrestricted by bony or other non-muscular limitations (Gajdosik 2001). Following the application of sustained longitudinal loading (typically >30 seconds: Behm &

Chaouachi 2011), the MTU has been shown to exhibit a significant viscoelastic stress relaxation response (Magnusson et al. 2000). This viscoelastic behaviour appears to be the result of both mechanical and neural adaptations (Guissard & Duchateau 2004). The adaptations manifest themselves as hysteresis and creep (Linke & Leake 2004), where the reduction in MTU stiffness may explain immediate (elastic) changes in passive joint ROM (Magnusson et al. 1997).

Alongside decreased MTU stiffness, the mechanisms responsible for chronic (plastic) increases in ROM are also attributed to increases in stretch tolerance (Magnusson et al. 1996). Strategies to influence soft-tissue mobility through exercise prescription are not just limited to passive stretching. 'Stretching' variations such as proprioceptive neuromuscular facilitation and active/dynamic exercises are all effective methods of increasing flexibility and muscle extensibility (Page 2012). In addition, resistance training (with evidence specifically supporting the use of eccentric strength training) is an effective method of influencing the length–tension relationship in soft tissue (O'Sullivan et al. 2012).

Motor Control and Pain

The presence of musculoskeletal pain often creates deficits in motor control (ability to coordinate movement and posture); this will not only affect tissue loading, but could also contribute to deficits in general features of motor output such as poor strength and endurance; the patient essentially becomes less efficient. The impact of pain on motor coordination could be at a local (peripheral) level with the failure of activation or delay in activation of specific muscles. For example, quadriceps function is significantly disrupted with any knee injury or pathology, with the presence of this arthrogenic inhibition creating issues with activation and overall force development/muscular capacity. Similar relationships have been found in the deep muscles of the spine in the presence of low-back pain, and the rotator cuff with shoulder joint pain or structural damage.

Equally the failure in motor coordination could be at a global (central) level and result in, for example, an antalgic gait. Antalgic or pain-avoiding gait patterns initially develop as an adaptive strategy to avoid placing load on the injured structure to minimize any pain. Often these gait patterns become counterproductive and actually create more load and stress within tissues, both perpetuating the injury and potentially increasing the risk of developing further injuries. Consider an individual walking on a plantar flexed foot following injury to the lateral ankle ligaments. If this gait is maintained it rapidly creates a situation where the patient has lost ankle dorsiflexion ROM, leading to an increased compensatory foot pronation or knee valgus in midstance to maintain gait; there is inappropriate quadriceps control of knee extension (the knee is held in flexion by overactive hamstring muscles); and the patient fails to hip extend fully, which creates reduced activity in the gluteal muscles (further impacted upon by increased hamstring activity), resulting in suboptimal control of frontal and transverse plane loads. All this could happen simply because the patient does not maintain a simple heel–toe gait pattern, which actually does not load the lateral ankle complex in the first place!

In the presence of pain, suboptimal motor control is driven by simplification – the cortex typically switches to simple stability mechanisms, where maladaptive movement patterns can result in considerable secondary consequences both locally and remotely to the original injury. When assessing the patient following injury the clinician needs to consider how the sensorimotor system is impacting on the patient's presentation. The strategy of the movement/muscle activation can create conditions which lead to excessive loading of the tissues. Examples could include: compromised activation leading to muscle atrophy so the muscle can no longer meet the demands of the task; inaccurate sensory information leading to inaccurate control; movement which now involves too much (excessive movement and instability) or too little variability (excessive stiffness and rigidity). This can often lead to a situation where the original reason for the patient developing injury and pain may be different from the reason it is maintained. To complicate this situation further, though the initial traumatic load or the suboptimal mechanics from less than ideal sensorimotor strategy may be the initial stimulus for tissue damage and pain, other mechanisms could become involved in the creation of persistent pain and altered sensorimotor control. Central sensitization, cognitive and psychological factors can significantly impact on sensorimotor control. The abhorrent processing of nociceptive input through the processes of peripheral and central sensitization can have a direct effect on motor output; likewise kinesiophobia (fear of movement) and catastrophizing (exaggeration of the impact of an action) will also change the way the individual moves and so how tissues are loaded. In improving the patient's movement the focus should therefore be on rehabilitating not only the biomechanical and physiological issues, but also the psychological ones.

The Role of Proprioception in Motor Control

The term proprioception is best used when referring to the detection of one or all of the following sensations:

- position and movement of joints (joint position sense)
- sensation of force and contraction
- sensation of orientation of body segments as well as of the body as a whole.

Most experts believe that the muscle mechanoreceptors are the primary source of this proprioceptive information, especially in the middle ranges of motion, with ligamentous receptors only contributing towards the extremes of motion. This has implications for rehabilitation, where joint inflammation and loss of ROM could change the nature, accuracy and reliability of information from the ligamentous receptors, whilst muscle atrophy could likewise change information from the muscle receptors. It is unclear though whether proprioception can actually be trained in the strictest sense, that is, altering the physiological function of the mechanoreceptors themselves. What can be achieved, however, is an improvement in the efficiency of signal processing, increase in the use of convergent feedback from other receptors and development of triggered (automatic subconscious) reactions, all of which could lead to improved proprioceptive acuity.

The nervous system uses three sources of sensory information in order to maintain postural stability (hold the body's centre of mass within or close to its base of support):

- somatosensory (or proprioceptive) feedback
- vestibular feedback
- visual feedback.

When developing a rehabilitation programme consideration should be given to fully and progressively challenging all these systems, in order to prepare the patient fully for return to unrestricted activity. In order to understand the level of challenge required, it is critical to understand the levels of deficit the individual may have; therefore, valid and reliable means of testing are needed.

Clinical Testing for Proprioceptive Deficits

Testing for Postural Stability

When testing for postural stability the two most common tests which can easily be replicated clinically are the balance error scoring system (BESS) and the star excursion balance test (SEBT). These assess slightly different aspects of static balance, with BESS probably being more a test of static balance stability and SEBT dynamic balance dissociation.

Balance Error Scoring System. This test assesses the number of errors occurring during a 20-second static hold in a variety of positions (stances). The BESS test has three stances: double-leg stance (hands on pelvis and feet together), single-leg stance (standing on one leg with hands on pelvis) and tandem stance (non-dominant (or non-injured limb) foot behind the dominant foot) in a heel-to-toe fashion. The stances are performed on both a firm and foam surface with eyes closed. The errors are counted during the 20-second trials. Typical errors to be scored are opening eyes, lifting forefoot or heel, abducting the hip by more than 30° or failing to return to the test position in more than 5 seconds. Bell et al. (2011) produced a systematic review of the test's reliability, validity and sensitivity, concluding overall that the test was good to excellent in all of these areas. In Iverson and Koehle's (2013) paper, they provide normative data for this test across a range of ages and both genders.

Star Excursion Balance Test. Participants perform the test by standing in the middle of a testing grid of eight lines, placed at 45° to each other; they then reach with one foot as far as possible along the different grid lines, and then return to the starting position. The measure of dynamic postural control movement dissociation is inferred from how far a participant has reached whilst maintaining balance. When undertaking the test there appears to be a significant learning effect, with Munro and Herrington (2010) establishing that SEBT scores are reliable after the fourth trial. The test has been shown to be a reliable measure, has validity to identify balance deficits in patients with a variety of lower-limb injuries and is sensitive to changes generated with training (Gribble et al. 2012).

Testing for Joint Position Sense

This test involves assessing joints' accuracy at identifying and replicating joint positions. Knee and shoulder (tested in 90° abducted position) joint position sense (repositioning accuracy) should improve as the knee moves towards full extension and the shoulder towards full lateral rotation in the abducted position, so it is important to test joint position sense in both a mid and relatively (though not fully) end-range position (Herrington et al. 2009; Relph & Herrington 2016). The tests can be undertaken either using photography and then analysing the angles (via angle-measuring software) or using goniometry (ideally from a smartphone app). The process is essentially the same: the subject, with eyes closed or blindfolded, has the joint moved passively to a target angle (this angle is measured); the position is held for 5 seconds and then the limb is returned to the start position. The individual is then asked to try to reproduce the joint angle actively, this attempt is measured, and the difference between target and actual is the patient's joint position sense, with smaller being better and typical errors being less than 5°.

Considerations When Rehabilitating to Regain Proprioceptive Acuity

Progressively Challenging Static Balance

On the surface static balance exercises to minimize postural sway seem relatively simple to train, in that the patient just needs to practise standing on two then one leg, thus reducing the base of support. The question is: how is this activity to be progressed in a way which challenges but does not overload the system, resulting in excessive muscle co-contraction and rigidity? If we first consider the starting position, standing flat-footed with an extended knee, we can simply add more challenge to the system here by standing up on to the toes or standing with the knees flexed, for example; both will increase postural sway and so increase the challenge on the sensorimotor control mechanisms. Which progression is chosen will be dictated by the goal (i.e. focusing challenge on the ankle or the hip–knee). The surface the individual stands on potentially provides further challenge, where standing on a yielding soft surface presents a greater challenge than a hard floor so is a logical progression. Challenging the visual or vestibular systems adds further challenge (e.g. rotating the head slowly from side to side whilst trying to maintain a static limb position or closing the eyes whilst undertaking a balance task).

Movement Dissociation Training

Movement dissociation is the ability to move one part of the body whilst keeping another part still. For example, kicking a ball requires good movement dissociation skill, where the stance leg needs to stay still during performance of the motor task. Training movement dissociation is a progression from static balance training; Riemann and Schmitz (2012) found only limited association between static balance and movement dissociation tests. It would appear necessary that, once the patient has progressed through static balance and can balance on soft surfaces at a variety of joint angles whilst having a visual or vestibular challenge applied, the next progression would be to start to undertake movement dissociation activities. These tasks could include standing on one leg and catching or throwing a ball or kicking it, or undertaking movements of the trunk or other leg whilst maintaining limb position.

Movement Control in Motor Skill Learning

Skill acquisition is the process which is followed to acquire new skills. The skill is considered to be acquired when particular criteria can be fulfilled. The skills should be able to be demonstrated consistently, alongside appropriate mobility and movement efficiency in the task undertaken. It is no use if the individual can only perform a single strategy in an isolated circumstance. For example, the recruitment of the transversus abdominis muscle is often cited as critical in the motor control of the spine, but the act of recruiting this muscle in isolation is only a small part of the bigger picture of integrating its action into functional tasks (Spencer et al. 2016). Motor learning is measured by assessing an individual's performance with the consideration of three distinct factors:

1. acquisition: the initial performance of a new skill
2. retention: the ability to replicate the movement after a time delay in which the skill is not practised

3. transfer: the ability to perform a similar, although different, movement to the original task demonstrated in the acquisition phase.

The motor skill which is being undertaken is then defined in terms of the size of the movement involved (which may vary from gross to fine) and the stability of the environment in which it is performed (which may be very closed with considerable internal control or very open with considerable external influences and variability). In addition, the skill may be very discrete, with clear start and end points, or may be continuous.

How practice is undertaken has a significant impact on the ability to acquire, retain and transfer any particular skill, so practice needs to be optimized to improve requisition and retention. Practice could involve undertaking the whole or only part of the skill task. Whole practice relates to practising the entire movement from the start to the end point while part practice refers to segmenting the movement into specific areas to focus upon. To identify the optimal approach the movement must be analysed based on the number of segments involved in the task and also the extent that the segments influence subsequent actions. For instance, continuous tasks are reliant upon the previous movement and thus should be practised as a whole (e.g. running), where breaking down the movement into segmented activities (initial contact, midstance and propulsion phases) is unlikely to be as successful as practising the skill as a whole. Skills consisting of a number of coupled movements may be best broken down into separate components – for example, the power clean Olympic lift is often taught in segments before sequencing the whole movement.

Extrinsic versus Intrinsic Training Feedback Cues

Feedback can be provided both internally and externally. Internal feedback is often referred to as the knowledge of performance and is a major component in motor skill learning; however, an excessive focus on internal feedback can have limitations, as will be discussed later. External feedback (augmented feedback) can come from various sources, for example, visual demonstrations or using a mirror, verbal instruction or physical elements such as manual guidance. Augmented feedback can greatly improve an individual's ability to learn a skill;

however, consideration of the content, timing and frequency of the feedback is important. Verbal augmented feedback aims to provide supplementary information regarding knowledge of performance and results of the movement, both of which are critical to skill learning. Knowledge of performance is related to the execution of the movement, typically the quality of the movement. Conversely, knowledge of results pertains to the actual outcome of the movement – whether it is successful or not.

Often feedback is very descriptive in style. It is often better to engage with individuals via questioning to understand the style of feedback which works best for them. Presenting feedback through open questions which encourage individuals actively to problem solve deficiencies related to their movement is likely to be most effective. Additional considerations relate to the specificity of the information – are you focusing on the movement as a whole or individual segments that need focusing on? Is the information intending to result in an internal focus of attention or an external focus of attention?

Feedback can be provided at different times either during or after the movement and at different intervals. Concurrent feedback has previously been thought to be beneficial in immediately preventing a problem; however, research suggests that concurrent augmented feedback ('in action') can actually impede motor skill learning (retention and transfer) because the individual becomes reliant on such information. Equally, post-practice feedback can hinder learning if the frequency of feedback causes the recipient to become passive in problem-solving movement errors. Feedback should question individuals' beliefs about the performance, not just give them information overload about the performance. Thus, as the skill is developed augmented feedback should be reduced.

Guidance for Providing Feedback

- Provide feedback only when the magnitude of the error is very large (or very small).
- Use a reducing feedback schedule as training progresses.
- Allow the individual athlete/patient to have control over the areas receiving feedback.
- Use summary feedback after a number of attempts rather than after individual attempts.

Modelling is when actions are reproduced based on observing another. Demonstrations are a very effective method of providing an individual with information about the general movement pattern, especially when related to movement sequences and velocities that would be challenging to verbalize accurately. However, care must be taken to demonstrate the movement correctly, as evidence suggests that observed movements are readily adopted, whether they are the correct form or not. This demonstration can also be provided through video of the task. Even when the demonstration is less than perfect, when carefully thought through, modelling using a less than perfect model can prove beneficial in promoting the client to problem solve and identify how the movement pattern can be improved.

Another form of feedback is manual guidance. Manual guidance relates to physically moving individuals so that they can experience proprioceptive feedback associated with the correct movement. However, care should be taken not to overrely on this approach as individuals (as with augmented feedback) could become overly reliant on the support of the practitioner rather than identifying strategies themselves. This method of support is effective in the early stages of motor learning, although it needs to be reduced as learning progresses.

When performing a movement the individual can focus either internally or externally. Internal focus of attention relates to the movement and positioning of the body; this could include focusing on contracting the bicep while lifting a barbell. Conversely, an external focus of attention relates to focusing on the effect of the movement, so in the same example this would be the movement of the barbell. A range of research has identified that in skill learning and execution adopting an external focus of attention is beneficial. Examples have included greater movement efficiency, reduced muscle activity, greater accuracy of movement and increased force when using an external focus; however a recent systematic review has questioned the evidence base (Herrington & Comfort 2013). Language must be carefully considered to use instructions which promote an external focus of attention.

In the context of injury, Benjaminse et al. (2015) provide an excellent review of the use of feedback in relation to anterior cruciate ligament injury prevention programmes, while Agresta and Brown (2015) provide another on running gait retraining. These provide great examples of how using the appropriate feedback has positive outcomes.

Adding Complexity to Movement Skill Training

The learning process that individuals utilize to acquire movement skill has been proposed to have three stages: cognitive, associative and autonomous. The cognitive stage is characterized by a conscious attempt to determine what exactly needs to be done, step by step, involving considerable repetition of the same task. The associative phase starts when the basic movement pattern has been acquired. The movement outcome is now more reliable, consistent, automatic and economical. Once this is accomplished, more attention can be directed to other aspects of performance. After extensive practice, the performer reaches the autonomous phase, which is characterized by fluent and seemingly effortless motions. Movements are accurate, very consistent and efficiently produced. The skill is performed largely automatically at this stage, and movement execution requires little or no attention. It is commonly believed that directing the athlete's attention to step-by-step components of a skill is necessary during the early stages of acquisition. Gaining cognitive control (explicit knowledge) of the task is a necessary phase that athletes must go through. It is in this stage that the athlete practises a new skill over and over to reach the autonomous stage, so-called automatic movement control. However, repetition of the same movement patterns may be a suboptimal method compared to utilizing pattern variations, which can stimulate the brain to find optimal solutions to unanticipated events more effectively. What follows is a discussion of how to incorporate these greater levels of complexity into training.

The fundamental aim of any motor skill learning programme is to achieve transference of the skill into sport (or activity of daily living) performance (dynamic correspondence). A lot of training programmes undertake work at or on the conscious (cognitive) level, relying on closed skill activities carried out in a block order. Typically this involves repeated practising of the closed skill, that is, the same movement tasks, undertaken in stable predictable environments, most often carried out at a pace determined by the participant. To reflect the motor skill requirements of sports and even life more appropriately, motor skill training programmes need to have progressively increasing complexity where more open skill (non-planned skills/tasks) elements become incorporated in a more and more random fashion once the closed skill tasks have been mastered. This leads to practices that are initially controlled and self-paced, allowing participants to understand and learn the specifics of the appropriate movement patterns in environments that are predictable and static to allow them to plan their movements in advance (closed skill practice). The practices then need to progress to incorporate more random elements, where the environment becomes unpredictable and performers need to adapt their movements in response (open skill practice). During the whole of the practice practitioners need to consider the appropriate feedback and cues which they use to maximize the skill development, as discussed above. An example of developing skill through this process is reported in the paper of Herrington and Comfort (2013), illustrated in Figs 10.5 and 10.6 (see below).

Considerations When Rehabilitating to Regain Motor Control Skill

Research indicates that the level of load placed on the musculoskeletal system is different despite doing the same task, when a sport-specific context is applied. For example, Dempsey et al. (2012) found knee loads were significantly increased during a landing task when the participants had to catch a ball during the task. This simple more 'functional' addition shows how much greater loading stress could occur in the random chaotic environments presented by sport participation or even a patient walking around the shops on a busy Saturday afternoon. The final stages of rehabilitation, if we are truly going to have full neuromuscular control of the task in hand, must therefore train them to cope with these random chaotic environments. This is as relevant for an 80-year-old with an arthritic knee as an elite sportsperson; both will be exposed to risk of further, recurrent or other injury if not able to cope with these environmental demands.

Certain fundamentals are required in order to engage in motor control rehabilitation. Patients must have adequate strength, work capacity (WC), proprioceptive acuity and ranges of movement for the task to be undertaken; otherwise these become the rate limiters to their progression. As detailed above, motor skill control begins with practice in a closed skill block

manner with both internal and external feedback cues, so for instance, this might involve doing repetitive single-leg squats in front of a mirror, attempting to maintain good limb alignment. Once the task is mastered in that context, then it can be challenged by increasing complexity (task demand) by performing a step landing, for example, still as a closed skill, but requiring far greater control because of the increased forces involved. This might further be challenged by stepping on to different surfaces or from different heights. Once each of these tasks has been mastered individually, then they could be undertaken together, which adds variability to the global task of step landing; patients have to land from a variety of heights on to a variety of surfaces, so they cannot preplan to the same extent, hence the task becomes more open. Then further complexity could be added by including perturbation, which makes the situation even more random. So at the end of this little training progression patients would be able to demonstrate good motor control skill of the task of step landing off a variety of heights of step on to a variety of surfaces whilst potentially being pushed off balance (perturbed) – that should teach them how to cope with the shops on a Saturday afternoon! The progressions through closed and open skill training are illustrated in Figs 10.5 and 10.6 (see below).

FUNDAMENTALS OF STRENGTH TRAINING AND ADAPTATION

This section identifies the underpinning knowledge required to understand the fundamentals of strength and work capacity (WC) training and then discusses how these concepts could and should be applied when rehabilitating the injured patient. The development of exercise prescriptions tailored to specific outcomes is discussed.

Exercise Prescription by Intention, Adaptation and Physical Outcome

The comprehensive restoration of physical abilities during rehabilitation is fundamental in the attainment of athletic performance and mitigation of injury risk on return to sporting activity, but equally this construct could be applied to maximizing functional capacity in activities of daily living. In order to achieve this, those rehabilitating the patient need to identify both the current capabilities of the patient and the injured tissue and the patient's 'end goals' (i.e. the nature and level of stress the tissue [and individual] will have to cope with in order to perform). Critically, different exercises produce different effects on neuromuscular performance and effective rehabilitation is underpinned through a clear understanding of exercise specificity and targeted adaptation, where intended physical outcome (e.g. mobility, motor control, strength) dictates the nature of exercise prescription. The practitioner needs to balance carefully the requirement to reestablish physical qualities and address modifiable (hypothesized) factors contributing to injury causation (described by Wainner et al. [2007] as regional interdependence), alongside the loading capacity of the healing tissue and the inherent physical attributes of each individual patient. The entry point or baseline for loading in rehabilitation will be discussed later in the chapter.

Defining Work Capacity and Strength

Discrepancies between load tolerance and requirements for performance are a critical determinant in rehabilitation efficacy. Progressive tissue overload through targeted resistance training and appropriate manipulation of training variables (i.e. exercise selection, tempo, intensity, volume, rest and frequency of performance) enables the practitioner to facilitate optimized improvements in strength and capacity whilst avoiding deleterious loading, which could result in tissue failure or reinjury.

Work Capacity

WC is synonymous with local muscular endurance (Ratamess et al. 2009) and can be defined as the ability to produce or tolerate variable intensities and durations of work (Siff 2003). WC is a training outcome where the accumulation of training over many weeks and months results in chronic local adaptation to muscle, tendon and metabolic biogenesis. This chronic local adaptation increases the ability of the system to produce more work during repeated efforts and allows the local musculature to tolerate (or demonstrate resilience to) a larger training volume of work. By comparison, strength endurance (high-intensity endurance) has been described as a performance outcome test completed in isolation, whereby the goal is to achieve a specific amount of work at a given intensity, such as maximum number of repetitions at 50% of one repetition maximum (1RM) or at a specific submaximal load, with less emphasis placed on the physiological adaptation required for WC development. As a result, strength endurance can be used as a proxy measure of WC or as a training variable within WC. Through specific WC training, the patient is able to produce, transfer, absorb or dissipate (and recover from) repeated or sustained submaximal forces, providing a platform of 'general physical preparedness' for the development and performance of specific strength qualities. The American College of Sports Medicine resistance training guidelines suggest that light to moderate loads (40–60% of 1RM) be performed for high repetitions (>15) using short rest periods (<90 seconds) two to three times per week to develop local muscular endurance.

Muscular Strength

Muscular strength can be defined as the ability to produce force, with maximal strength being the largest force the musculature can produce (Stone et al. 2004).

Rate of Force Development

Rate of force development (RFD) has been defined as the rate of rise of contractile force at the beginning of a muscle action and is time-dependent (Aagaard et al. 2002). Functionally, globally coordinated RFD augments external power production during maximal velocity movements (e.g. sprinting, kicking, jumping or throwing) or creates segmental 'stiffening' against yielding forces (e.g. bracing against an external impact). The production of force/torque and stiffness depends on morphological and neurological factors from the neuromuscular system. Morphological factors include cross-sectional area, muscle pennation angle, fascial length and fibre type (Cormie et al. 2011). Neurological factors include motor unit recruitment, firing frequency, motor unit synchronization and intermuscular coordination (Cormie et al. 2009). Strength development in highly trained individuals typically utilizes higher loads corresponding to a repetition range of a 1–6RM using 3–5-minute rest periods between sets, as much as 4–5 days per week. The loads required in untrained individuals are comparatively low, where a repetition range of an 8–12RM or higher, 2–3 days per week, is sufficient to create an increase in maximal strength. Lighter loads (0–60% RM) performed at a fast contraction velocity with a multijoint emphasis are appropriate for enhancing RFD/external power production (Ratamess et al. 2009).

EXERCISE PROGRESSION WITHIN RELOADING REHABILITATION

This section explains how to develop a needs analysis for patients, breaking this down into appropriate stages, setting appropriate goals to demarcate the ability to progress to the next stage and monitoring the effect of load on both the injured tissue and the individual. This section will also consider how to regain 'fitness', that is, chronic capacity in the injured tissue and the individual to reduce the risk of recurrence. Finally it will look at the decision making around the return to performance.

A concise, comprehensive format detailing progression of exercise rehabilitation for musculoskeletal injuries is lacking within the research and professional literature. Of the limited examples, it is worth considering the papers of Ralston (2003) on the RAMP principle and Herrington et al. (2013) on anterior cruciate ligament reconstruction rehabilitation; which offer insight into a comprehensive process which could be applied generically to all injuries. This section outlines a structure from which an exercise rehabilitation framework for musculoskeletal injury can be built. A previous section (Reloading in rehabilitation) outlined the underpinning theory as to why progressive appropriate loading is essential in the development of tissue tolerance to load and how this knowledge underpins exercise rehabilitation.

Performance Needs Analysis

A successful outcome of rehabilitation is when the individual is able to return fully to whatever tasks s/he wishes to participate in without limitation and at no greater risk of further injury to the previously damaged tissues. In reality however this is highly unlikely, with previously injured tissues often constraining performance. Part of the reason this happens might be that the individual has not been adequately prepared for return to full activity. When planning any rehabilitation programme it is critical to understand what the 'end goal' is. That is, what is the nature of the activities the individual wishes to return to? Once the performance

---

BOX 10.1

COMPONENTS OF AN ACTIVITY-SPECIFIC NEEDS ANALYSIS

- Sport, role and position
  - What is the person's role/position within activity/sport?
- Performance duration
  - What is the total duration of the person's whole performance?
  - What is the duration and frequency of training sessions?
- Activity duration
  - Is the activity continuous or does it involve bursts of varying intensity and duration?
- Activities
  - What is involved? Jumping, landing, sprinting, change of direction, kicking, throwing, lifting, carrying?
- Involvement of impact/contact/collisions
- Distances covered and directions moved in
- Predominant muscle groups
- Predominant muscle actions
- Flexibility and range of movement demands
- Motor skill requirements

---

needs are established, it is important to define the physical abilities underpinning the performance of each activity (Box 10.1). Detailed consideration of mobility and motor control qualities has been described in an earlier section and readers should also consider the maintenance, restoration and development of cardiovascular qualities within the rehabilitation process. What follows is a conceptual model of how to load the tissues progressively, that is, how to deliver a progressive loading programme to bring about appropriate adaptations within the tissue and reestablish loading tolerance underpinning the mechanical demands of the target activity. The language used within this section will often refer to the athlete and sport, but the concepts and underpinning philosophy could equally be applied to any individual wishing to return to any activity of daily living or work task. Box 10.1 identifies typical information required to assess the activity-specific needs of an individual.

Progressing Load and Function (Entry Criteria for Progression)

When designing a rehabilitation programme the first stage is to assess the problem; this involves two elements.

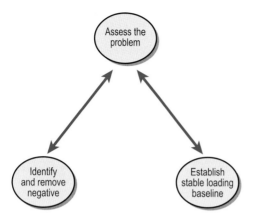

FIG. 10.3 ■ Stage 1 in developing an exercise rehabilitation programme.

One is to establish a clear definitive diagnosis of the problem; the establishing of a clinical diagnosis is covered elsewhere within this text. Here we will concentrate on the second element, which is defining the 'problems' associated with the injury (Fig. 10.3).

The status of the injured tissue is the primary consideration. How much load can the injured tissue tolerate? With some injuries this would appear obvious, where it might be assumed that an acute muscle/ligament/tendon injury would have zero tolerance of load when damaged, or would they? Even these injured structures can often generate or tolerate a level of force (albeit low). It is essential that the level of load the tissues can tolerate is clearly identified. For example, if a tendon can only tolerate low repetitions of body weight loads then it is critical that activities such as walking are restricted or the relative load reduced by using walking aids (e.g. crutches) or a walking boot. Equally, if the tendon only becomes irritated and painful after running for 8 km, it would be inappropriate to stop the individual from running entirely as this is likely to cause significant atrophy of the tissue. Likewise, for muscle, if a 5-kg weight, for example, can be lifted without issue, then that would be the starting point for loading. Significant muscle atrophy can occur within 5–14 days of inactivity (Wall et al. 2013), so it is imperative that the minimum activity an athlete can perform is established so that atrophy related to underactivity and disuse is reduced to an absolute minimum.

In addition to allowing the application of 'safe' loads, all extraneous loads which could stress the tissue need to be identified. The second element of this stage is therefore to identify and remove negative external (and internal) forces and factors promoting continued trauma. This could involve the use of gait aids, tape and braces or modification/restriction of certain elements of training. Equally it could involve the modification of movement patterns, which create asymmetrical loads on the tissues, which may represent an ongoing goal throughout the rehabilitation process.

Once the starting point for rehabilitation has been established then the exercises themselves can be developed. Whilst undertaking the rehabilitation programme, the athlete needs to be monitored within each session, daily and weekly, for specific markers which may indicate that the tissue is becoming stressed by the level of loading. The athlete's quality of performance and response to loading are monitored continuously throughout the rehabilitation process. This information provides intelligence to ascertain whether the level of exercise is appropriate (the moving baseline level) and whether the movement patterns are appropriate, which indicates whether external (extra) loading is being controlled with the use of appropriate movement patterns. Methods for monitoring the patient are discussed later in this section.

When introducing the programme it is important to get the initial load right. If the load is too high then there is the potential for further tissue damage, but equally if the level is too low, it could cause tissue atrophy and set the patient back and prolong the rehabilitation period unnecessarily. Understanding how the tissue responds to the loads applied is a critical element of ongoing exercise rehabilitation programming and prescription. The control of pain is also essential; pain can cause muscle inhibition, alter sensory feedback and

BOX 10.3
KEY ISSUES WHEN RELOADING THE INJURED TISSUES

- What is the stable baseline load?
- Has the loading level start point been established?
- What forces stress the injured structure?
- Which forces and loads do not stress the injured structure?
- For ligaments, have the direction and magnitude of injurious force been defined?
- For muscle and tendon, has the nature of contraction load, force velocity and length–tension relationship implications been defined?
- For articular surfaces, define the direction and magnitude of injurious forces and the impact of malalignment?

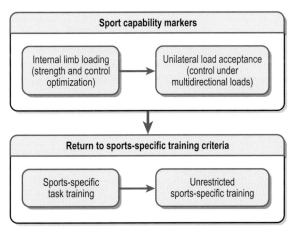

FIG. 10.4 ■ Typical exercise progression.

alter movement patterns, all of which would limit the effectiveness of the exercise programme. Box 10.2 identifies key elements in setting up and the progression of the exercises chosen.

Tissue Function and Exercise Specificity

When developing specific exercise programmes, the relationship between the role of the injured tissue and the target activity or activities must be carefully considered. Box 10.3 highlights the key issues when reloading the injured tissue.

Tissue Loading

As discussed, when reloading the injured tissue the first consideration is the level of load it can tolerate. Depending on the tissue injury-specific factors which need to be accounted for in the plan for progressive reloading (highlighted in Fig. 10.4; see below), a starting level of load is established, from which exercises can be progressed. Two critical interrelated concepts need to be considered within the rehabilitation exercise progression plan: Wolf's law and the SAID (specific adaptation to imposed demand) principle. According to Wolf's law injured tissues are stressed and so stimulated to heal and adapt according to the forces that are applied to them. The SAID principle similarly states that tissue adapts to the specific stress applied to them. The implication of this information is simply that the tissue must be (eventually) exposed to the loads and stresses involved in the sports and activities that the patient wishes to participate in.

It has already been identified that, if tissue is unloaded, it atrophies and its tolerance to load is decreased, so the imperative factor to prevent reinjury is to make sure the tissue is strong enough to tolerate the loads it will be exposed to during sporting or functional activity. In order to achieve this, a progressive exposure plan must be developed. For muscle that is relatively easy, the load the muscle has to lift and lower can be progressively increased. But even here the situation is not that straightforward. The length–tension and force–velocity relationships must be incorporated into the plan; the muscle must not only generate progressively greater forces but do it at different lengths, during different types of muscular contraction and contraction velocities. Tendon loading would have to follow a similar pattern with the added complication of decisions regarding the impact of tensile versus torsional or compressive loading. Moreover, articular and osseous injuries require gradually increased exposure to axial (compressive) loading, whilst minimizing exposure to torsional and shear loading.

When considering the progression of loading for a ligament, initially the most stressful direction of load would need to be identified and avoided with focus on controlling the forces which move the joint in that direction. Gradually, the joint movements would need to be focused towards the stressful direction, to load the ligament and facilitate adaptation in order to restrict movement in that direction, or laxity and unrestrained movement will persist. In addition, mechanical stimulus in the direction of maximum ligamentous tension is needed to generate proprioceptive 'knowledge' of what movement in the stressful position 'feels like'. This increased awareness helps facilitate appropriate reactive muscle action to restrict pathological loading. If the movement is constantly avoided, when it does occur, the body will not know how to react, increasing the risk of reinjury. Furthermore, if the structure is biologically weaker (from limited load exposure) the potential damage may be significantly greater.

Task-Specific Training

In addition to specifically reloading the injured tissue, a holistic approach needs to be taken towards management of the athlete. There are two main considerations. Firstly, whilst undergoing rehabilitation individuals have the potential to detrain globally with regard to the 'fitness' required to perform their sport. This must be avoided or minimized because of its performance implications; and because an athlete who is poorly conditioned is more likely to get injured. Secondly, progressing the athlete through specific capability markers towards unrestricted sports-specific training will increase the success of a graduated loading programme.

Fig. 10.4 describes a typical progression for rehabilitation, where the athlete initially starts with controlled exercises, often described as closed-chain exercises (though the inclusion of open-chain exercises may be appropriate); some example progressions are outlined in Fig. 10.5. The intent is to develop the fundamental WC and strength qualities underpinning sport-specific progression. When specific capability markers are achieved, the athlete would then progress to load acceptance tasks (landing on the limb and moving towards running). When the athlete is accepting load

in multiple directions and running without issues, sport-specific elements can be added based on the sport activity needs analysis. These elements need to consider directions and durations of loading which reflect those in the sport (with the addition of specific technical and tactical elements such as kicking or catching a ball during the task, etc.) and may include open skill and random training when fatigued to reflect end of game situations (Fig. 10.6).

The guiding principle of the sport-specific training element of the rehabilitation programme is to reload athletes in a manner which fully meets the needs of the sport they wish to return too. This process would work equally well for a return to activities of daily living and work; the example used here just happens to be sport. A key factor is to ensure the athlete's chronic capacity

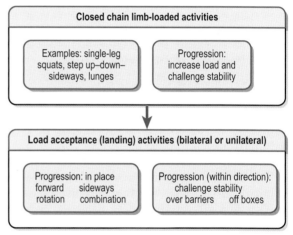

FIG. 10.5 ■ Closed skill exercise progression. *(After Herrington & Comfort 2013.)*

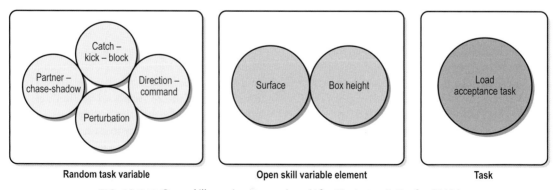

FIG. 10.6 ■ Open skill exercise progression. *(After Herrington & Comfort 2013.)*

is increased to a sufficient level that any acute increase in load should not significantly overload the system. It is important to understand fully the demands placed on individuals in order to ensure they are fully prepared for a return to unrestricted activities. The process of regaining and measuring chronic capacity is described below. Once individuals are able to carry out all relevant tasks whilst fatigued (with sport-specific elements incorporated where appropriate), they would then be commenced on unrestricted sport-specific training. Again, comprehensive monitoring is required to assess the tissue reaction during the return to the training phase.

Monitoring the Effect of Rehabilitation Exercise Load

Pain, stiffness and swelling can be used to determine exercise progression as these factors will relate to the loading stresses placed on the tissues and will provide an indirect measure of any tissue inflammation which has been generated as a result of tissue trauma.

Pain

Pain can be monitored using numeric rating scales, for example, on a scale of 0–10, with 0 equalling no pain and 10 equating the worst pain imaginable. This is more useful when placed in a specific context; for example, where 2/10 might be described as the level of discomfort typically experienced following a 'hard' training session (i.e. delayed-onset muscle soreness). Likewise it is more sensitive to link pain scores to specific events rather than a generic question, for example, rating pain following a rehabilitation session or whilst performing a specific task, such as squatting, walking or going downstairs. Similarly, diurnal variation in pain is typically more sensitive, where rating pain in the evening may identify build-up of inflammatory products in the tissue over the day as a result of repetitive overload. Using numeric rating scales has been shown to be sensitive to changes in pain which affect function (Krebs et al. 2007), with a reduction or increase by 1 point being regarded as the minimal clinically important change (Salaffi et al. 2004). Any change in score from the previous day is noted and significant increases in postrehabilitation scores (>1) which do not resolve by the evening are likely to indicate overload.

Stiffness

Stiffness or resistance to movement of the tissue, especially the next morning, is a strong indicator of an overloaded tissue demonstrating signs of inflammatory stress. A simple scale can be used to monitor stiffness in the morning on rising; again, this works best if linked to a physical task, for example, squatting, sitting, going downstairs, as appropriate. A typical scale could be:

0 = free movement
1 = some restriction
2 = significant restriction
3 = unable to move as too painfully restricted.

Swelling

Swelling is an obvious overt sign of inflammation. Here the change in swelling is likely to be a more sensitive measure than merely the presence or absence of swelling itself. So assessment of swelling should take place following activity and in the morning and evening. The goal would be that swelling does not vary over the day or between days, however; if postexercise it had increased, this would have ideally resolved by the evening. If it had not resolved by the next morning, then subsequent loading may have to be modified until the situation is resolved. Circumferential measurements are possible in the periphery to be used as a monitoring tool for this aspect of response to exposure monitoring.

Regaining Chronic Capacity

Despite considerable work investigating which factors predict the occurrence of injury (and reinjury), little is still known, apart from the fact that previous injury is the greatest predictor of all the variables currently investigated. This poses the question: is it that the tissue is perpetually weak due to 'poor healing' and unable to tolerate the loads it is exposed to, or is it that the tissue has not been exposed to sufficient loading during the rehabilitation process in order to bring about the required adaptation to cope with the return to sport demands? If the latter is the case, then the levels of load applied during rehabilitation need careful consideration. The application of load during rehabilitation has been discussed above; however, an element which was not covered was the frequency with which these loads need to be applied. The occurrence of injury would appear to be related to the application of loads in excess of what the tissue is capable of withstanding. This indicates that a relative increase in load from these chronic levels could predispose tissue stress; Blanch and Gabbett (2016) called this the acute–chronic load ratio.

The acute–chronic ratio relates to the amount of training the athlete has completed during the rehabilitation period, compared with the amount required when in full training. This ratio is calculated by comparing the acute load (i.e. training performed during the current week) with the chronic load (i.e. the training performed over the last 4 weeks, for example). Training load could be calculated from either external workload, such as kilometres ran/amount of weight lifted and/or internal load such as minutes exercised multiplied by a perceived exertion rating. Once calculated, an acute–chronic workload of 0.5 would indicate that an athlete had undertaken only half as much workload in the most recent week as in the previous 4 weeks, whereas a ratio of 2.0 would indicate that the athlete was undertaking twice as much work in the current week as the previous 4 weeks. It has been reported that acute–chronic workload ratios of greater than 1.5 indicate a significant elevation in the injury risk profile (Blanch & Gabbett 2016). The work in this area indicates that the athlete must have a gradual increase in workload eventually to match the demands required to complete in full unrestricted activities. For example, it is easy to see how an athlete recovering from a hamstring strain would be at elevated risk of reinjury on return to game play following a period of time off (or very restricted) high-speed running, despite being able to sprint painfree. Similarly, the patient with osteoarthritis of the knee who has been off her feet with a cold or flu returning to full activity could equally suffer an increased risk of problems with her sudden spike in acute–chronic workload ratio.

Return to Performance: Decision Making and Measuring Effectiveness

Return to performance/play efficacy is measured across three key elements: actually returning to play (whatever 'play' is – sport, work or walking around the shops on a Saturday); competence (i.e. returning to play at the same competence level or better); and sustained performance over time. Attainment across all three factors presents a significant challenge to the practitioner and

provides context to research measuring successful rehabilitation/intervention by 'returning to play' alone. Return to play decision making is often very challenging; clinicians are required to advise when it is 'safe' to resume sports participation, or at the very least, provide information to enable patients to make informed decisions regarding the advantages and disadvantages of returning to sporting activity. The information presented must include a balanced interpretation of the health risks associated with a return to play (i.e. the risk of reinjury, or sustaining a new injury) alongside the predicted consequences (which may be minor, significant or even serious/life changing). Whilst a precise calculation of risk/consequence is impossible, the practitioner must provide a reasoned hypothesis based on available knowledge and previous experience. The perceived risk is also amplified or dampened according to the nature of the intended return (e.g. sport, position and role) and the available options to mitigate the threat of further injury (e.g. modified training, the use of padding/ strapping). The following section highlights the key considerations for medical practitioners involved in return-to-play decision making.

As described in detail in this chapter, rehabilitation is not determined by attainment of a temporal or time-based prognosis. Whilst injury prognostics are inevitably part of the practitioner's role, and often the first question asked by athletes and coaches following injury, rehabilitation must be considered as a progressive, criterion-based journey from injury to return to play. It is an interdisciplinary process, where collaboration and collective integration between the support team, coach/parent and athlete are paramount. This optimized approach ensures that: the physical qualities underpinning sporting performance (i.e. mobility, motor control, WC and strength/RFD) are fully restored and, where available, mapped against profiling data captured prior to the injury; and the athlete is progressively exposed (and adapts) to the physical and psychological demands of the sport. Quantification of performance parameters in training and competition provides important information during the rehabilitation process. Methods of capturing workload data may be relatively simple or highly complex and can be measured in a variety of different ways. External loads relate to physical work (e.g. distance ran, weight lifted, number and intensity of sprints) and are accompanied by an internal load relating

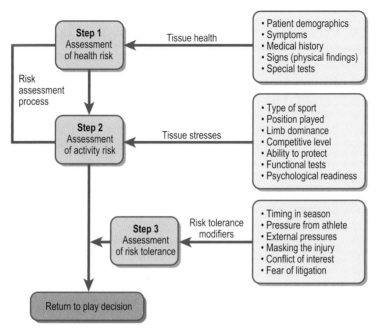

FIG. 10.7 ▪ Strategic Assessment of Risk and Risk Tolerance (StARRT) framework.

to the physiological or perceptual response (e.g. ratings of perceived exertion and heart rate) (Gabbett 2016). This information helps practitioners comprehend the biomechanical and physiological stresses during training and competition; and provides performance benchmarks to inform functional reintegration and return-to-play criteria based on historical data analysis.

The comprehensive rehabilitation journey ends with a successful and sustained return to unrestricted training, at which stage the athlete is passed 'fit' to return to competition. In this sense, the athlete's response to a traditional field-based 'fitness test' becomes redundant. Unfortunately, however, optimized rehabilitation planning often becomes complicated by external factors such as the athlete's fundamental desire to return, time constraints (i.e. the competition schedule), financial incentives or pressure from parents, coaches and the media. In such cases, the practitioner is faced with a difficult decision regarding the appropriateness of a return to play. The Strategic Assessment of Risk and Risk Tolerance (StARRT) assessment, described by Shrier (2015), introduces a strategic approach underpinning return-to-play decisions in sport. This approach helps practitioners to reason opinions and advice offered to

patients in a consistent and transparent way. The model in Fig. 10.7 organizes key information and interactions between factors associated with tissue health (e.g. medical history, symptoms, objective clinical testing) and tissue stress (e.g. type of sport, position played, psychological readiness) to determine the risk of participation. Importantly, risk is then placed in the context of risk tolerance: the clinician's (and athlete's) threshold for an acceptable risk. For example, it might be considered that a 20% chance of reinjury to the lateral ankle ligaments is an acceptable risk in order to compete at the Olympic Games, especially if the risk can be mitigated with the use of strapping/bracing. Conversely, however, the potential consequences of allowing an athlete with suspected concussion to return to play are so severe (regardless of risk tolerance modifiers), the risk assessment unreservedly exceeds risk tolerance, and the decision should be not to return to play. Whilst the medical team perform an essential role informing the decision-making process, input from the interdisciplinary team is crucial to determine whether the athlete is ready to return at the level of intensity (and frequency) required to sustain the performance outcomes within the target activity.

SUMMARY

The primary goals when rehabilitating any musculoskeletal injury are to maximize the patient's potential level of function postinjury whilst minimizing the risk of injury recurrence or secondary injury or other comorbidities. These goals are true whether rehabilitating an Olympic athlete or an octogenarian with a degenerate hip, and the fundamental processes are also the same. A thorough assessment of the presenting problems, the patient's capability (at the injured tissue and global levels) and the patient's end goals is the starting point. From there the injured tissue and the patient globally are exposed to progressively more challenging loads in order to generate adaptation in these systems, so that the capabilities of the tissue and the individual are improved in such a way as to move the person closer to the overarching treatment goals. A comprehensive understanding of the concepts underpinning rehabilitation planning and delivery provides the foundation for successful return to performance. 'Performance' is not a term reserved for those interested in sporting activity; indeed, meaningful tasks are determined by patients' desire to return to any activity they deem important – this is the outcome measure. The outcome may or may not present a realistic objective, however; the process must always start with a clear and detailed understanding of the physical, physiological and biomechanical demands of the intended target activity. This performance analysis enables the practitioner to consider what physical qualities underpin performance in the context of the clinical assessment/diagnosis, function of the injured tissue and current physical status. The analysis is driven by both the impact of the injury and by factors contributing to injury aetiology. Rehabilitation planning then details the reloading journey and the intervention required to attain progressive, criterion-based goals throughout the process.

Successful rehabilitation requires targeted intervention, defined and measured by the intended outcomes. Pain management is paramount, and provides a primary focus particularly during the initial stages of management, but, wherever possible, the approach should proactively avoid the deleterious effects of offloading. Skilled movement control training provides the basis for optimizing load distribution and mechanical efficiency but can only be achieved on the foundation of adequate tissue mobility and the ability to produce and absorb force – ultimately, the patient must develop tolerance to load through careful exposure and chronic adaptation. The skill of rehabilitation is therefore the prescription of highly individualized exercises/physical activities defined by an intended outcome and physical adaptation (exercises are not defined by name, equipment used or the place where they are performed). As patients are functionally reintegrated towards their target activity, the practitioner must be certain that the individual has the appropriate physical qualities to underpin the demands of each progressive task. If achieved, the transition back to performance is optimized with maximum efficiency and minimum risk of further injury.

REFERENCES

Aagaard, P., Simonsen, E.B., Andersen, J.L., et al., 2002. Increased rate of force development and neural drive of human skeletal muscle following resistance training. J. Appl. Physiol. 93, 1318–1326.

Agresta, C., Brown, A., 2015. Gait retraining for injured and healthy runners using augmented feedback: using augmented feedback: a systematic literature review. J. Orthop. Sports Phys. Ther. 45, 576–584.

Behm, D.G., Chaouachi, A., 2011. A review of the acute effects of static and dynamic stretching on performance. Eur. J. Appl. Physiol. 111, 2633–2651.

Bell, D., Guskiewicz, K., Clark, M., et al., 2011. Systematic review of the balance error scoring system. Sports Health 3, 287–295.

Benjaminse, A., Welling, W., Otten, B., et al., 2015. Novel methods of instruction in ACL injury prevention programs, a systematic review. Phys. Ther. Sport 16, 176–186.

Blanch, P., Gabbett, T., 2016. Has the athlete trained enough to return to play safely? The acute:chronic workload ratio permits clinician to quantify a player's risk of subsequent injury. Br. J. Sports Med. 50, 471–475.

Cormie, P., McBride, J.M., McCaulley, G.O., 2009. Power–time, force–time, and velocity–time curve analysis of the countermovement jump: impact of training. J. Strength Cond. Res. 23, 177–186.

Cormie, P., McGuigan, M.R., Newton, R.U., 2011. Developing maximal neuromuscular power: part 1 – biological basis of maximal power production. Sports Med. 41, 17–38.

Dempsey, A., Elliott, B., Munro, B., et al., 2012. Whole body kinematics and knee moments that occur during an overhead catch and landing task in sport. Clin. Biomech. (Bristol, Avon) 27, 466–474.

Dye, S., 2005. The pathophysiology of patellofemoral pain. Clin. Orthop. Relat. Res. 436, 100–110.

Gabbett, T., 2016. The training–injury prevention paradox: should athletes be training smarter and harder? Br. J. Sports Med. 50, 300–303.

Gajdosik, R.L., 2001. Passive extensibility of skeletal muscle: review of the literature with clinical implications. Clin. Biomech. (Bristol, Avon) 16, 87–101.

Gribble, P., Hertel, J., Plisky, P., 2012. Using star excursion balance test to assess dynamic postural control deficits and outcomes in lower extremity injury: a literature and systematic review. J. Athl. Train. 47, 339–357.

Guissard, N., Duchateau, J., 2004. Effect of static stretch training on neural and mechanical properties of the human plantar flexor muscles. Muscle Nerve 29, 248–255.

Herrington, L., Comfort, P., 2013. Training for prevention of ACL injury: incorporation of progressive landing skill challenges into a programme. Strength Cond. J. 36, 59–65.

Herrington, L., Horsley, I., Rolf, C., 2009. Evaluation of shoulder joint position sense in professional rugby players. Phys. Ther. Sport 11, 18–22.

Herrington, L., Myer, G., Horsley, I., 2013. Task based rehabilitation protocol for elite athletes following anterior cruciate ligament reconstruction: a clinical commentary. Phys. Ther. Sport 14, 188–198.

Hodges, P.W., Moseley, G.L., 2003. Pain and motor control of the lumbopelvic region: effect and possible mechanisms. J. Electromyogr. Kinesiol. 13, 361–370.

Iverson, G., Koehle, M., 2013. Normative data for the balance error scoring system in adults. Rehabil. Res. Pract. 1, 1–5.

Khan, K., Scott, A., 2009. Mechanotherapy: how physical therapists' prescription of exercises promotes tissue repair. Br. J. Sports Med. 43, 247–252.

Krebs, E., Carey, T., Weinberger, M., 2007. Accuracy of the pain numeric rating scale as a screening test in primary care. J. Gen. Intern. Med. 22, 1453–1458.

Langevin, H.M., Sherman, K.J., 2007. Pathophysiological model for chronic low back pain integrating connective tissue and nervous system mechanisms. Med. Hypotheses 68, 74–80.

Linke, W.A., Leake, M.C., 2004. Multiple sources of passive stress relaxation in muscle fibres. Phys. Med. Biol. 49, 3613–3627.

Magnusson, S.P., Simonsen, E.B., Aagaard, P., et al., 1996. A mechanism for altered flexibility in human skeletal muscle. J. Physiol. 497, 291–298.

Magnusson, S.P., Simonsen, E.B., Aagaard, P., et al., 1997. Determinants of musculoskeletal flexibility: viscoelastic properties, cross-sectional area, EMG and stretch tolerance. Scand. J. Med. Sci. Sports 7, 195–202.

Magnusson, S., Aagaard, P., Simonson, E., et al., 2000. Passive tensile stress and energy of the human hamstring muscles in vivo. Med. Sci. Sports Exerc. 10, 351–359.

Mueller, M., Maluf, K., 2002. Tissue adaptation to physical stress: a proposed 'Physical Stress Theory' to guide physical therapy practice, education and research. Phys. Ther. 82, 383–403.

Munro, A., Herrington, L., 2010. Between session reliability of the star excursion balance test. Phys. Ther. Sport 11, 128–132.

O'Sullivan, K., McAuliffe, S., Deburca, N., 2012. The effects of eccentric training on lower limb flexibility: a systematic review. Br. J. Sports Med. 46, 838–845.

Page, P., 2012. Current concepts in muscle stretching for exercise and rehabilitation. Int. J. Sports Phys. Ther. 7, 109–119.

Ralston, D., 2003. The RAMP system: a template for the progression of athletic injury rehabilitation. J. Sports Rehabil. 12, 280–290.

Ratamess, N.A., Alvar, A., Evetoch, T.K., et al., 2009. American College of Sports Medicine position stand. Progression models in resistance training for healthy adults. Med. Sci. Sports Exerc. 41, 687–708.

Relph, N., Herrington, L., 2016. The effects of knee direction, physical activity and age on knee joint position sense. Knee 23, 1029–1034.

Riemann, B., Schmitz, R., 2012. The relationship between various modes of single leg postural control assessment. Int. J. Sports Phys. Ther. 7, 257–266.

Sahrmann, S., 2002. Diagnosis and treatment of movement impairment syndromes. Elsevier Health Sciences, St Louis, MO, pp. 12–13.

Salaffi, F., Stancati, A., Silvestri, C., et al., 2004. Minimal clinically important changes in chronic musculoskeletal pain intensity measured on numerical rating scale. Eur. J. Pain 8, 283–291.

Shrier, I., 2015. Strategic Assessment of Risk and Risk Tolerance (StARRT) framework for return-to-play decision-making. Br. J. Sports Med. 49, 1311–1315.

Siff, M.C., 2003. Supertraining. Supertraining Institute, Denver, CO, pp. 32–33.

Spencer, S., Wolf, A., Rushton, A., 2016. Spinal exercise prescription in sport: classifying training and rehabilitation by intention and outcome. J. Athl. Train. 51, 613–628.

Stone, M.H., Sands, W.A., Carlock, J., et al., 2004. The importance of isometric maximum strength and peak rate-of-force development in sprint cycling. J. Strength Cond. Res. 18, 878–884.

Vleeming, A., Albert, H.B., Östgaard, H.C., et al., 2008. European guidelines for the diagnosis and treatment of pelvic girdle pain. Eur. Spine J. 17, 794–819.

Wainner, R.S., Whitman, J.M., Cleland, J.A., et al., 2007. Regional interdependence: a musculoskeletal examination model whose time has come. J. Orthop. Sports Phys. Ther. 37, 658–660.

Wall, B., Dirks, M., van Loon, L., 2013. Skeletal muscle atrophy during short term disuse: implications for age related sarcopenia. Ageing Res. Rev. 12, 898–906.

INDEX

Page numbers followed by "*f*" indicate figures, "*t*" indicate tables, and "*b*" indicate boxes.